Statistical Research Methods for Dermatologists and Plastic Surgeons

Kyu-Ho Yi

Statistical Research Methods for Dermatologists and Plastic Surgeons

Springer

Kyu-Ho Yi, MD, PhD
Medical Research Inc.
Seoul, Korea (Republic of)

ISBN 978-981-95-5667-0 ISBN 978-981-95-5668-7 (eBook)
https://doi.org/10.1007/978-981-95-5668-7

This Springer imprint is published by the registered company Springer Nature Singapore Pte Ltd.
The registered company address is: 152 Beach Road, #21-01/04 Gateway East, Singapore 189721, Singapore

Contents

1 What Is Research?

1.1 Definition and Purpose of Research

Scientific methods are objective, observable, and probabilistic approaches used to acquire new knowledge. These methods are considered reliable, unbiased, and systematic. Objectivity refers to the ability of a third party to reproduce similar results under comparable conditions, using the same subjects, procedures, and methods. Through scientific methods, we can generalize phenomena or determine whether a result is due to chance.

Even scientific methods have limitations. First, not all questions in life can be addressed through science. For instance, questions such as "Does a creator exist?", "What is the purpose of life?", or "Is there an afterlife?" cannot be answered scientifically, not because they are unimportant, but because they cannot be objectively observed or measured. Even a near-death experience, while subjectively real, cannot be objectively verified by others. Second, the results obtained through scientific methods can still be of low quality. If the researcher holds biases, the study is poorly designed, or errors are introduced, the findings may be meaningless or even misleading, leading to mistrust.

Research can thus be defined as a process of applying scientific methods to seek answers to specific questions. It involves actively identifying a research problem, collecting, analyzing, and interpreting data in a systematic way to find the best possible solution. It goes beyond simply reviewing existing literature.

For example, when a student discovers a new fact and records it, this may seem like research, but it is not. That activity is better described as fact-finding or information-gathering. Research involves deriving meaning from such data, not just listing them. It is a process of re-examining or searching again through scientific methods to confirm facts. Therefore, the purpose of research is to uncover unknown truths and to expand the boundaries of knowledge.

1.2 Research Literature and Related Terminology

In general, a thesis refers to a master's degree, a dissertation refers to a doctoral thesis, and a research paper is used to describe scholarly articles. In academic journals, research papers and reports are generally referred to as articles, which include original articles, review articles,[1] and case reports. An original article presents new findings derived from original research. A review article summarizes and synthesizes existing data or publications, and is often solicited by editorial boards from established scholars in the field. Peer-reviewed journals refer to academic jour-

[1] Hill (1999), Baker et al. (2001), and Robertson and Baker (2001).

K.-H. Yi, *Statistical Research Methods for Dermatologists and Plastic Surgeons*,
https://doi.org/10.1007/978-981-95-5668-7_1

nals that employ a system in which submitted manuscripts are evaluated by experts in the field, called reviewers, to assess the quality and validity of the research prior to publication.

1.3 Categories of Research in Cosmetic Dermatology and Plastic Surgery

1. *Survey*

Survey research involves collecting a large amount of data on a specific topic and using descriptive statistics to highlight key findings. This type of research typically serves the following purposes:

First, it aims to describe a phenomenon of interest. For example, how many patients undergo facial contouring or double chin reduction procedures? The data may be examined by age group, gender, socioeconomic status, medical history, occupation, or length of treatment.

Second, it seeks to explore a problem area in more detail. If, for instance, facial contouring procedures are most common among individuals in their 40s and 50s, further research may examine whether this trend is related to age-related fat accumulation, bone structure, sun exposure, or hormonal changes. Investigating whether the underlying causes are lifestyle-related, genetic, or environmental can provide useful insights.

Third, survey research can help identify trends over time from past to present. For example, has demand for acne scar treatments increased over the past 10 years? If so, is this trend expected to continue? In that case, research may shift toward identifying optimal treatment protocols, post-procedure care, or patient education for long-term improvement.

In some cases, hypothesis testing may not be appropriate for survey research. Correlational or experimental research is required for hypothesis testing.

2. *Experimental Study*

Experimental research tests whether the relationship between two variables exists as predicted by a hypothesis. To examine this, one variable is manipulated, and the other variable is measured. The researcher must carefully design the experiment and control other variables. The results are analyzed through statistical testing, and when the experiment is properly conducted, it can provide useful answers regarding causal relationships.

However, experimental research has several limitations. The procedures are often complex and time-consuming. Additionally, it can be difficult to conduct experiments when ethical issues are involved. For example, in a study examining the effects of a widely accepted scar revision treatment on patients with hypertrophic facial scars, assigning one group to receive the treatment and another group to receive no treatment raises ethical concerns. The researcher may be held ethically responsible for withholding a beneficial treatment from the untreated group. In such cases, it is difficult to find a way to conduct the experiment without ethical conflict. In situations like this, a correlational design may serve as an alternative.

3. *Correlational Designs*

In correlational research, it is difficult to explain causality; only hypotheses about relationships between variables can be tested. This is because, in correlational studies, researchers cannot artificially manipulate patients or treatment variables. Instead, the research is conducted under natural conditions as they exist. Therefore, the conclusions drawn from correlational studies cannot be regarded as definitive evidence. In correlational research, one might examine whether a high score on one variable is associated with a high score on another, or whether a high score on one variable is related to a low score on another.

1.4 Classification of Research Papers in Academic Journals of Cosmetic Dermatology and Plastic Surgery

Based on Robertson's (1995) classification of research articles in the journal *Physical Therapy*, the following types can be adapted to suit research in cosmetic dermatology and plastic surgery.

1. *Group Experimental Design*

In this design, comparisons are made between treatment groups, and subjects are randomly assigned to each group. Statistical analysis is always used to interpret the results.

2. *Quasi-Group Comparison*

In quasi-group comparison studies, comparisons are made between groups, but random assignment is not employed. The independent and dependent variables are clearly defined, and there is an intent by the researcher to manipulate the variables. Statistical analysis is conducted to evaluate outcomes.

3. *Single-Subject Design*[2]

This design applies experimental methodology to a single case. A baseline is established, followed by repeated measurements during the intervention phase. Then, the baseline measurement is repeated, and the intervention phase may be repeated again. Results are often presented in graphical form and are either visually analyzed or statistically tested.

4. *Survey*

Survey studies use interviews or questionnaires to gather information, such as attitudes or observed data. There is no attempt to manipulate variables.

[2]Backman et al. (1997).

5. *Case Study*

Case studies involve an in-depth investigation of one or more cases. These may describe specific treatment methods in cosmetic dermatology or plastic surgery, or other relevant medical management. Numerical data may or may not be included in such reports (Choi et al. 2024; Ormseth et al. 2023).

6. *Correlational Study*

Correlational studies examine relationships between variables. Statistical methods such as Pearson's correlation coefficient or Spearman's rank correlation are used. Like other nonexperimental designs, there is no attempt to control or manipulate variables (Zhang et al. 2018).

Sometimes, research is also categorized by the time sequence of observation:

1. Cross-Sectional Study: A type of observational study that collects data at a single point in time to investigate a current condition.
2. Longitudinal Study: A study that observes changes in a group over time, also known as a cohort study.
   (a) Prospective Study: A study that investigates events or outcomes from the starting point of the research and into the future.
   (b) Retrospective Study: A study that investigates data in the direction of the past from the point at which the study is initiated.

1.5 Steps of the Research Process

1. *The research process can be divided into five stages*

   First, formulating a researchable problem
   Second, developing a research method to address the problem
   Third, collecting data
   Fourth, analyzing, interpreting, and reviewing the data
   Fifth, drawing conclusions and disseminating the findings

Table 1.1 The research process

1. Problem Identification	(1) Formulating a researchable problem (2) Establishing hypotheses (3) Operationalizing variables
2. Research design and planning	(1) Selecting a research design (2) Defining the population and sampling (3) Choosing measurement methods (4) Conducting a pilot study
3. Data collection	
4. Data analysis	(1) Processing the data (2) Analyzing the data (3) Interpreting the results
5. Dissemination of findings	(1) Writing, submitting, and publishing the research paper

A more detailed breakdown of these stages is shown in Table 1.1.

2. *Considerations When Selecting a Research Problem*

First, the topic should be of genuine interest to the researcher. It must engage the researcher's curiosity and serve as a source of motivation.

Below are some examples of researchable questions:

- Example 1: Is LED light therapy more effective than cryotherapy in reducing post-procedure swelling?
- Example 2: What is the most effective relaxation technique to reduce anxiety in patients with Type A personality traits before cosmetic surgery?
- Example 3: Do compression garments help reduce the risk of thrombosis after liposuction?
- Example 4: Is facial neuromuscular stimulation effective in improving muscle tone in patients with mild facial nerve paralysis?

To formulate such research questions, it is essential to read extensively within the field of interest.

Through reviewing related literature, the researcher may begin to identify controversial topics.

Examples may include:

Whether repeated botulinum toxin injections for masseter hypertrophy result in long-term functional changes

The effectiveness and safety of radiofrequency microneedling, particularly in terms of long-term skin response

The impact of neuromodulator treatment on facial asymmetry and its possible effects on neuroplasticity

Second, once a broad research problem has been identified, the problem should be clearly and specifically defined. Table 1.2 provides an example of how to refine a general problem into detailed sub-questions.

Third, the researcher must possess adequate knowledge and skills to address the research problem effectively.

Fourth, the feasibility of solving the problem should be considered. Topics that are too complex or overly broad should be avoided.

Fifth, it is important to assess whether the necessary equipment, technology, and facilities are accessible to carry out the research.

Sixth, the budget and timeline required to conduct the research must be realistically evaluated.

No matter how creative or compelling a research idea may be, if it does not meet the criteria listed above, it will be difficult to carry out the study successfully.

Table 1.2 Example of research question refinement

Main problem (global problem)
How can skin elasticity be effectively improved through non-invasive procedures?
Subproblems
(1) *Type of treatment*
Q1: Among radiofrequency, ultrasound, and microneedling, which modality is most effective in improving skin elasticity?
Q2: Does each modality demonstrate treatment specificity depending on skin depth or region?
(2) *Treatment parameters and influencing factors*
Q1: How many treatment sessions are required to achieve significant improvement? (e.g., 1, 3, 5, or 7 sessions?)
Q2: What is the optimal treatment interval for maintaining skin improvement? (e.g., weekly vs. biweekly?)
Q3: What energy levels are most effective for radiofrequency devices? (e.g., 20 W, 40 W, 60 W, etc.)
Q4: How many passes per treatment area produce the best results?
Q5: Does treatment efficacy differ depending on the anatomical site (e.g., cheek vs. jawline)?
Q6: Does the use of a topical anesthetic affect treatment outcomes or patient perception?
Q7: Does combining microneedling with platelet-rich plasma (PRP) enhance the results compared to microneedling alone?
Q8: Does skin hydration level prior to treatment influence the degree of skin tightening achieved?
Q9: Does pre-conditioning with antioxidant serums improve post-treatment outcomes?
Q10: Does the addition of neuromuscular electrical stimulation post-treatment lead to greater skin firmness?

3. *Challenges in Research on Human Behavior*

It is difficult to conduct research on human behavior because feelings, motivations, and emotions are rarely consistent each time a person participates in a study. There are also considerable individual differences among participants, and it is rare to find individuals who behave consistently regardless of the passage of time. In most cases, human behavior changes as it interacts with the surrounding environment. Sometimes, the research process itself may influence the subject's behavior. For example, a person who is aware of being observed may behave differently than they would under normal circumstances. Additionally, certain human characteristics, such as intelligence, learning motivation, and satisfaction, are difficult to define with complete precision. Even when these concepts are defined, they are often difficult to quantify, and challenges remain in collecting objective evidence. Issues related to honesty, measurement accuracy, and research ethics are also ongoing concerns in studies involving human behavior.

1.6 Literature Review

The purposes of conducting a literature review are as follows:

First, to understand the current state of research. By analyzing previous studies, researchers can broaden their perspective, avoid duplication, and identify comparative data.

Second, to explore approaches to problem-solving. Reviewing existing research can reveal strengths and weaknesses, suggest areas for improvement, and help identify measurement tools, research strategies, and appropriate statistical methods.

Third, to establish the theoretical foundation and hypotheses of the study. It allows researchers to uncover the origins of the research problem and examine various theories and perspectives.

Fourth, to assist in generating and refining research questions.

Fifth, to evaluate the feasibility of conducting the study. By learning from the experiences of previous researchers, one can better understand technical or practical challenges.

Ultimately, a literature review helps researchers build a solid theoretical background for their study, determine whether their research is original or a replication, and expand their understanding of the methodologies necessary to carry out the research.

1. *Procedure for Conducting a Literature Review*

(1) *Compiling a List and Collecting Sources*

Before computers became widely available, literature reviews were often conducted manually. Researchers would use index cards available in the library to record details of books, such as the author, title, edition, place of publication, publisher, and year of publication, and then summarize key information on reading cards. For journal articles, the author's name, article title, journal name, volume, issue, year, and page numbers would be recorded. A common strategy was to first locate review articles, then examine their reference lists to identify original articles of interest. When writing a research paper, it is generally recommended to cite primary sources (original articles) rather than secondary sources.

Today, with the widespread use of computers, researchers often organize literature by topic-specific folders or categorize contents within a file (e.g., Introduction, Methods, Discussion) to streamline future writing. Reference lists can be recorded alongside. This digital method is far more time-efficient and organized than handwritten notes. Many libraries now have online databases, making it possible to locate relevant materials simply by entering keywords. Well-known reference management tools include RefWorks and EndNote, as well as Mendeley, which is commonly used to organize and annotate academic papers. Common academic databases and search platforms are listed in Table 1.3.

Most references can now be accessed through online search engines. In the medical field, one of the most widely used bibliographic resources is Index Medicus, which remains a primary tool for literature retrieval.

For nursing and allied health fields, the CINAHL database (Cumulative Index to Nursing and Allied Health Literature) is widely used. CINAHL includes not only nursing journals but also sources in physical therapy, occupational therapy, cardiopulmonary technology, respiratory therapy, social services, and other health-related disciplines.

Most medical databases are organized using Medical Subject Headings (MeSH), developed by the U.S. National Library of Medicine. Utilizing MeSH terms makes it easier to conduct targeted searches.

In addition, most research articles include keywords, which also serve as useful tools for locating relevant literature.

(2) *Index Medicus*

In the past, before computers were widely accessible, researchers relied on printed resources such as Index Medicus to locate relevant literature. Today, most libraries are fully digitized, and literature searches are typically conducted using online computer systems. In addition to using online databases like International Nursing Index or Physiotherapy CATS (Current Awareness Topic Search), researchers can also access literature through a library's reference information system.

One of the most prominent and widely used citation databases is the Science Citation Index (SCI), developed by the Institute for Scientific Information (ISI) in the United States, and first published in 1960. SCI provides comprehensive information on which scientific papers have been cited, when, where, and by whom, across disciplines such as medicine and the natural sciences. SCI indexes more than 3500 leading scientific journals worldwide and allows users to determine how often a specific paper, book, or patent has been cited, and by which other publications.

SCI is available in various formats including print, CD-ROM, CD-ROM with abstracts, magnetic tape, web access, and online platforms. An expanded version known as SCI Expanded

Table 1.3 Database search

Title	Database search
MEDLINE	PubMed is a free search engine that provides access to MEDLINE, the largest bibliographic database for medical literature. It includes more than 12 million articles from over 4600 journals. http://www.ncbi.nlm.nih.gov/Pubmed
Cochrane library	A leading resource for systematic reviews and meta-analyses in evidence-based medicine, including surgical and dermatological interventions. https://www.cochranelibrary.com
KoreaScience:	Provides free pdf files of registered articles. http://koreascience.or.kr
Google scholar	A freely accessible web search engine that indexes scholarly articles and academic sources across various disciplines. http://scholar.google.com
MedRIC:	Searches domestic medical journals, provides abstract information and full text. http://kmbase.medric.or.kr
KoreaMed:	Provides English bibliographic information and abstracts of articles published in Korean medical journals. The format is similar to that of PubMed. http://www.koreamed.org
KISS	Provides full-text access to Korean academic journal articles. http://search.koreanstudies.net
National Assembly Electronic Library Original Database	Offers access to full-text databases of all domestic publications including books, journals, theses, and academic papers. http://www.nanet.go.kr
KERIS	Provides access to full texts of academic journals from domestic academic societies and university research institutes, and to overseas doctoral dissertations (DDOD). Medical science databases such as PML are also accessible. http://www.riss4u.net
NDSL	Offers integrated search across international electronic journals, including those from ScienceDirect, Blackwell, LWW, and EBSCOhost. http://www.ndsl.kr/index.do
EBSCO	Integrated platform for accessing international electronic journals. http://ejournals.ebsco.com
ProQuest	CINAHL journals and PML journals. http://www.umi.com/pqdauto
Scopus	The world's largest abstract and citation database covering the fields of science, technology, medicine, and social sciences. http://www.scopus.com/
Web of science	A citation indexing database that has provided access to bibliographic and citation information for over 100 years. http://isiknowledge.com

(SCIE) was introduced through magnetic tape, adding approximately 2100 journals to the original 3500 indexed titles (as of 1999). The web-accessible version is referred to as SciSearch, which includes an additional 1900 journals beyond the original SCI collection. For the social sciences, a parallel citation database called the Social Science Citation Index (SSCI) is used. Journals with a high citation rate (impact factor) are selected for inclusion in the SCI database through a formal review process. In academic settings, particularly in Korea, journals indexed in SCI are regarded as internationally recognized scholarly journals.

The impact factor refers to the frequency with which a single article published in a journal is cited during a specific year or within a given period. It is often used as a proxy to evaluate the overall quality and influence of a journal. It is calculated as the average number of citations in the target year to articles published in the 2 years preceding that year.[3]

For example:

Number of articles published in *Journal of Biological Chemistry*:

1995: 4635 articles
1996: 4949 articles
Total articles (1995 + 1996): 9584
Total citations in 1997 to those articles:
From 1995: 38,028 citations
From 1996: 28,706 citations
Total citations in 1997: 66,734
Impact Factor of 1997 = 66,734 ÷ 9584 = 6.963

The combined results of impact factor evaluations are published annually in a report known as the Journal Citation Reports (JCR).

To find information on specific journals, SCI listings, or official journal abbreviations, researchers can visit https://www.google.com and search for "Web of Science." Autocomplete suggestions will appear, making it easy to navigate to the correct database and perform literature searches.

(3) *Information Retrieval Using MEDLINE CD-ROM*

MEDLINE stands for MEDLARS on Line, and it is a comprehensive biomedical literature database managed by the National Library of Medicine (NLM) in the United States. It includes the contents of Index Medicus, Index to Dental Literature, and the International Nursing Index, and features bibliographic information and abstracts from selected journals in fields such as public health, medicine, dentistry, and nursing. Using the MEDLINE CD-ROM, researchers can perform subject-based searches, author searches, journal title searches, and combine search results using logical operators. The retrieved results can be viewed, saved, printed, or stored on a diskette. Today, free internet-based access to MEDLINE is also available. To locate a free MEDLINE site, simply go to a web search engine (e.g., https://www.google.com) and enter the keywords: free+medline, then press Enter.

(4) *Interlibrary Loan Request*

The interlibrary loan (ILL) system is a service based on agreements between libraries to share resources and documents. When a researcher needs a domestic article that is not available at their institution's library, they can consult the Union List of Medical Periodicals and fill out a document delivery request form. The form should include complete bibliographic information along with the requester's contact details. Once submitted to the library's reference services, the requested document can be delivered via postal mail or fax.

(5) *Using the Cumulative Index of Academic Journals*

Many academic journals include a cumulative index in their December issue, listing all articles published throughout the year by subject and by author. Nowadays, most journals are available online, where abstracts are typically accessible for free. However, full-text access often requires a subscription or additional payment.

(6) *Using Electronic Journals (E-Journals)*

Most university and institutional libraries offer electronic journal access, allowing users to read the full text of academic articles for free. To view full-text documents in e-journals, users generally need to have Adobe Acrobat Reader installed on their computer.

The following is a list of major journals and databases frequently used in the fields of cosmetic dermatology and plastic surgery (Tables 1.4, 1.5, and 1.6).

(7) *How to Use PubMed*

Let us explore how to conduct a literature search using PubMed. First, access the PubMed platform either by searching for it through an

[3] Si-Kyung Noh (2000).

Table 1.4 Representative journals in cosmetic dermatology and plastic surgery

Cosmetic Dermatology Journals
British Journal of Dermatology
Clinical and Experimental Dermatology
Clinical, Cosmetic and Investigational Dermatology
Dermatologic Surgery
Dermatologic Therapy
International Journal of Dermatology
JAMA Dermatology
Journal of Cosmetic and Laser Therapy
Journal of Cosmetic Dermatology
Journal of Dermatological Science
Journal of the American Academy of Dermatology
Journal of the European Academy of Dermatology and Venereology
Lasers in Surgery and Medicine
Skin Research and Technology
The Journal of Clinical and Aesthetic Dermatology
Plastic Surgery Journals
Plastic and Reconstructive Surgery
Aesthetic Plastic Surgery
Aesthetic Surgery Journal
Annals of Plastic Surgery
European Journal of Plastic Surgery
Facial Plastic Surgery & Aesthetic Medicine
JAMA Facial Plastic Surgery
Journal of Craniofacial Surgery
Journal of Plastic, Reconstructive & Aesthetic Surgery

Table 1.5 Korean journals in cosmetic dermatology

Journal of Investigative Cosmetology
The Korean Journal of Aesthetics
Korean journal of aesthetics and cosmetics society
Journal of the Korean Society of Cosmetology
Korean Journal of Dermatology
The Aesthetics

Table 1.6 Korean journals in plastic surgery

Archives of Aesthetic Plastic Surgery
Archives of Craniofacial Surgery
Archives of Plastic Surgery
Journal of Cosmetic Medicine

internet search engine or by navigating through your institution's library website. For direct access, type the URL: http://www.ncbi.nlm.nih.gov/pubmed/ into your web browser to reach the PubMed homepage (Fig. 1.1).

On the PubMed Services page, click Clinical Queries, where you can search for Systematic Review articles (Fig. 1.2). Enter your keyword(s) in the Search field and click Search. For example, if you are interested in laser resurfacing, type laser resurfacing and click the search button (Fig. 1.3).

A total of 1021 related articles are retrieved, but only five are displayed per page by default. If a title appears relevant, you can click on it to view the abstract. For example, click on the fifth article titled "Establishing an animal…" to view its details (Fig. 1.4).

The abstract of the article will appear on the screen. By clicking on the author names, you can view other articles written by the same authors. Under the Related Citations section, articles on similar topics are listed. Clicking on any of these titles will take you directly to the abstract of that article.

If your institution's library provides full-text access, the article may be available in PDF or HTML format.

In some cases, you may also have the option to request the full text through a document delivery service.

From the PubMed homepage, click on MeSH Database to access the Medical Subject Headings (MeSH) system (Fig. 1.5). To learn how to use it, you can click Tutorials on the left side of the homepage, where instructional videos are available (Fig. 1.6).

On the MeSH search page, enter skin resurfacing and click Search. PubMed will display a list of relevant Medical Subject Headings. From the list, click on "skin resurfacing, plasma" (Fig. 1.7).

The results page will appear. Click on the term "adverse effects" to narrow the search scope, then click Add to search builder on the right side of the screen (Fig. 1.8).

Click Search PubMed to display the search results. This executes a search limited to articles related to both "skin resurfacing, plasma" and "adverse effects" (Fig. 1.9).

As a result of the refined search, 12 articles are retrieved, with 10 articles displayed per page (Fig. 1.10). To view an abstract, simply click on the title of the corresponding article.

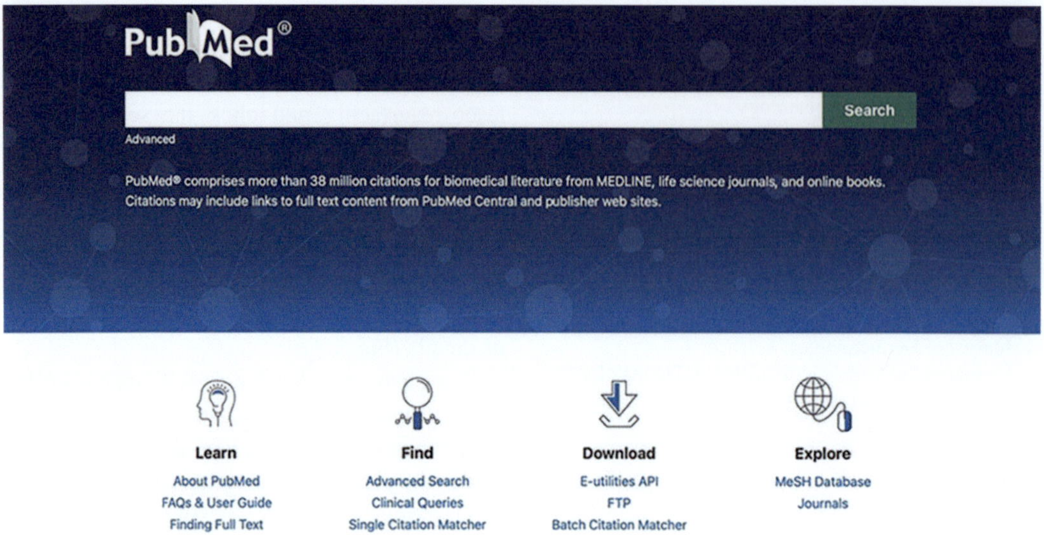

Fig. 1.1 Initial view of the PubMed homepage upon first visit

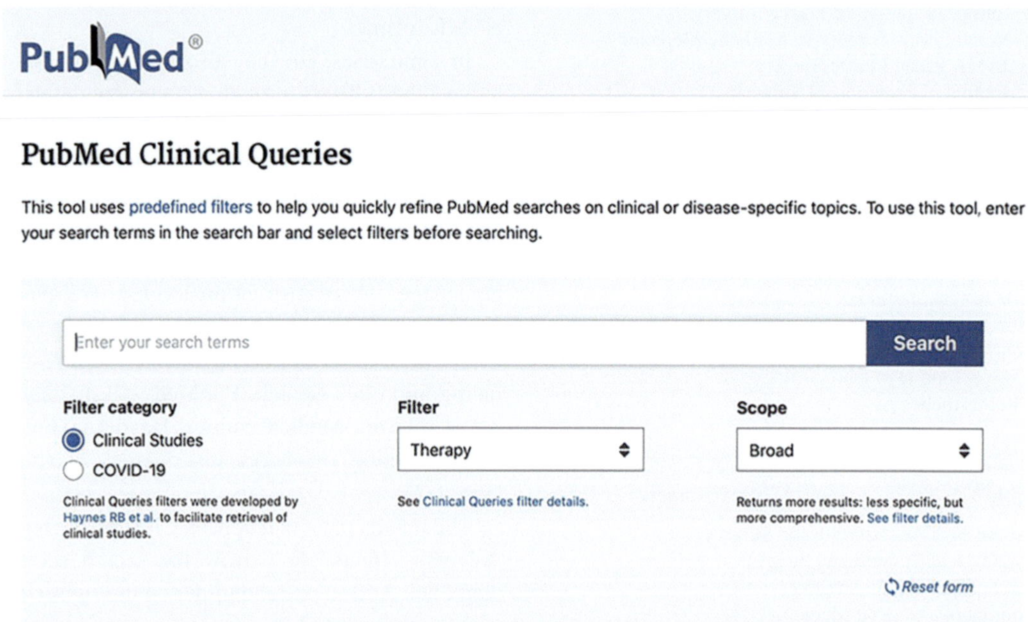

Fig. 1.2 Interface displayed after selecting “Clinical Queries” on the PubMed website

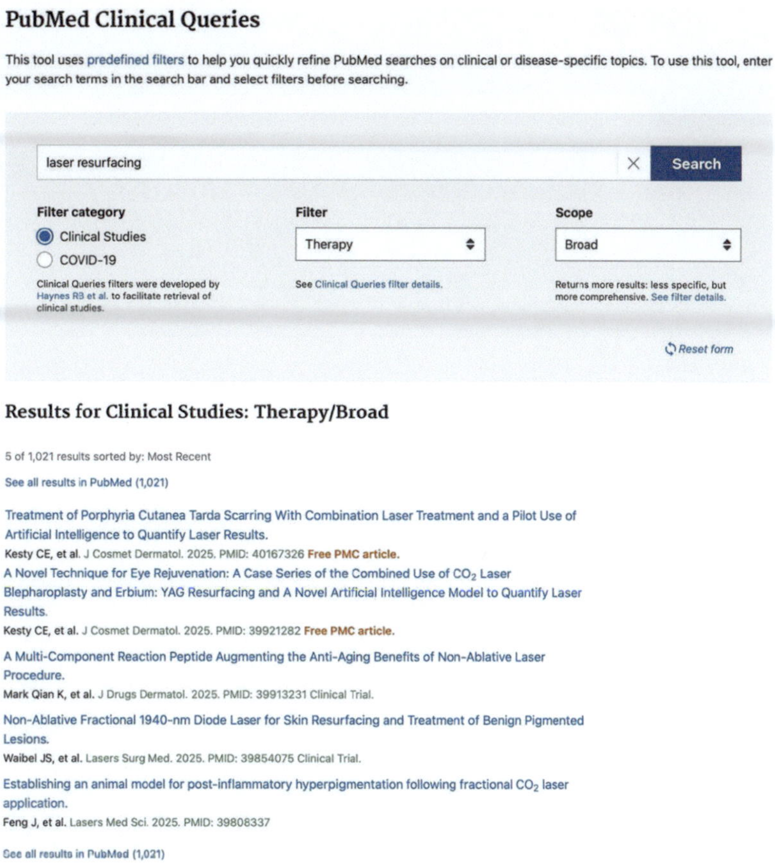

PubMed Clinical Queries

This tool uses predefined filters to help you quickly refine PubMed searches on clinical or disease-specific topics. To use this tool, enter your search terms in the search bar and select filters before searching.

laser resurfacing | Search

Filter category
Clinical Studies
COVID-19
Clinical Queries filters were developed by Haynes RB et al. to facilitate retrieval of clinical studies.

Filter
Therapy
See Clinical Queries filter details.

Scope
Broad
Returns more results: less specific, but more comprehensive. See filter details.

Reset form

Results for Clinical Studies: Therapy/Broad

5 of 1,021 results sorted by: Most Recent

See all results in PubMed (1,021)

Treatment of Porphyria Cutanea Tarda Scarring With Combination Laser Treatment and a Pilot Use of Artificial Intelligence to Quantify Laser Results.
Kesty CE, et al. J Cosmet Dermatol. 2025. PMID: 40167326 Free PMC article.

A Novel Technique for Eye Rejuvenation: A Case Series of the Combined Use of CO_2 Laser Blepharoplasty and Erbium: YAG Resurfacing and A Novel Artificial Intelligence Model to Quantify Laser Results.
Kesty CE, et al. J Cosmet Dermatol. 2025. PMID: 39921282 Free PMC article.

A Multi-Component Reaction Peptide Augmenting the Anti-Aging Benefits of Non-Ablative Laser Procedure.
Mark Qian K, et al. J Drugs Dermatol. 2025. PMID: 39913231 Clinical Trial.

Non-Ablative Fractional 1940-nm Diode Laser for Skin Resurfacing and Treatment of Benign Pigmented Lesions.
Waibel JS, et al. Lasers Surg Med. 2025. PMID: 39854075 Clinical Trial.

Establishing an animal model for post-inflammatory hyperpigmentation following fractional CO_2 laser application.
Feng J, et al. Lasers Med Sci. 2025. PMID: 39808337

See all results in PubMed (1,021)

Fig. 1.3 PubMed search for "laser resurfacing" as an example

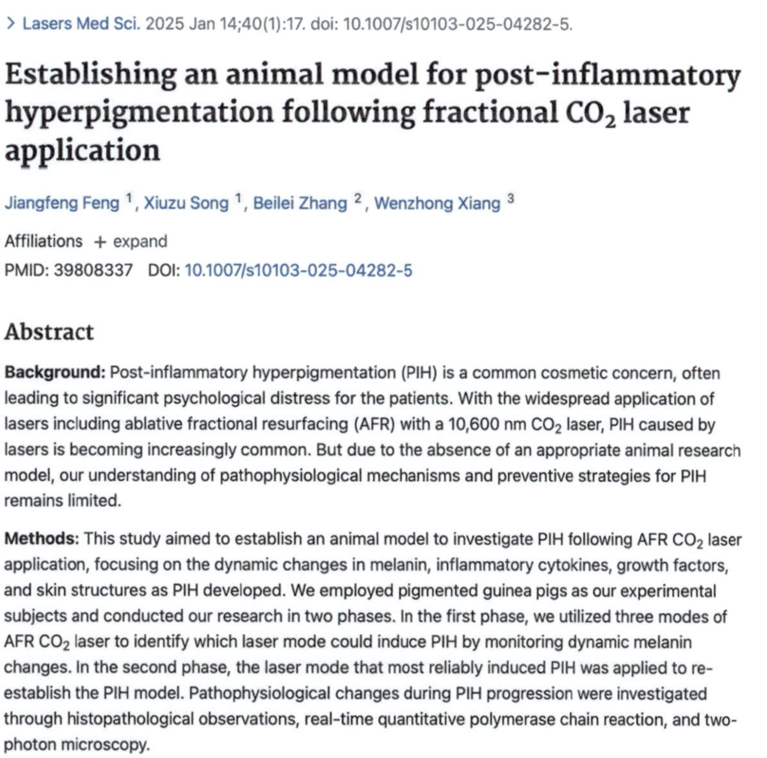

> Lasers Med Sci. 2025 Jan 14;40(1):17. doi: 10.1007/s10103-025-04282-5.

Establishing an animal model for post-inflammatory hyperpigmentation following fractional CO_2 laser application

Jiangfeng Feng [1], Xiuzu Song [1], Beilei Zhang [2], Wenzhong Xiang [3]

Affiliations + expand

PMID: 39808337 DOI: 10.1007/s10103-025-04282-5

Abstract

Background: Post-inflammatory hyperpigmentation (PIH) is a common cosmetic concern, often leading to significant psychological distress for the patients. With the widespread application of lasers including ablative fractional resurfacing (AFR) with a 10,600 nm CO_2 laser, PIH caused by lasers is becoming increasingly common. But due to the absence of an appropriate animal research model, our understanding of pathophysiological mechanisms and preventive strategies for PIH remains limited.

Methods: This study aimed to establish an animal model to investigate PIH following AFR CO_2 laser application, focusing on the dynamic changes in melanin, inflammatory cytokines, growth factors, and skin structures as PIH developed. We employed pigmented guinea pigs as our experimental subjects and conducted our research in two phases. In the first phase, we utilized three modes of AFR CO_2 laser to identify which laser mode could induce PIH by monitoring dynamic melanin changes. In the second phase, the laser mode that most reliably induced PIH was applied to re-establish the PIH model. Pathophysiological changes during PIH progression were investigated through histopathological observations, real-time quantitative polymerase chain reaction, and two-photon microscopy.

Fig. 1.4 Detailed view of a selected article from the PubMed search results

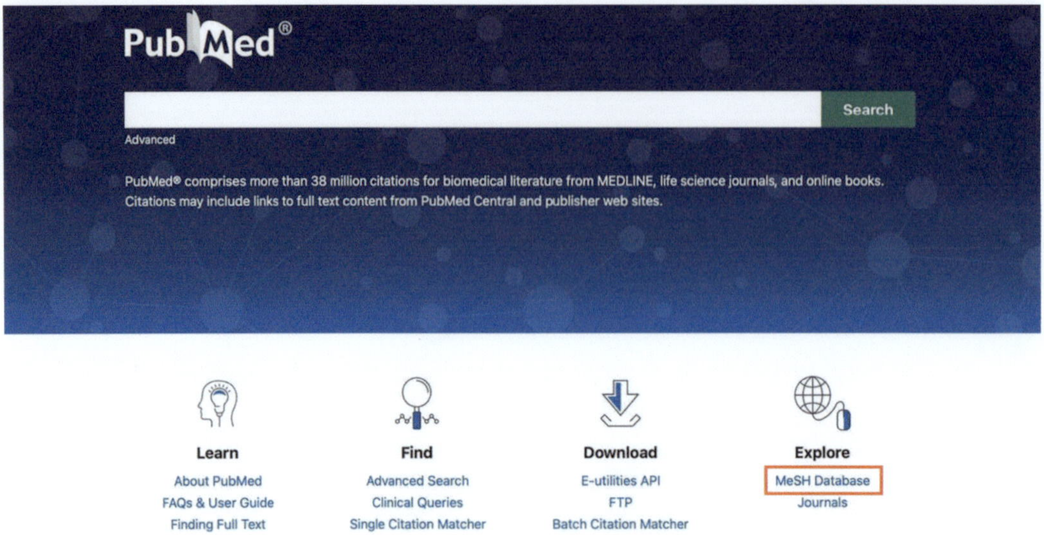

Fig. 1.5 PubMed homepage with the MeSH Database access point highlighted in red under the "Explore" section

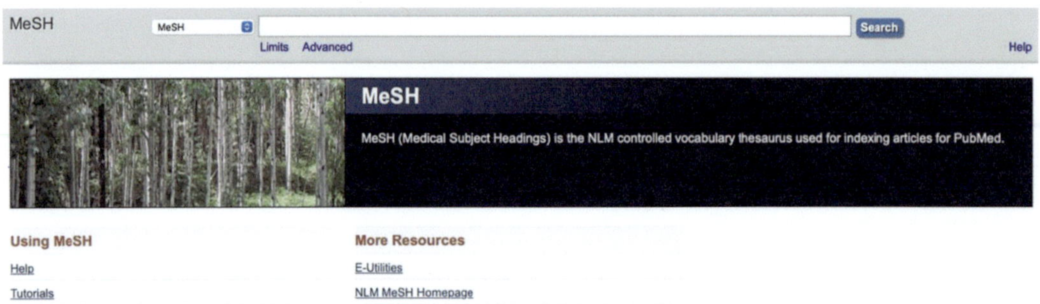

Fig. 1.6 Interface displayed after selecting the MeSH Database from the PubMed homepage

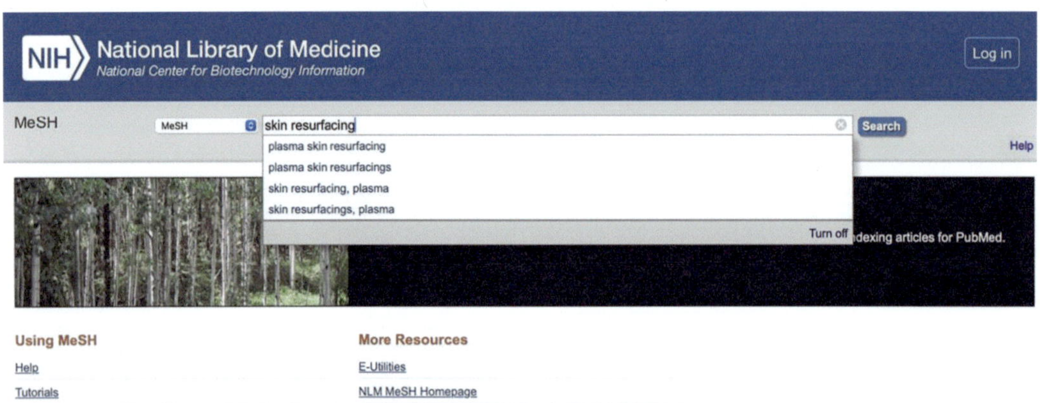

Fig. 1.7 Example of a MeSH Database search using the query "skin resurfacing, plasma"

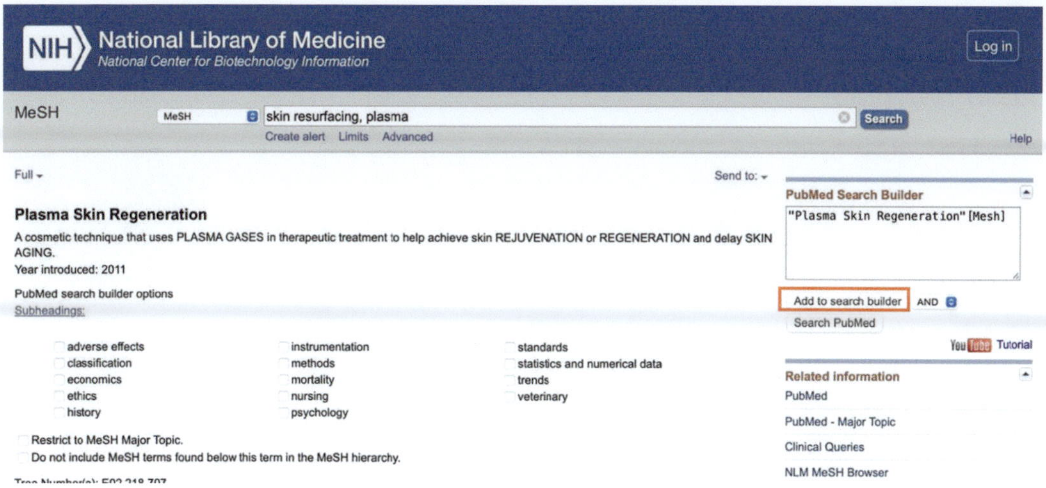

Fig. 1.8 Example of adding a MeSH term to the PubMed Search Builder using the "Add to search builder" function

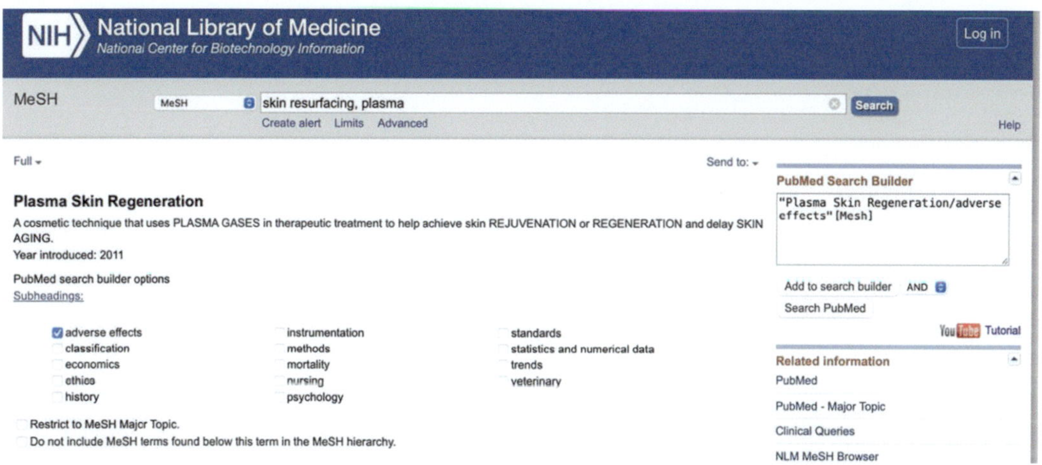

Fig. 1.9 Refining the PubMed search by including the subheading "adverse effects" from the MeSH term "plasma skin regeneration"

Meanwhile, from the PubMed homepage, the PubMed Single Citation Matcher allows users to locate specific articles using information such as journal title, author name, publication year, or keywords (Fig. 1.11).

If you wish to find the article on facial rejuvenation authored by Dr. Rohrich RJ, enter the relevant information into the appropriate fields and click Search (Fig. 1.12).

The search results will then appear as shown in Fig. 1.13.

From the PubMed homepage, you can use the Journals in NCBI Databases tool to look up the full title and details of a journal when only an abbreviation is known. For example, if you come across the abbreviation *Plast Reconstr Surg*, click Journals in NCBI Databases, enter *Plast Reconstr Surg*, and select Plastic and Reconstructive Surgery from the list of results. Then, click Search to access detailed information about the journal (Fig. 1.14).

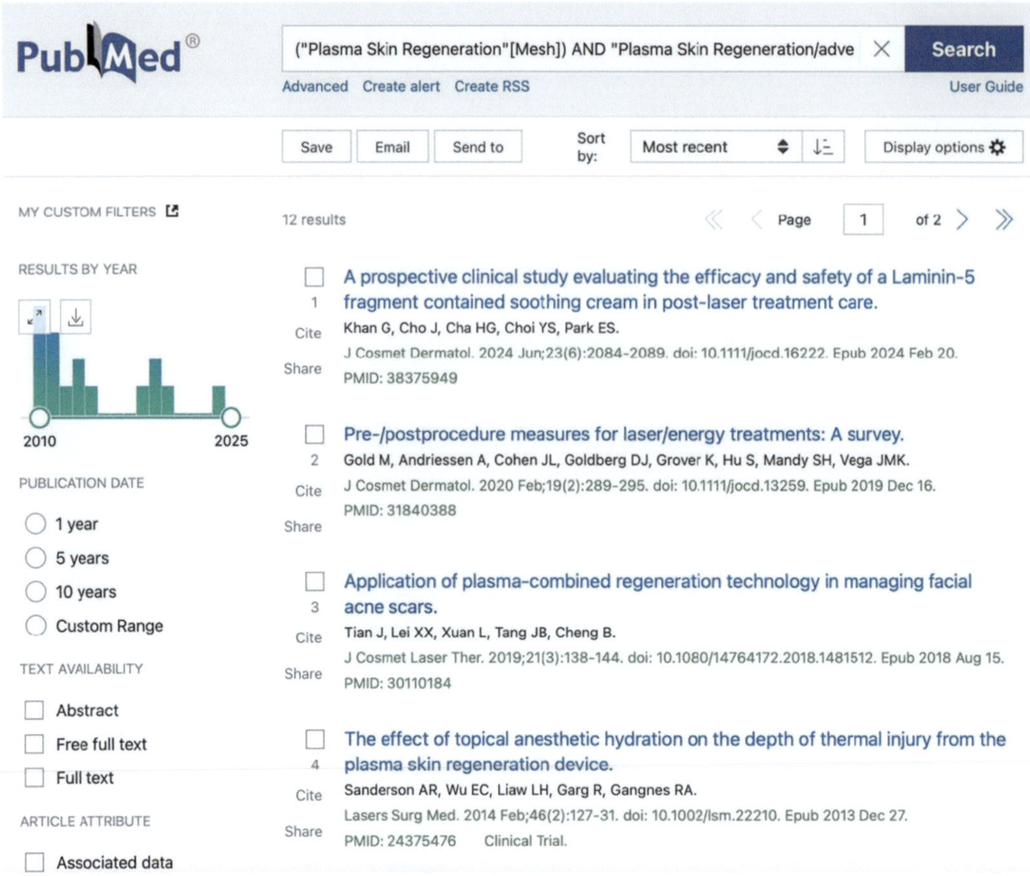

Fig. 1.10 PubMed search results generated by executing the MeSH-based query for "plasma skin regeneration/adverse effects"

If you wish to save the retrieved abstract, click on the Send to option. From there, you can choose to export the information as Text, File, Printer, Clipboard, or send it via E-mail (Fig. 1.15).

From the PubMed homepage (https://www.ncbi.nlm.nih.gov/pubmed), click Advanced Search to open the search builder. By clicking the downward arrow next to All Fields, you can narrow your search by specifying filters such as author, date, journal, or language, allowing for more targeted results (Fig. 1.16).

When entering search terms, using Boolean operators can help refine and optimize your search. For example, in the main PubMed search bar, entering botulinum toxin AND wrinkle treatment will retrieve articles that include both terms as shared topics. If you enter botulinum toxin OR wrinkle treatment, PubMed will return all articles that contain either of the terms, which may include many irrelevant results. On the other hand, entering botulinum toxin NOT adverse effects will exclude articles that mention adverse effects, narrowing the results to those more relevant to your interest. You can also combine multiple Boolean operators. For instance, using laser AND acne AND resurfacing will return only articles that address all three terms together (Figs. 1.17 and 1.18).

To explore recent research trends on a specific topic, it is helpful to review systematic or narrative review articles. For example, if you want to find review articles on the use of microneedling for treating acne scars, you can enter: "acne scars" AND microneedling AND Review[ptyp], which will filter the results to review articles on that topic (Fig. 1.19).

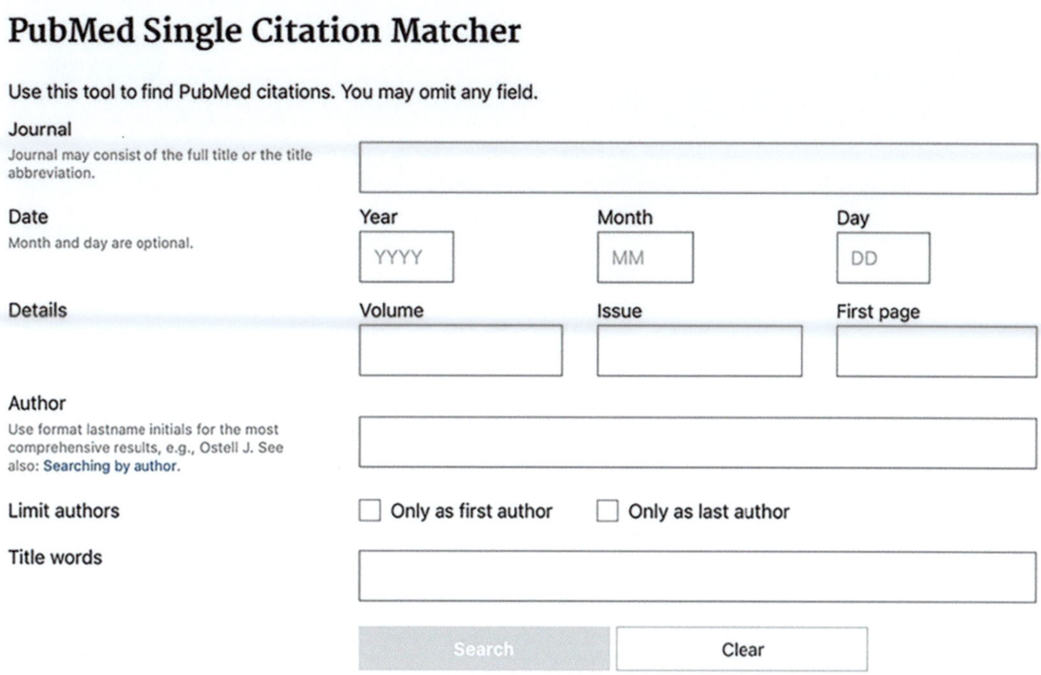

Fig. 1.11 Interface of the PubMed Single Citation Matcher

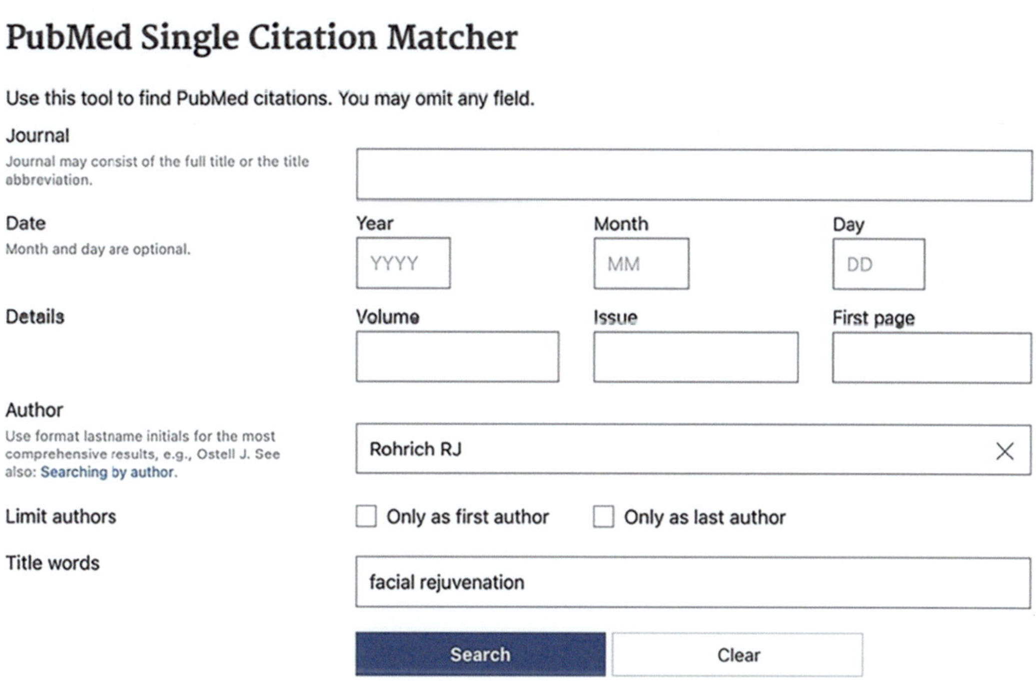

Fig. 1.12 Example of using the PubMed Single Citation Matcher to search for articles authored by Rohrich RJ with "facial rejuvenation" as title keywords

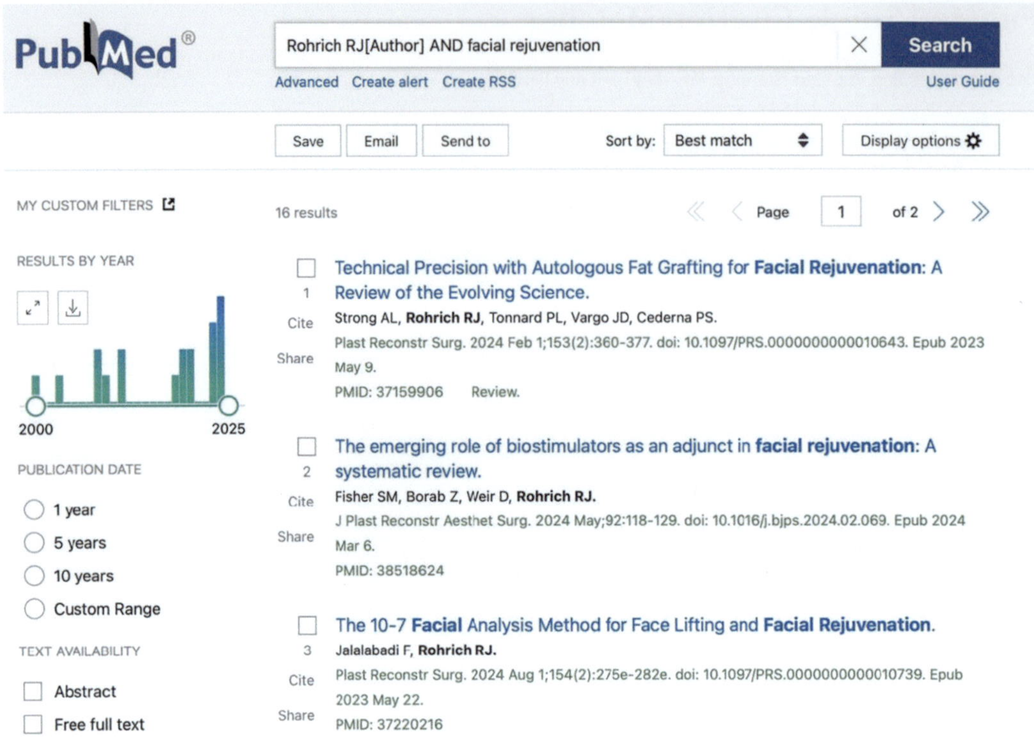

Fig. 1.13 Search results displayed after using the PubMed Single Citation Matcher with author "Rohrich RJ" and title keyword "facial rejuvenation"

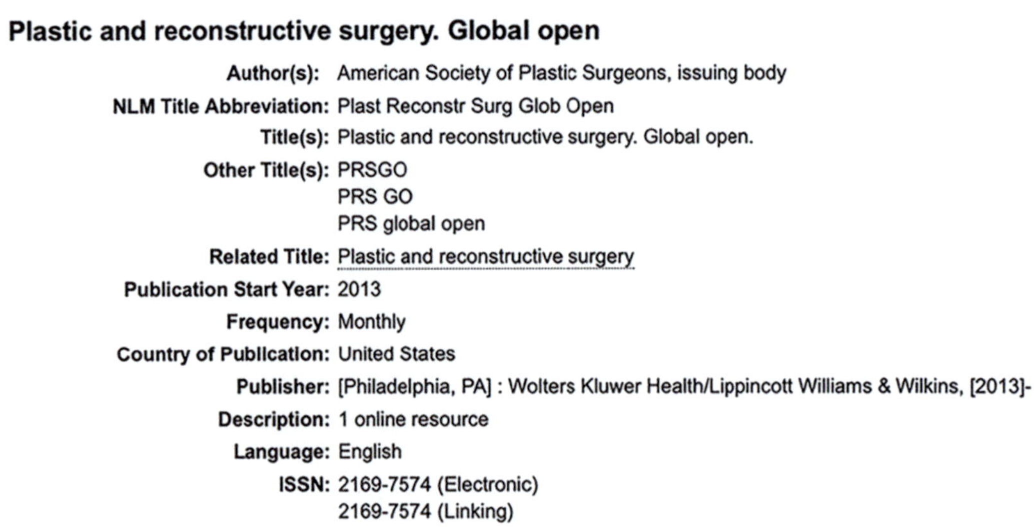

Fig. 1.14 Using the "Journals in NCBI Databases" tool to look up the full title and details of a journal from its abbreviation "Plast Reconstr Surg"

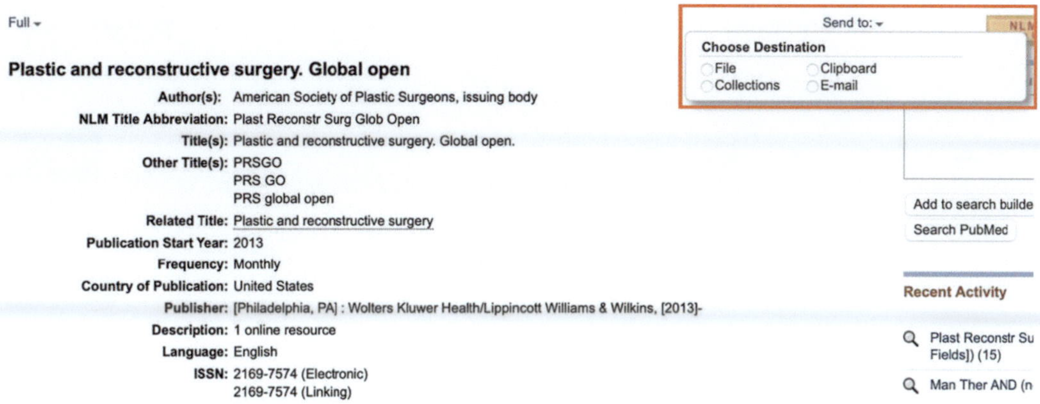

Fig. 1.15 Options available under the "Send to" feature in PubMed for exporting or saving retrieved abstracts

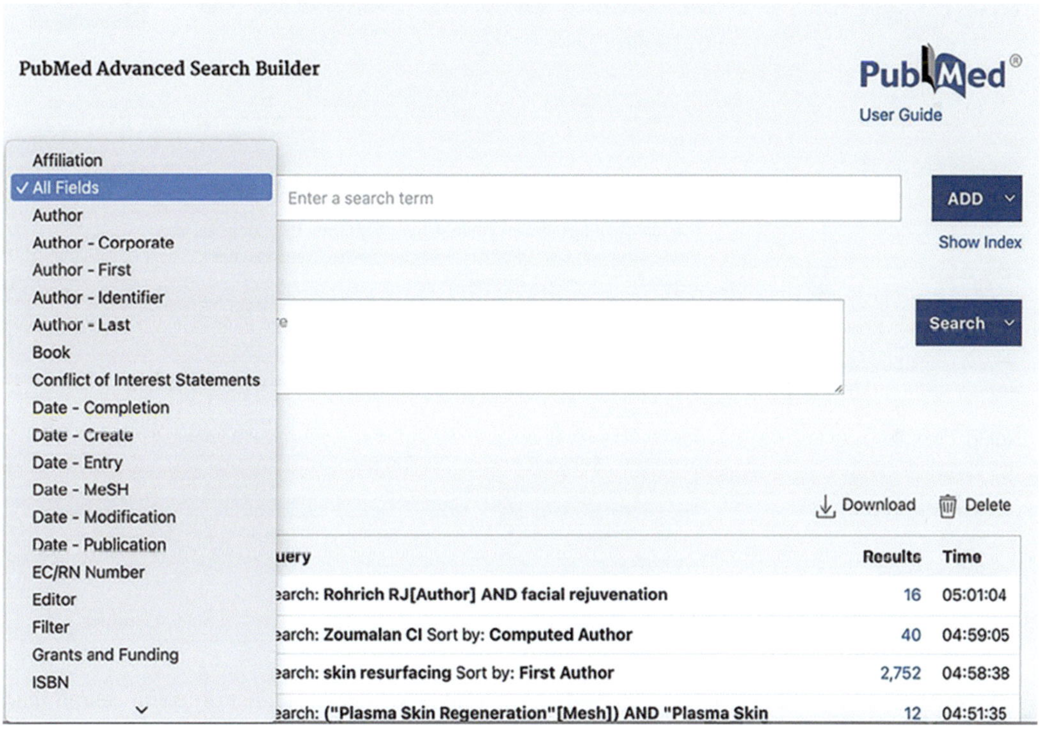

Fig. 1.16 Using the Advanced Search builder in PubMed to apply field-specific filters for a more targeted search

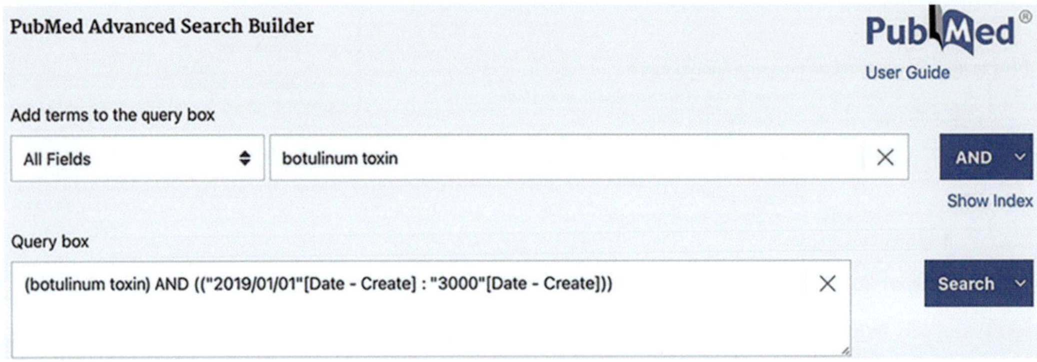

Fig. 1.17 Example of a customized search query created using the PubMed Advanced Search Builder with field-specific filters

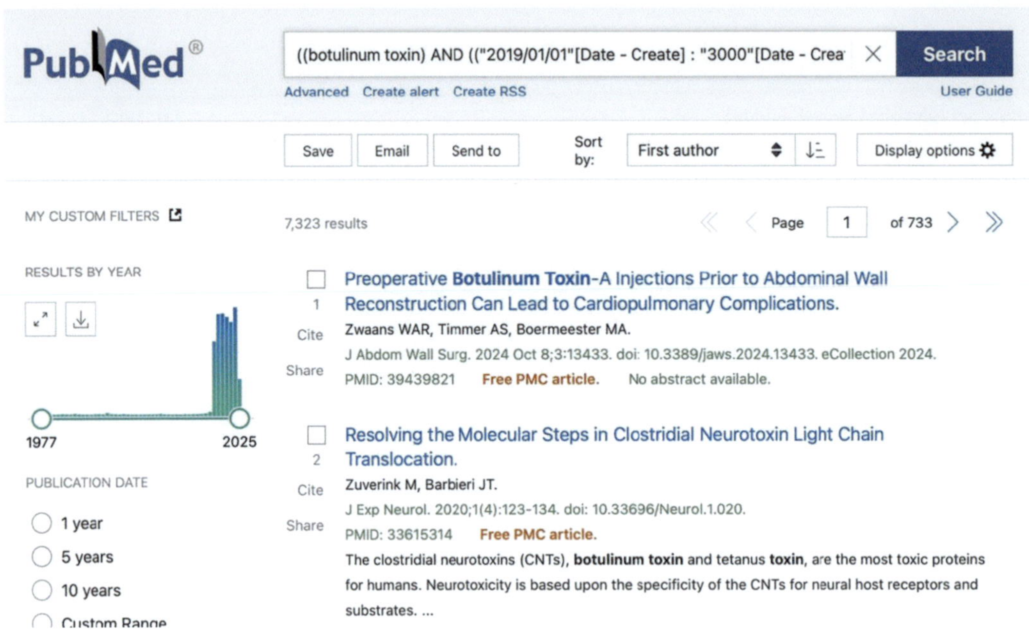

Fig. 1.18 PubMed search results generated from a structured query built using the Advanced Search Builder

If you wish to search for articles published in a specific year, you can use the date tag. For example, entering "acne scars" 2018[dp] will retrieve articles published in 2018 that include the term *acne scars* in the title or abstract (Fig. 1.20).

In addition, truncation symbols such as * or $ can be used to expand search results.

For instance, searching for "dermatolog* will return articles that include terms such as *dermatology*, *dermatologist*, or *dermatological*.

Table 1.7 displays a list of useful search field tags to refine your PubMed queries.

(8) *How to Use RISS*

RISS (Research Information Sharing Service), operated by the Korea Education and Research Information Service (KERIS), is a useful platform for accessing a wide range of academic resources. By visiting http://www.riss.kr, users can search and obtain materials such as master's

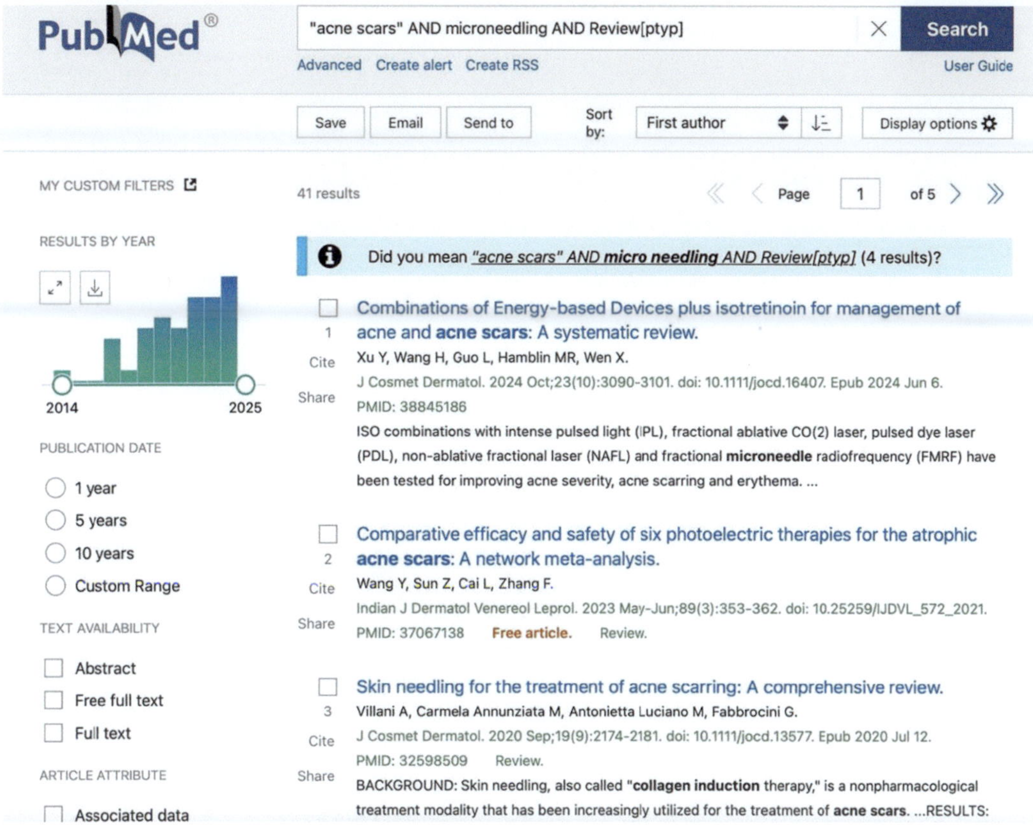

Fig. 1.19 Focused search strategy for identifying review literature on a specific clinical topic in PubMed

and doctoral theses, domestic and international journal articles, books, open lectures, and research reports (Fig. 1.21).

Enter "skin aging" in the search bar and click Search, or explore the categories such as Theses, Journal Articles, Academic Journals, or Books. The system will return documents with titles containing the term skin aging (Fig. 1.22).

By clicking View Full Text, you can access the article in PDF format. If you wish to narrow your search results, click Advanced Search in the search bar (Fig. 1.23).

In Advanced Search, users can refine their queries by specifying fields such as title, author, keywords, publication year, language, subject category, and indexing status.

(9) *How to Use the Cochrane Library*

The Cochrane Collaboration is a nonprofit, independent organization that provides systematic reviews in the field of evidence-based medicine. Access to the Cochrane Library is available through the National Center for Medical Information and Knowledge (http://library.nih.go.kr). To use this service, users must first register on the website (Fig. 1.24). Then, from the top menu, click Resources, select WebDB, and click Cochrane Library (Figs. 1.25 and 1.26).

By entering "Laser therapy" in the search bar, you can access related systematic review articles (Fig. 1.27).

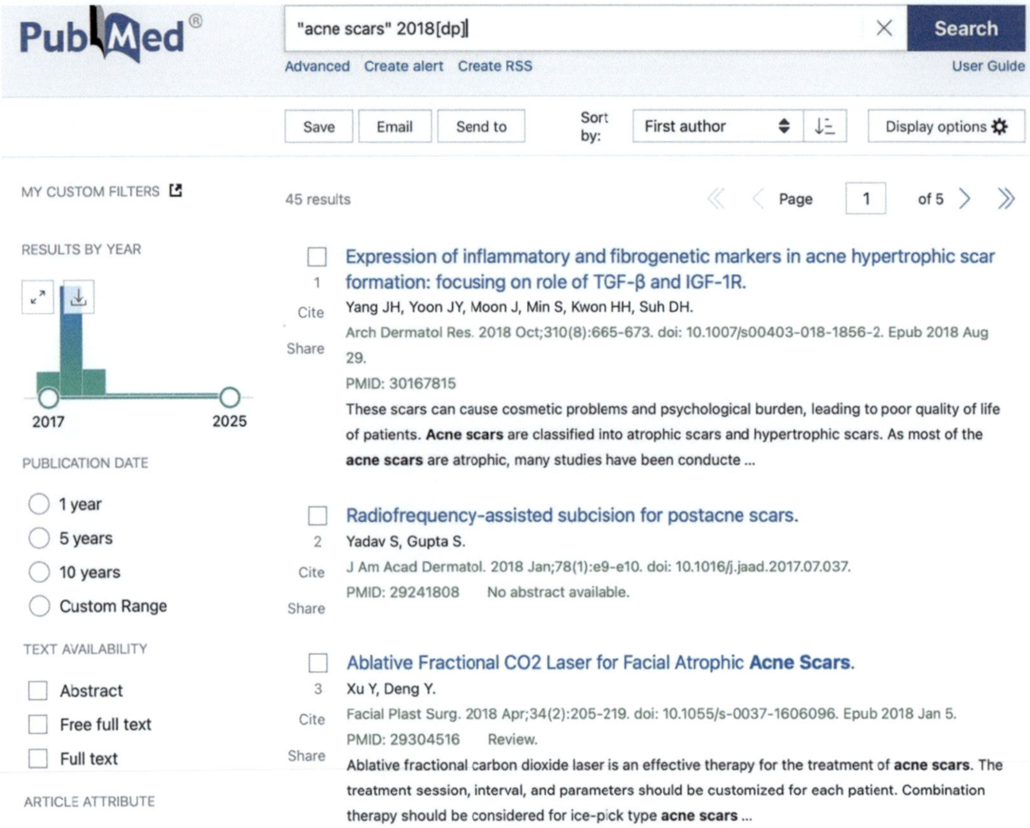

Fig. 1.20 Year-specific search for articles on "acne scars" using 2018[dp] in PubMed

Table 1.7 Commonly used search field tags in PubMed and their functions

Field	Field tag	Description	Example usage
Affiliation	[AD]	First author's institutional name	Yonsei University[ad]
Author	[AU]	Author's name	Yi CH[au]
Journal title	[TA]	Full title or ISSN of the journal	0028–4793[ta]
Language	[LA]	Language of the article	Korean[la]
Place of publication	[PL]	Country where the journal was published	Korea[pl]
Title	[TI]	Keywords in the article title	Asthma[ti]
Year	[DP]	Year of publication	2015[dp]

A total of 170 systematic reviews examining laser therapy are retrieved.

Click on the entry titled Laser therapy for treating hypertrophic and keloid scars to view its details (Fig. 1.28).

To view the abstract in Korean, click the Korean option in the abstract section (Fig. 1.29).

If you wish to read the full article, click View PDF at the top right corner of the screen (Fig. 1.30).

You can scroll down to read the content directly on the screen. To download the PDF file, click the PDF icon located at the top right corner.

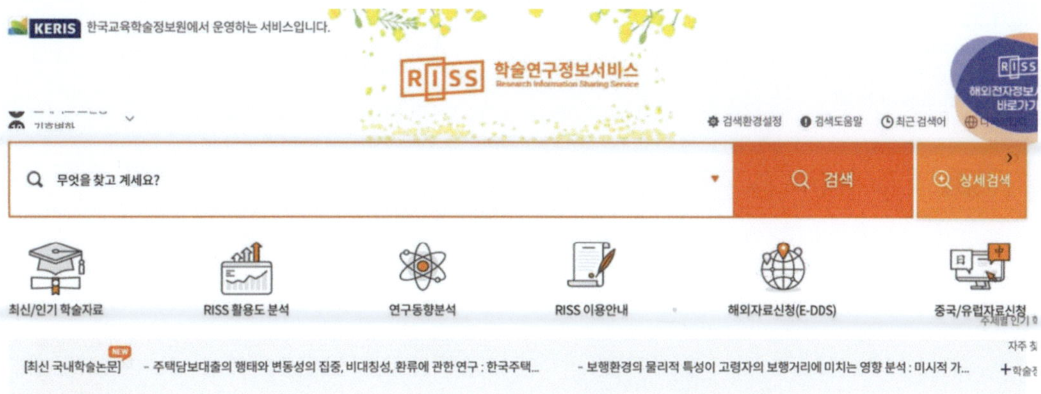

Fig. 1.21 Main interface of the RISS website used for accessing academic resources in Korea

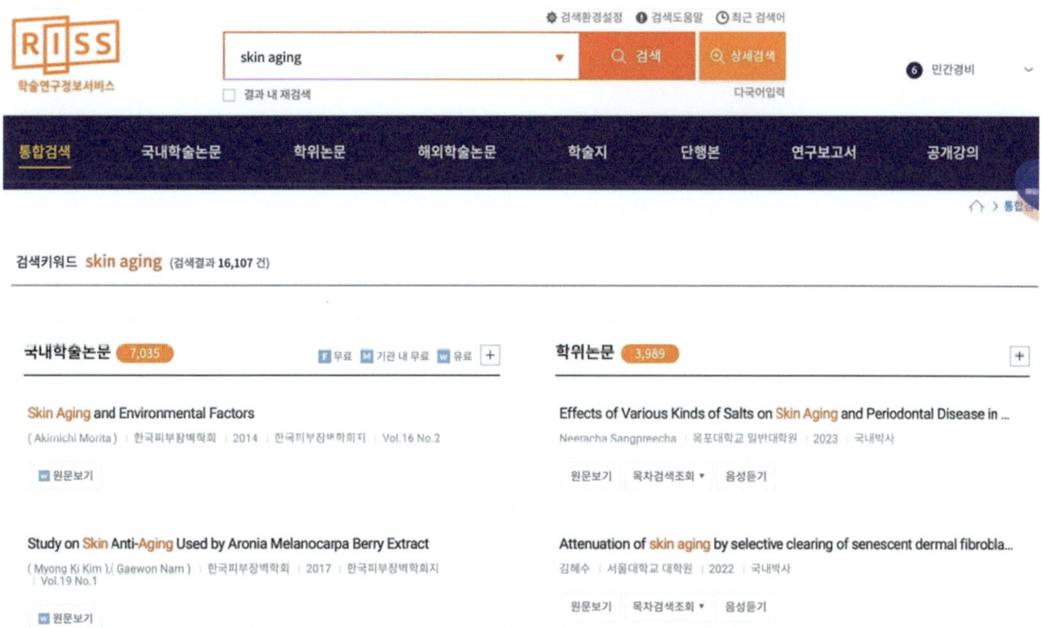

Fig. 1.22 Example of RISS search results for the keyword "skin aging"

From the Cochrane Library homepage, clicking Browse allows users to search for systematic reviews by subject category (Fig. 1.31).

Clicking Advanced Search provides access to features such as search filters, search history, and MeSH-based searching (Fig. 1.32).

By selecting Search Manager, users can build and combine complex search strategies. The example below shows multiple searchable terms related to laser therapy (Fig. 1.33).

To view the search results, click the button next to the MeSH term, where the total number of results is displayed (Fig. 1.34).

Fig. 1.23 Advanced Search interface in RISS with the option to access full-text articles in PDF format

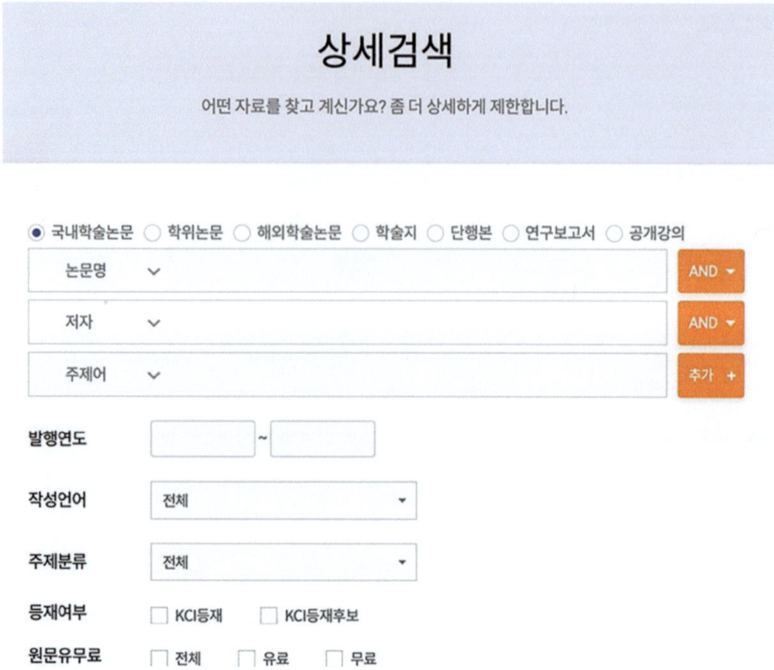

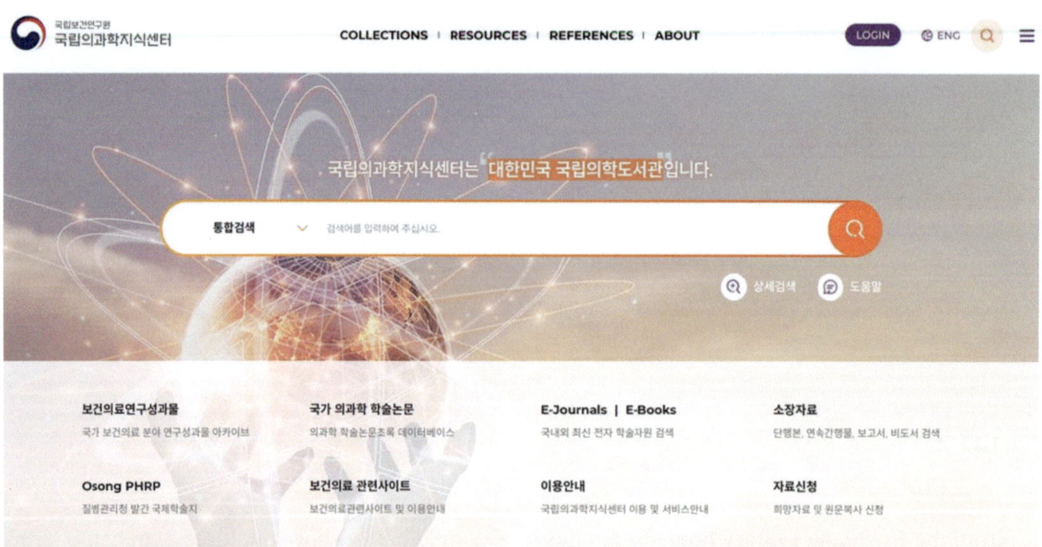

Fig. 1.24 Homepage of the National Center for Medical Information and Knowledge used to access the Cochrane Library

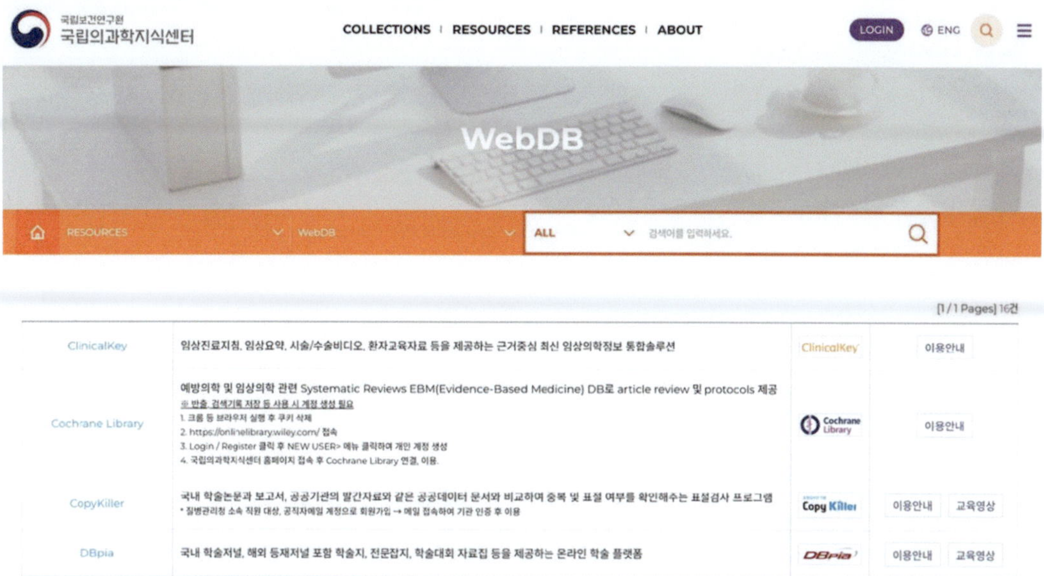

Fig. 1.25 List of available databases and tools under the "Resources" tab in the National Center for Medical Information and Knowledge

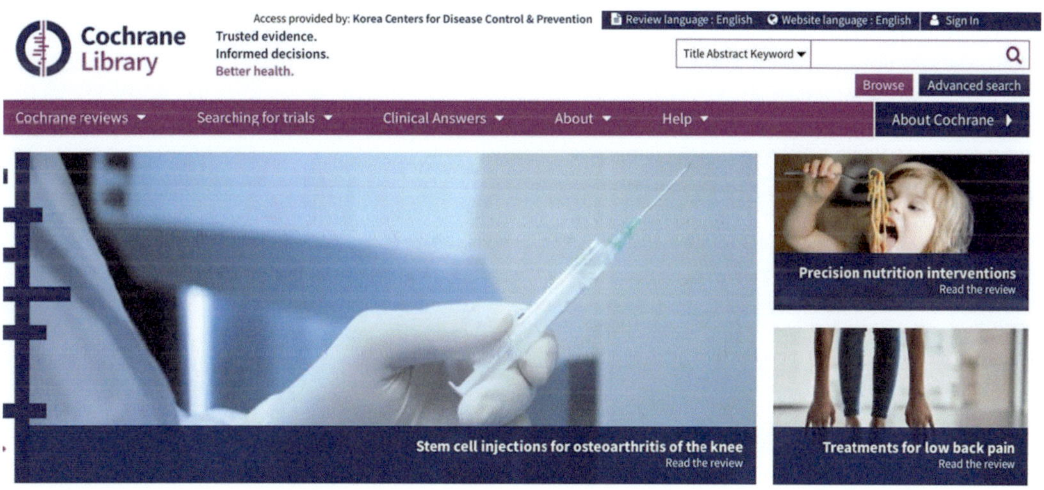

Fig. 1.26 Main interface of the Cochrane Library

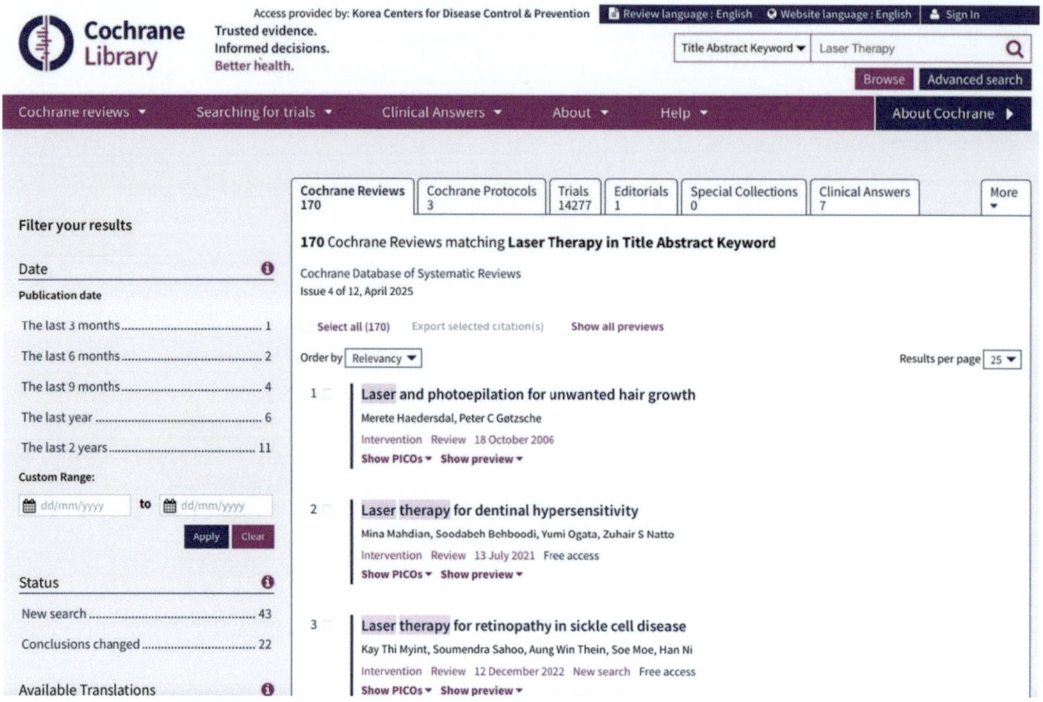

Fig. 1.27 Example of Cochrane Library search results for "Laser therapy," showing related systematic review articles

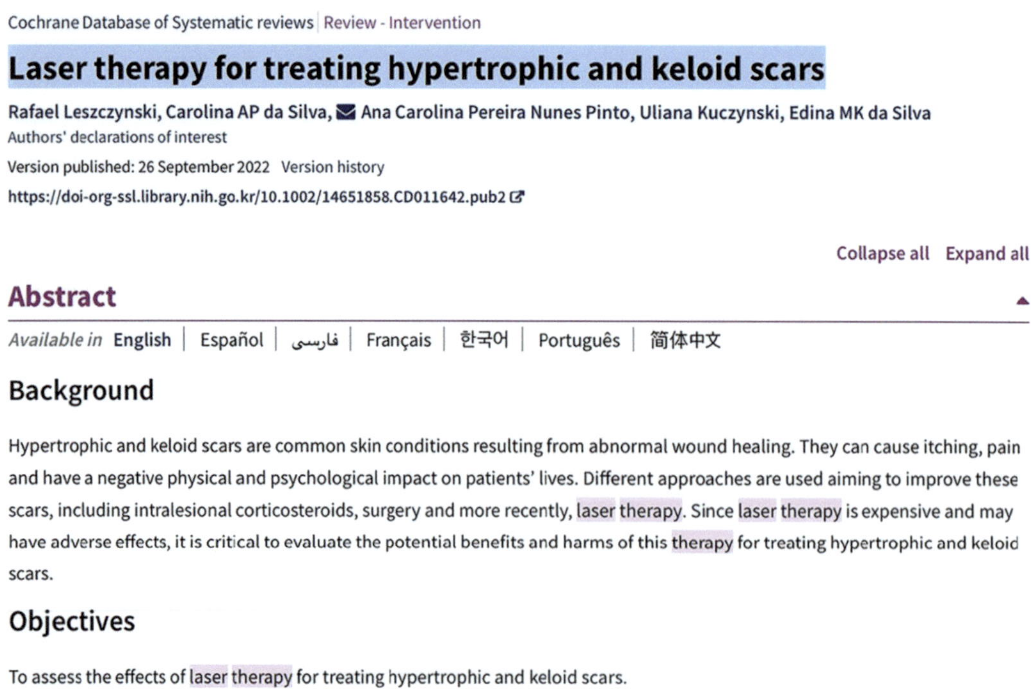

Fig. 1.28 Detailed view of a selected systematic review article on "Laser therapy" in the Cochrane Library

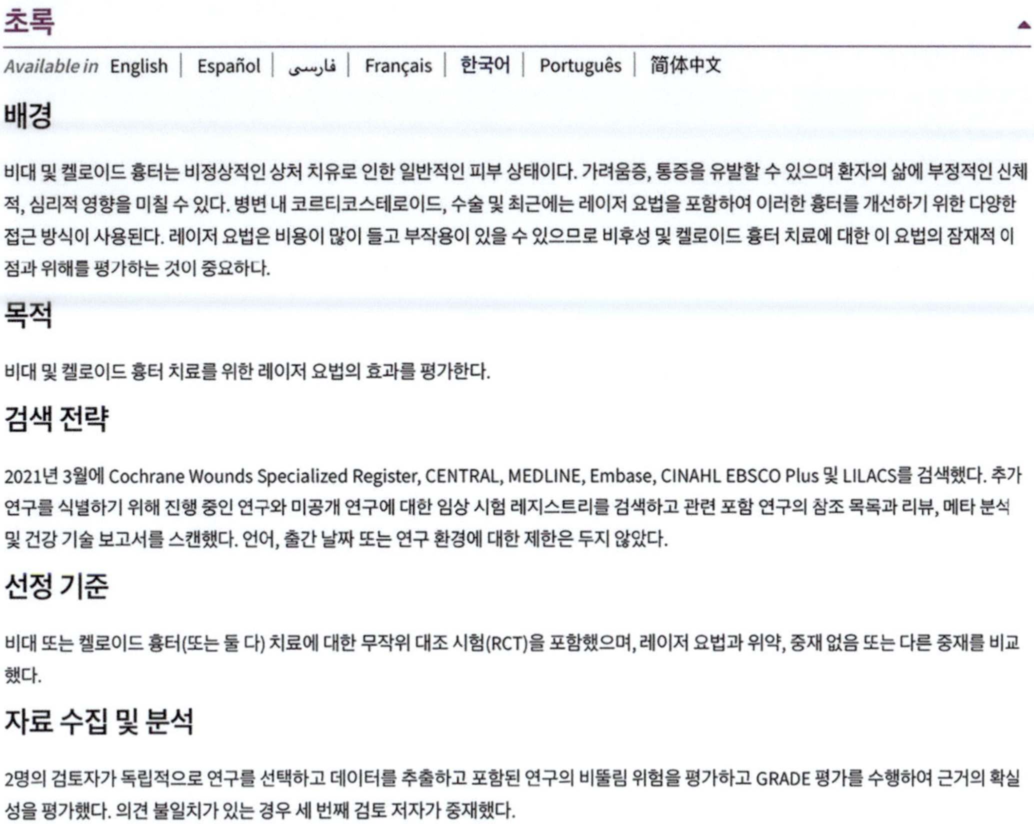

초록

Available in English | Español | فارسی | Français | 한국어 | Português | 简体中文

배경

비대 및 켈로이드 흉터는 비정상적인 상처 치유로 인한 일반적인 피부 상태이다. 가려움증, 통증을 유발할 수 있으며 환자의 삶에 부정적인 신체적, 심리적 영향을 미칠 수 있다. 병변 내 코르티코스테로이드, 수술 및 최근에는 레이저 요법을 포함하여 이러한 흉터를 개선하기 위한 다양한 접근 방식이 사용된다. 레이저 요법은 비용이 많이 들고 부작용이 있을 수 있으므로 비후성 및 켈로이드 흉터 치료에 대한 이 요법의 잠재적 이점과 위해를 평가하는 것이 중요하다.

목적

비대 및 켈로이드 흉터 치료를 위한 레이저 요법의 효과를 평가한다.

검색 전략

2021년 3월에 Cochrane Wounds Specialized Register, CENTRAL, MEDLINE, Embase, CINAHL EBSCO Plus 및 LILACS를 검색했다. 추가 연구를 식별하기 위해 진행 중인 연구와 미공개 연구에 대한 임상 시험 레지스트리를 검색하고 관련 포함 연구의 참조 목록과 리뷰, 메타 분석 및 건강 기술 보고서를 스캔했다. 언어, 출간 날짜 또는 연구 환경에 대한 제한은 두지 않았다.

선정 기준

비대 또는 켈로이드 흉터(또는 둘 다) 치료에 대한 무작위 대조 시험(RCT)을 포함했으며, 레이저 요법과 위약, 중재 없음 또는 다른 중재를 비교했다.

자료 수집 및 분석

2명의 검토자가 독립적으로 연구를 선택하고 데이터를 추출하고 포함된 연구의 비뚤림 위험을 평가하고 GRADE 평가를 수행하여 근거의 확실성을 평가했다. 의견 불일치가 있는 경우 세 번째 검토 저자가 중재했다.

Fig. 1.29 Example of viewing the abstract in Korean by changing the language setting in the Cochrane Library

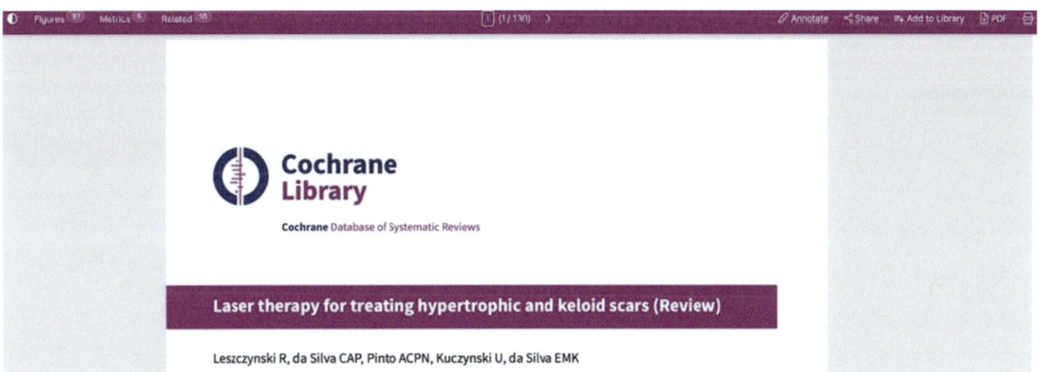

Fig. 1.30 Viewing the complete article in PDF format through the Cochrane Library interface

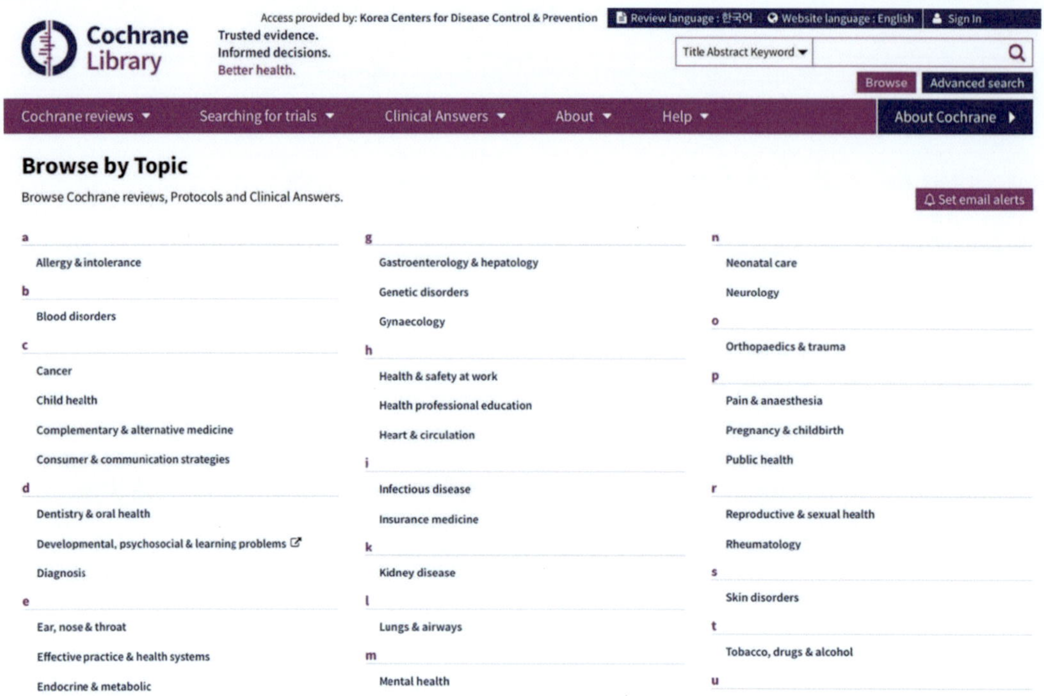

Fig. 1.31 Interface displayed after selecting the "Browse" option on the Cochrane Library homepage

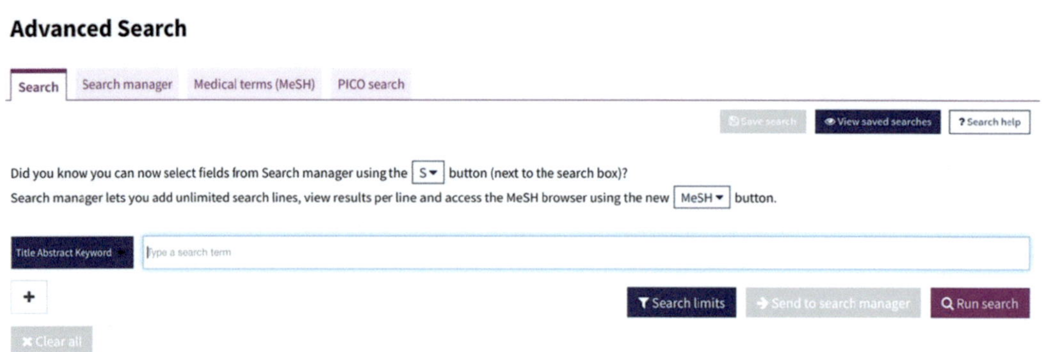

Fig. 1.32 Interface displayed after selecting the "Advanced Search" option on the Cochrane Library homepage

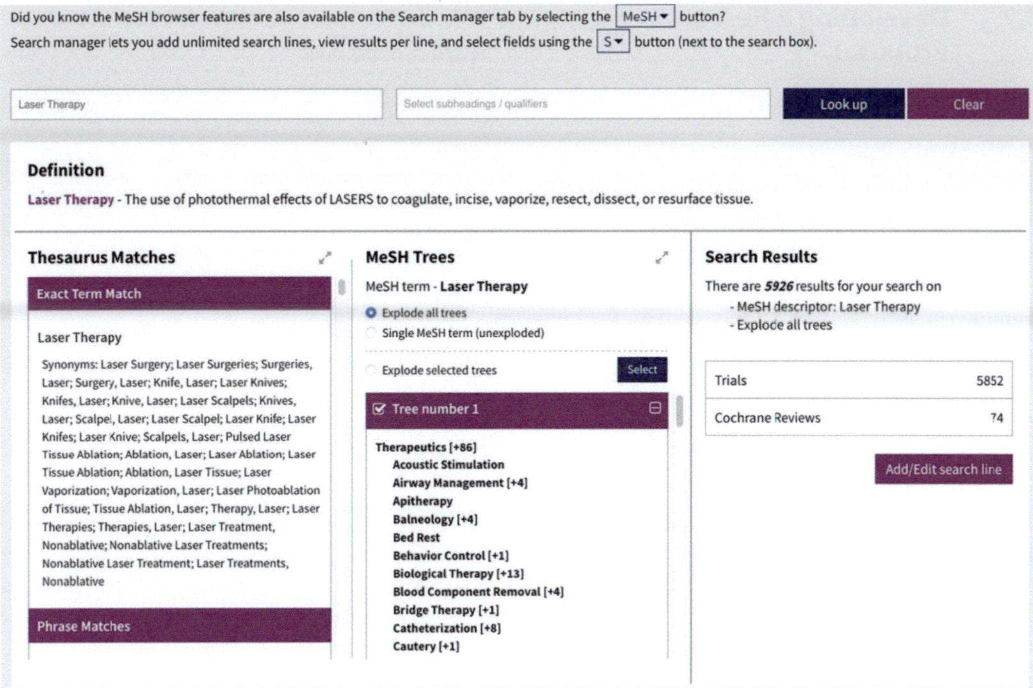

Fig. 1.33 Example of constructing a complex search strategy using the Search Manager in the Cochrane Library

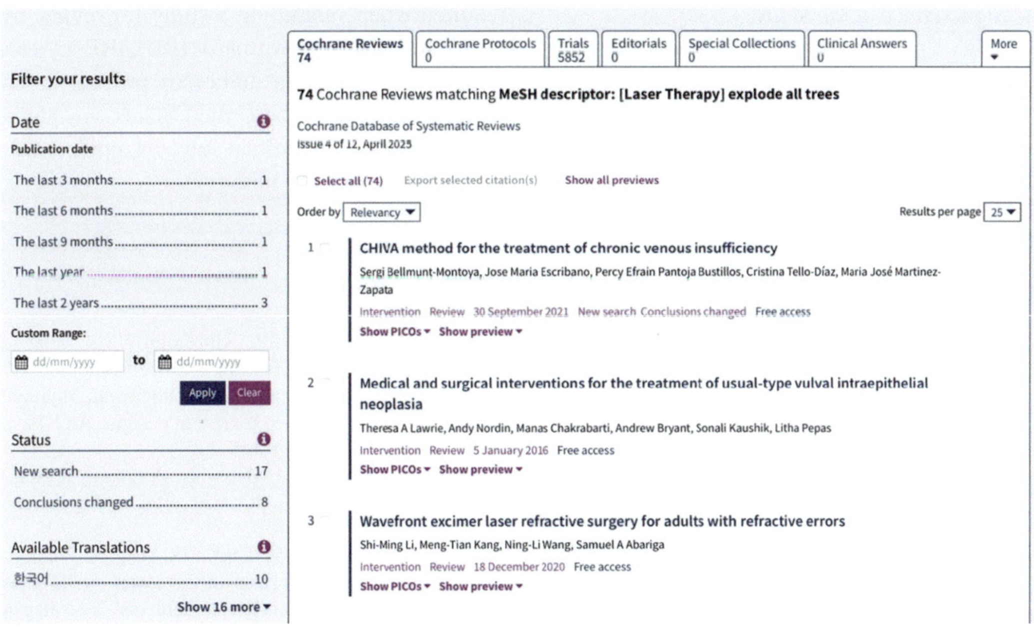

Fig. 1.34 Viewing search results in the Cochrane Library Search Manager

1.7 Developing a Research Proposal

1. *Title*

The title of a research proposal should clearly reflect the nature of the major problem or state a specific subproblem being investigated.

It does not need to be overly lengthy, but it should concisely and accurately convey the central focus of the study.

2. *Author(s) and Affiliation*

The principal investigator (PI) should be listed first, followed by co-authors in order of contribution. It is advisable to determine the order of authorship before the research begins.

3. *Purpose of the Study*

A brief and clear statement should be provided describing what the study aims to resolve.

4. *Significance of the Study*

Explain why addressing this research problem is important. Describe the potential theoretical or clinical implications if the problem is successfully addressed.

5. *Related Research or Background*

When reviewing related literature, present the information logically. You may also organize the review chronologically to demonstrate the scope of your literature review. This approach helps demonstrate the extent to which the researcher has reviewed the relevant literature. Be prepared to convince reviewers that the existing studies have not adequately addressed the research question. It is also important to show that the hypothesis being tested has not yet been examined, or that existing findings are inconclusive or controversial. If technical flaws are present in past research, it is more appropriate to discuss them in the Discussion section of the paper. If the proposed study addresses a novel problem that has not been previously investigated, cite the literature that is most closely related to the topic.

Table 1.8 Required components of a research proposal

① Purpose of the study
② Key findings or issues presented in previous studies
③ Characteristics of the sample; inclusion and exclusion criteria
④ Recruitment methods and procedures for obtaining informed consent
⑤ Research design
⑥ Research procedures
⑦ Potential risks associated with the study
⑧ Procedures to minimize risk and ensure confidentiality
⑨ Risk–benefit assessment
⑩ Incentives offered to participants
⑪ Sources of data: whether data are preexisting or will be newly collected through the study
⑫ Informed consent form

6. *Essential Components of a Research Proposal*

Table 1.8 outlines the key components required when submitting a study for review by an Institutional Review Board (IRB). IRB reviewers evaluate whether a study may proceed based on these criteria. In the United States, any study involving human or animal subjects must receive IRB approval prior to initiation.

References

Backman CL, Harris SR, Chisholm JM, Monette AD. Single-subject research in rehabilitation: A review of studies using AB, withdrawal, multiple baseline, and alternating treatment designs. Arch Phys Med Rehabil. 1997;78:1145–1153.

Baker K G, Robertson VJ, Duck FA. A review of therapeutic ultrasound: Biophysical effects. *Phys Ther.* 2001;81(7):1351–1358.

Choi M, Choi WY, Kim JM, Cheon JS, Yang JY. Foreign-body granuloma formation in the lower eyelid after injection of poly-D,L-lactic acid as a collagen stimulator: a case report. Arch Aesthetic Plast Surg. 2024;30(4):137–140.

Hill A. Phantom limb pain: A review of the literature on attributes and potential mechanisms. *Journal of Pain and Symptom Management*. 1999;17(2):125–142.

Si-Kyung Noh, An efficient evaluation method on the research achievements in science using the SCI & related DB, Master's thesis. Department of Library and Information Science, Chungbuk National University, 2000

Ormseth BH, Sarac BA, Westvik TS, Janis JE. The Value of Case Reports in Plastic Surgery: An Analysis of 68,444 Articles across Six Major Plastic Surgery Journals. Plast Reconstr Surg Glob Open. 2023 Jun 14;11(6):e5069.

Robertson VJ. A quantitative analysis of research in Physical Therapy. Phys Ther. 1995 Apr;75(4):313–327. https://doi.org/10.1093/ptj/75.4.313. PMID:7899489.

Robertson VJ, Baker KG. A review of therapeutic ultrasound: Effectiveness studies. *Phys Ther.* 2001;81(7):1339–1350.

Zhang JQ, Herman SB, Tepper OM, Garfein ES, Weichman KE. Rank and Research: The Correlation Between Integrated Plastic Surgery Program Reputation and Academic Productivity. *Ann Plast Surg*. 2018;80(5):553–560.

2 Research and Ethical Considerations

Researchers must maintain honesty and integrity throughout every stage of the research process, beginning with topic selection. While academic freedom allows researchers to explore any topic of interest, they must also consider the potential societal impact of their work. In clinical research, investigators bear ethical responsibility for the outcomes of their studies. This means that a study should be grounded in sound theoretical principles and carried out using an appropriate design and sample. Research that poses potential harm to participants is not only unethical but also unlikely to make a meaningful scholarly contribution.

During data collection, researchers should strive to minimize bias in measurement and observation. While it is impossible to eliminate all human bias, efforts must be made to control it as much as possible. Moreover, researchers must be honest and transparent during data analysis and reporting.

Statistical procedures must be performed properly, and it is unethical to manipulate data simply to achieve statistically significant results. Intentionally analyzing only those data that appear meaningful, while disregarding the rest, is a dangerous practice. Researchers must also be cautious of potential implicit or explicit pressure from sponsors—whether governmental, institutional, or corporate—to present favorable results.

Another ethical issue concerns authorship—specifically, how many contributors should be listed on the paper, and in what order. The first author is typically the individual who made the greatest contribution to the research. Other contributors should be listed in proportion to their involvement.

To avoid future conflicts, it is best to reach agreement on authorship order before the research begins. When additional assistance is received during the course of the study, a brief acknowledgment may be included at the end of the article.

For further guidance on research ethics, researchers are encouraged to consult two publications jointly issued by the Ministry of Education and Human Resources Development and the Korea Research Foundation: "An Introduction to Research Ethics" (2006) and "Case Studies on the Establishment of Research Ethics in Foreign Universitics" (2007).

2.1 Use of Control Groups

The use of placebo groups or control groups in experimental research often presents ethical challenges, particularly in medical and clinical studies. To evaluate the effectiveness of a treatment, researchers typically compare outcomes between a group receiving the intervention and another group receiving no treatment or a sham treatment. Such comparisons are used to determine whether a statistically significant difference

K.-H. Yi, *Statistical Research Methods for Dermatologists and Plastic Surgeons*,
https://doi.org/10.1007/978-981-95-5668-7_2

exists, thereby validating the therapeutic effect. However, this approach may raise ethical concerns, and some patients may refuse to participate if they know there is a chance they will not receive active treatment. For these reasons, many studies in fields such as aesthetic dermatology and plastic surgery tend to compare two or more active treatments, rather than including a non-treatment control group. In such cases, the primary research objective shifts to determining which treatment is more effective, rather than whether a treatment is effective compared to no intervention.

2.2 Protection of Human Rights in Clinical Research

All clinical research carries a fundamental commitment to protecting the rights and dignity of participants, beginning with the study design. In 1947, the Nuremberg Code was established in response to the unethical and often criminal human experimentation conducted by Nazi physicians on prisoners during World War II. The Code emphasizes that research involving human participants must only be conducted when voluntary consent has been obtained.

Researchers are obligated to fully inform participants of the purpose, procedures, potential discomforts, and possible risks of the study before seeking their consent. The Nuremberg Code also underscores the importance of researcher competence, stating that only scientifically qualified individuals should conduct human subjects research.

In 1964, the Declaration of Helsinki was adopted by the World Medical Association. This declaration states that if research participation offers no direct benefit or may cause harm to the subject, the participant must be clearly informed of such circumstances. Furthermore, written informed consent must be obtained from all participants, and approval must be secured from an Institutional Review Board (IRB) before research can proceed. A revised version, often referred to as Helsinki II, was introduced in 1975. For the first time, it required that research protocols be reviewed by independent researchers who are not involved in the study. It also specified that any study failing to comply with these ethical standards should not be accepted for publication in academic journals.

In the United States, all research involving human subjects must be conducted in accordance with the National Research Act of 1974 (PL-93-348). Under this law, research proposals must clearly describe the research question, its theoretical rationale, necessity, and significance. The study design must be appropriate for addressing the stated problem. Informed consent must be obtained from the participant or a legally authorized representative. Both the written research protocol and the informed consent form must be submitted to the Institutional Review Board for review and approval prior to the initiation of the study.

2.3 Informed Consent Form

The informed consent form consists of two main components: information and consent. Please refer to the example provided in the appendix.

2.4 Information Provided to Participants

1. *Sufficient Information Must Be Provided to Participants*

A written invitation to participate, the purpose of the study, the significance and value of participation—these elements must be clearly stated in the informed consent process. In addition, participants must be informed in advance about the expected duration of their involvement and what they may experience during the study. To ensure this, researchers are required to provide a thorough, sincere, and in-depth explanation of the study's objectives and procedures, both verbally and in writing.

The use of persuasive or misleading language to encourage participation must be avoided, as it can impair the participant's judgment. Although full disclosure of the study procedures may lead to bias or preconceived expectations among participants, in cases where the risk is minimal, an

Institutional Review Board (IRB) may permit the use of deception in research. Even in such cases, however, researchers are obligated to fully debrief participants after all data collection has been completed. For instance, participants placed in control or placebo groups without their knowledge must be informed of this fact once the study concludes.

The informed consent form must also describe any risks or discomforts, both direct and indirect, that may arise from participation. Researchers must develop and implement detailed plans to prevent or minimize these risks. For example, in studies involving laser resurfacing or microneedling, participants may experience temporary skin irritation or discomfort. Researchers should explain these risks in advance and ensure that appropriate post-treatment care protocols are in place to minimize adverse effects. For example, in studies involving chemical peels, participants may experience skin redness, tingling, or mild peeling as a response to treatment. To prevent excessive discomfort, researchers should include rest periods between sessions and ensure the use of appropriate post-treatment care, such as moisturizing. Potential benefits may also be included in the consent form; for instance, participants with acne scarring may experience visible improvement in skin texture following the intervention.

2. *Protection of Participant Confidentiality and Anonymity*

The confidentiality and anonymity of all research participants must be protected. This concern is especially relevant in survey-based studies, and researchers bear responsibility for ensuring that participant identities are not compromised when reporting the results. If the study involves video recording or photography, this must be clearly stated in the informed consent form.

3. *The Consent Form Should Be Written in Clear, Understandable Language*

The informed consent form must be written in a way that is clear and easy to understand. Technical or medical jargon should be avoided as much as possible. For example, instead of using a phrase like "intradermal injection of botulinum toxin into the frontalis muscle," it would be more appropriate to say "injecting a small amount of muscle-relaxing medicine into the forehead area to reduce wrinkles."

4. *Researchers Must Be Available to Answer Participant Questions at Any Time*

Researchers must respond honestly and thoroughly to any questions participants may have at any point during the study process.

2.5 Consent Elements

1. *Participation Must Be Voluntary*

Participants must give consent voluntarily. No penalties or disadvantages should occur if a participant declines to participate in the study. In certain cases, financial compensation may be offered in exchange for participation; however, even if compensation is provided, participants must not be held financially responsible if they choose to withdraw from the study at any point.

2. *When Participants Have Limited Decision-Making Capacity*

If participants have impaired cognitive function—such as those with psychiatric conditions, developmental disabilities, or intellectual impairments—the researcher must assess their mental capacity. If the participant is found not to be mentally competent, the consent must be obtained from a legally authorized representative or guardian. In the case of minors, informed consent must be obtained from a parent or legal guardian.

3. *Participants May Withdraw at Any Time*

Participants have the right to withdraw from the study at any time, for any reason, without penalty. Even after data collection has been completed, if a participant later chooses to withdraw, the corresponding data must be discarded.

2.6 Sample Informed Consent Form (Appendix)

An example of an informed consent form is provided in the appendix. All participants must receive and sign this consent form before participating in the study. The form must include the signatures of the researcher obtaining consent, the participant, and a witness. Both the participant and the researcher should retain a copy of the signed document.

2.7 Ethical Considerations in Publication

1. *Conflict of Interest*

A conflict of interest arises when authors, reviewers, or editors have relationships or interests that could compromise their ability to assess a manuscript objectively during submission, peer review, or publication.

For example, a reviewer may have a close personal connection with the author or be a direct academic competitor. A conflict may also exist when an author holds shares in a medical device company while submitting a study that evaluates a product developed by that company. The presence of any potential conflict of interest should be disclosed so that readers can take it into consideration when assessing the value of the paper.

Because potential bias is more difficult to detect in review articles or editorials compared to original research, some journals may choose not to accept non-original submissions from authors with significant conflicts of interest.

2. *Multiple Publication*

Researchers may sometimes feel tempted to divide data from a single study into multiple publications. However, artificially splitting related data into separate papers known as salami publication, bologna publication, or trivial publication is considered unethical. This practice violates research integrity and should be avoided by all authors.

3. *Double Publication*

Submitting a manuscript that has already been published or is under review elsewhere, or submitting essentially the same content to more than one journal, constitutes double publication. While it was once more common to translate and submit previously published papers from Korean to English journals, this is now considered a clear breach of ethical standards.

Most academic journals clearly state in their submission guidelines that manuscripts must not be under consideration or previously published elsewhere. Authors have a responsibility to avoid double submission. If they are uncertain whether their manuscript may constitute a duplicate or multiple publication, it is strongly recommended to consult the editor of the target journal and provide relevant documentation for clarification.

4. *Research Misconduct*

Research misconduct refers to acts of fabrication, falsification, or plagiarism committed during the planning, execution, review, or reporting of research results (Ministry of Education & Korea Research Foundation, *Introduction to Research Ethics*, p. 185, 2006).

1. Fabrication refers to making up data or research results that do not exist and recording or reporting them as if they were real.
2. Falsification means manipulating research materials, equipment, or processes, or altering or omitting data or results in a way that misrepresents the research record.
3. Plagiarism is the appropriation of another person's ideas, processes, results, or written work without proper authorization or attribution.

Common types of ethical misconduct related to publication practices are summarized in Table 2.1.

Table 2.1 Examples of misconduct in publication

Misconduct by authors
1. Describing data that do not exist or fabricating information.
2. Reporting data or findings known to be fabricated or manipulated.
3. Intentionally distorting or omitting evidence or data.
4. Misrepresenting data or findings.
5. Infringing on copyright, including plagiarism of others' original ideas or content.
6. Failing to include legitimate authors, thereby misrepresenting original contributors.
7. Listing individuals as authors who did not contribute to the work.
8. Submitting a manuscript to another journal when it has already been published elsewhere.
9. Submitting the same manuscript to multiple journals simultaneously.
Misconduct by reviewers
1. Providing false or misleading evaluations during the review process.
2. Intentionally delaying the review process for personal benefit.
3. Stealing research ideas or text from manuscripts under review.
Misconduct by editors
1. Fabricating or manipulating reviewer reports.
2. Providing false information to authors about the peer review process.
3. Using confidential information for personal gain.
4. Stealing research ideas or text from manuscripts under review.

3 Characteristics of Experiments

The most reliable scientific approach to test a hypothesis is the experiment. The primary goal of experimentation is to determine causal relationships between specific conditions or interventions and the outcomes being observed. For example, suppose we want to examine the effect of radiofrequency microneedling on reducing facial acne scars. If participants are also taking oral isotretinoin during the treatment period, any improvement in skin appearance might be influenced by both interventions. In this case, isotretinoin becomes a confounding variable, making it difficult to determine whether the effect was due to the microneedling itself, the medication, or a combination of the two. Furthermore, skin improvement could be the result of spontaneous healing or other cosmetic treatments the participant may have received concurrently. Experiments must therefore be carefully designed to control for such confounding variables. Although it is rarely possible to eliminate all confounders in clinical studies, experimental methods provide the strongest evidence to support causal relationships between variables.

3.1 Manipulation of Variables

Here, the term *manipulation* does not imply fabricating data, but rather handling variables in a structured and deliberate way. For example, if a researcher is interested in the effect of radiofrequency stimulation on improving skin laxity, participants can be assigned to either a treatment group or a control group. After a set period of time, changes in skin firmness are compared between the groups. In this case, the researcher applies the independent variable—radiofrequency—only to the treatment group, while the control group does not receive it. This process is referred to as manipulating a variable. An experiment may involve manipulating one variable or multiple variables at the same time.

Sometimes, a researcher may be interested in the influence of attribute variables such as sex, age, diagnosis, or behavioral traits. These types of independent variables cannot be manipulated by the researcher. Instead, participants are classified according to their preexisting characteristics. Therefore, studies that investigate the effects of one or more attribute variables cannot be considered true experimental designs. For example, one might compare skin hydration levels or collagen density across different age groups or between male and female participants. Such research is referred to as ex post facto,[1] meaning that key design elements are already determined before the study begins. Although ex post facto designs

[1] Latin for "from a thing done afterward." It refers to a type of nonexperimental research in which relationships between variables are examined using preexisting data or inherent attribute variables. Because of the nature of the data, the researcher has no opportunity to manipulate the variables.

K.-H. Yi, *Statistical Research Methods for Dermatologists and Plastic Surgeons*,
https://doi.org/10.1007/978-981-95-5668-7_3

allow researchers to examine relationships, they provide limited ability to control variables, making causal interpretations more difficult.

In some cases, researchers may combine attribute variables with manipulable variables in a single study. For instance, to examine the effects of age (an attribute variable) and chemical peel treatment (a manipulable variable) on skin brightness, participants may be grouped into four different age categories and then randomly assigned to either a treatment or control group. Because the researcher can manipulate at least one independent variable—in this case, whether or not the chemical peel is applied—the study is still considered experimental research.

3.2 Random Assignment

Once the sample is selected, it is important to ensure that the process of assigning participants to different groups remains randomized throughout. In random assignment, each participant must have an equal chance of being placed into any group, and the assignment must be free from personal judgment or bias. Random assignment is a fundamental feature of experimental research. If the groups can be assumed to be equivalent at the beginning of the experiment, then any observed differences at the end of the study can more confidently be attributed to the treatment effect. The concept of random assignment refers to the equal consideration of all groups, not to the idea that each individual in one group is exactly the same as those in another. Rather, it means that, when considering the group as a whole, the participants are roughly comparable across groups.

While randomization is frequently used in scientific research to achieve balance between groups, it does not always guarantee equivalence. For instance, it remains important to check whether the distribution of variables like gender or age is balanced across groups. Random assignment is a valuable tool to help achieve such a balance and reduce potential bias in group characteristics.

Let's consider an example: Suppose we want to compare the effects of two facial rejuvenation techniques on skin elasticity, using a third group as a control. A total of 45 participants are enrolled and randomly assigned into three groups of 15 participants each. Each participant is assigned a number from 1 to 45. Using a random numbers table, the researcher assigns participants alternately into Group 1, Group 2, and Group 3.

Here, Groups 1 and 2 receive different treatments, and Group 3 serves as the control group. By applying randomization techniques at each stage of the study, the researcher can enhance the study's validity and meet the essential requirements of experimental research.

One practical tool is the free website https://www.randomizer.org, where researchers can easily generate random samples (Fig. 3.1). For example, to select 10 participants from a pool of 100, input the range and number of selections, then click RANDOMIZE NOW! (Fig. 3.2).

Out of 100 participants, the system randomly selected ten individuals with the following numbers: 68, 10, 63, 14, 1, 59, 82, 43, 89, 55 (Fig. 3.3).

Now, let's try using the random assignment function. For example, if you want to randomly assign 40 participants into four groups of 10, you can proceed by entering the necessary values as shown in Fig. 3.4.

The results show that the first participant was randomly assigned to Group 4 (or Condition 4), the second participant to Group 3, the third to Group 2, and the fourth to Group 1 (Fig. 3.5). The remaining participants can be interpreted and assigned in the same manner. If you click DOWNLOAD on the results page, the file will be saved and can later be opened using a spreadsheet program such as Excel (Fig. 3.6).

Another useful website for random assignment and other statistical tools is **http://graphpad.com/quickcalcs/** (Fig. 3.7).

Click on Random Numbers (Fig. 3.8).

If you want to assign 10 participants to each of two groups, enter 10, 2, and 1 in the corresponding fields, as shown in the example below. Then, click DO it! to proceed (Fig. 3.9).

The result will appear as follows: among the 20 participants, the first individual is assigned to Group B, while the second and third individuals are assigned to Group A (Fig. 3.10). The remaining participants can be assigned to their respective groups in the same manner.

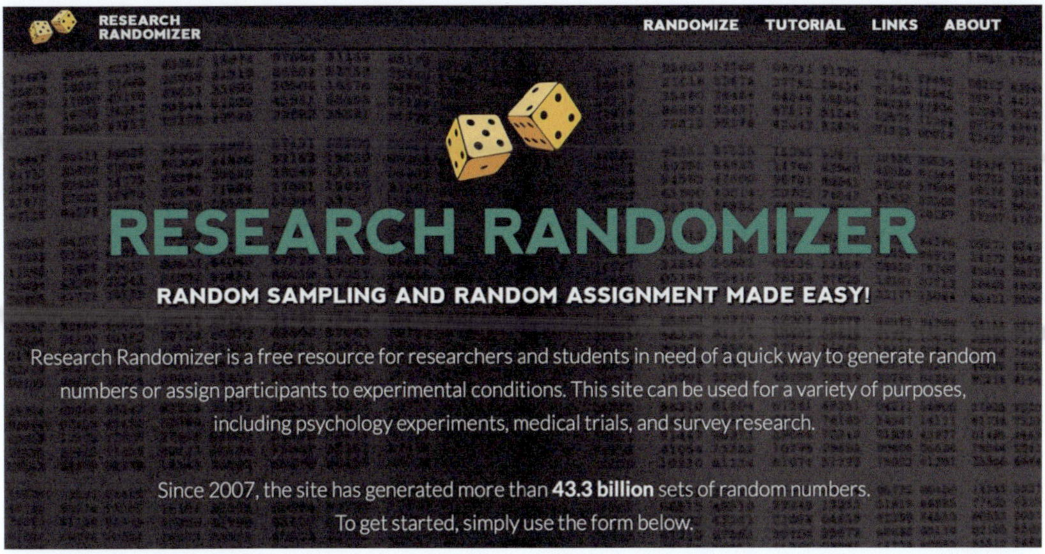

Fig. 3.1 Online randomization tool interface displayed upon accessing the Randomizer website

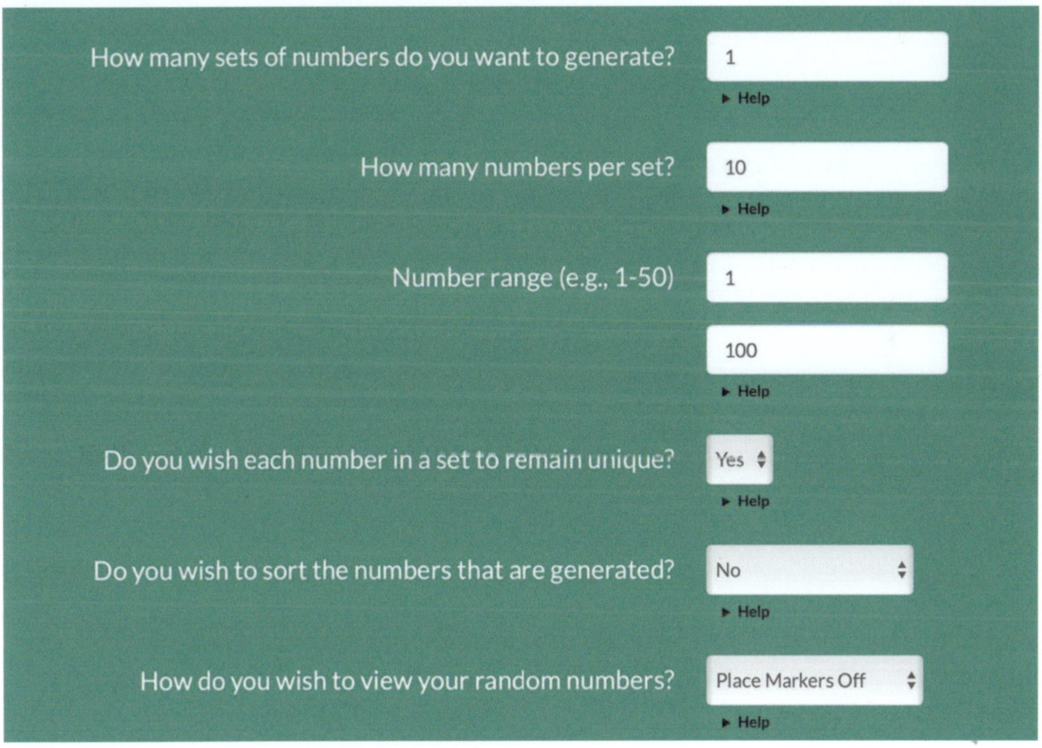

Fig. 3.2 Example of generating a random sample using the Random Sample Generator on the Randomizer website

If you want to randomly arrange the order of participants within each of the two groups, proceed as shown in Fig. 3.11.

Click Do it!, and the results will be displayed as follows. You will see that the participants in Group 1 and Group 2 have been randomly reordered within their respective groups (Fig. 3.12).

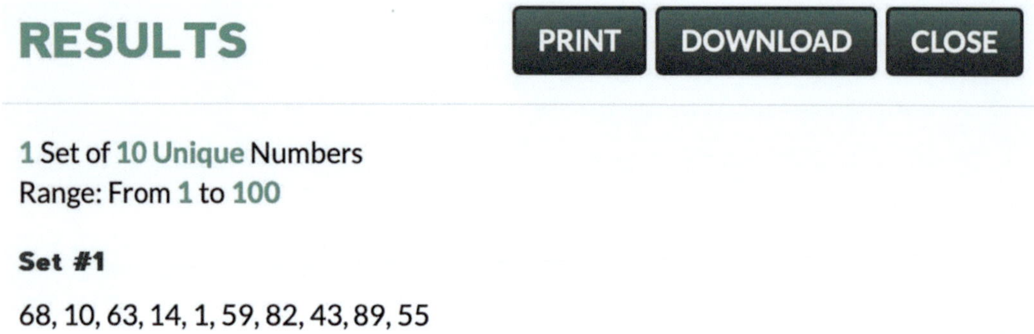

Fig. 3.3 Example of a random sample of 10 units generated on the Randomizer website

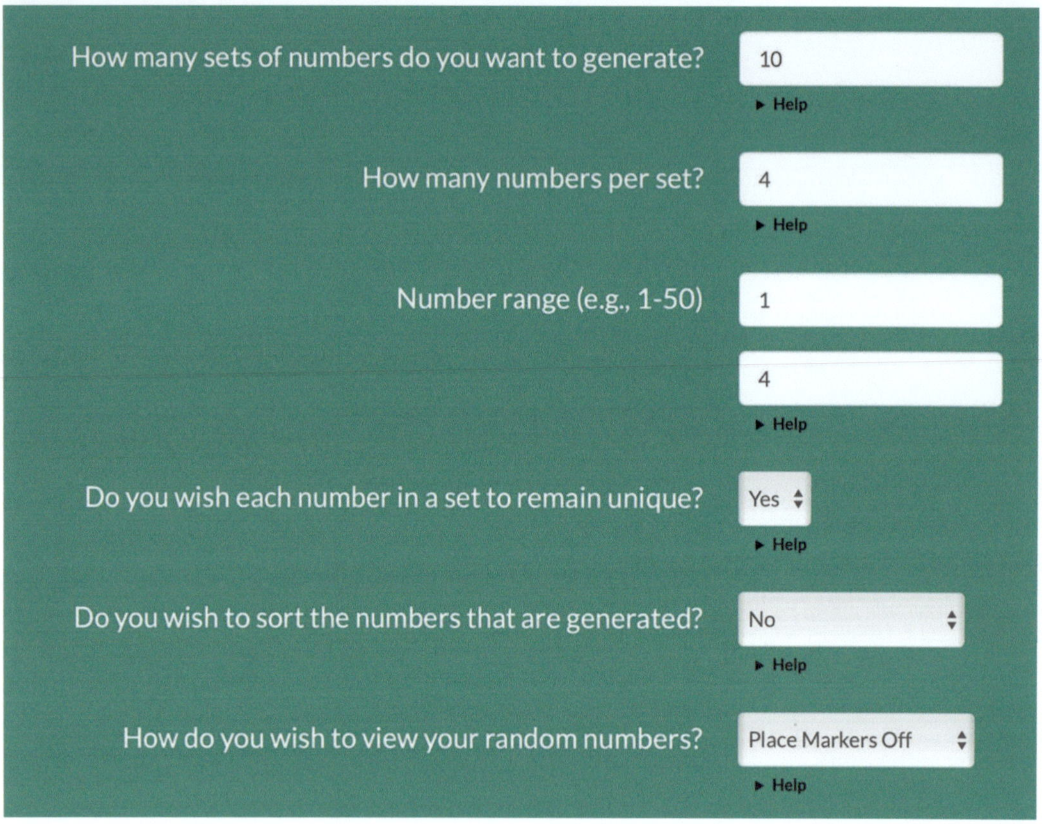

Fig. 3.4 Input screen for random assignment of 40 participants into four groups using the Randomizer tool

3.3 Control Groups

One of the most effective ways to eliminate the effects of extraneous variables is to use a control group. Participants in the control group may receive a new intervention, a placebo,[2] or no treatment at all, and are compared to those in the experimental group. For such comparisons to be valid, equivalence between the control and experimental groups must be established. If no change

[2]When patients with headaches are given a substance with no medicinal properties and are told it is a painkiller, a significant number report that their pain has actually subsided. This phenomenon is known as the placebo effect. Conversely, if patients are given the same inert substance but are told that it may cause headaches, some of them actually begin to experience pain. This is referred to as the nocebo effect, a term derived from the Latin word meaning "to harm."

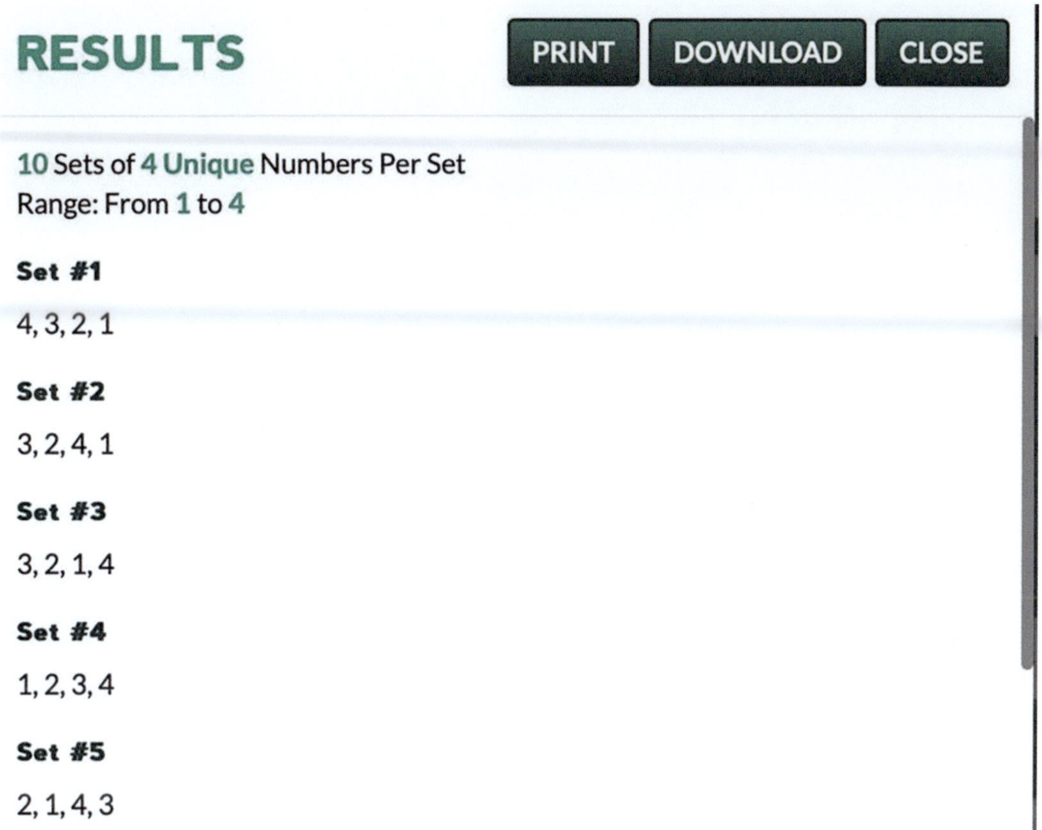

Fig. 3.5 Output of random assignment showing 40 participants distributed into four groups using the Randomizer tool

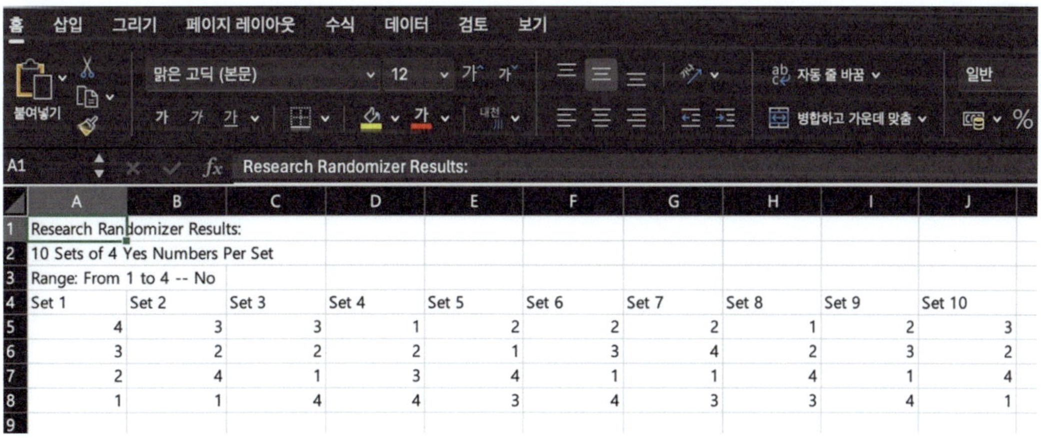

	A	B	C	D	E	F	G	H	I	J
1	Research Randomizer Results:									
2	10 Sets of 4 Yes Numbers Per Set									
3	Range: From 1 to 4 -- No									
4	Set 1	Set 2	Set 3	Set 4	Set 5	Set 6	Set 7	Set 8	Set 9	Set 10
5	4	3	3	1	2	2	2	1	2	3
6	3	2	2	2	1	3	4	2	3	2
7	2	4	1	3	4	1	1	4	1	4
8	1	1	4	4	3	4	3	3	4	1
9										

Fig. 3.6 Excel view of random assignment results generated using the Randomizer platform

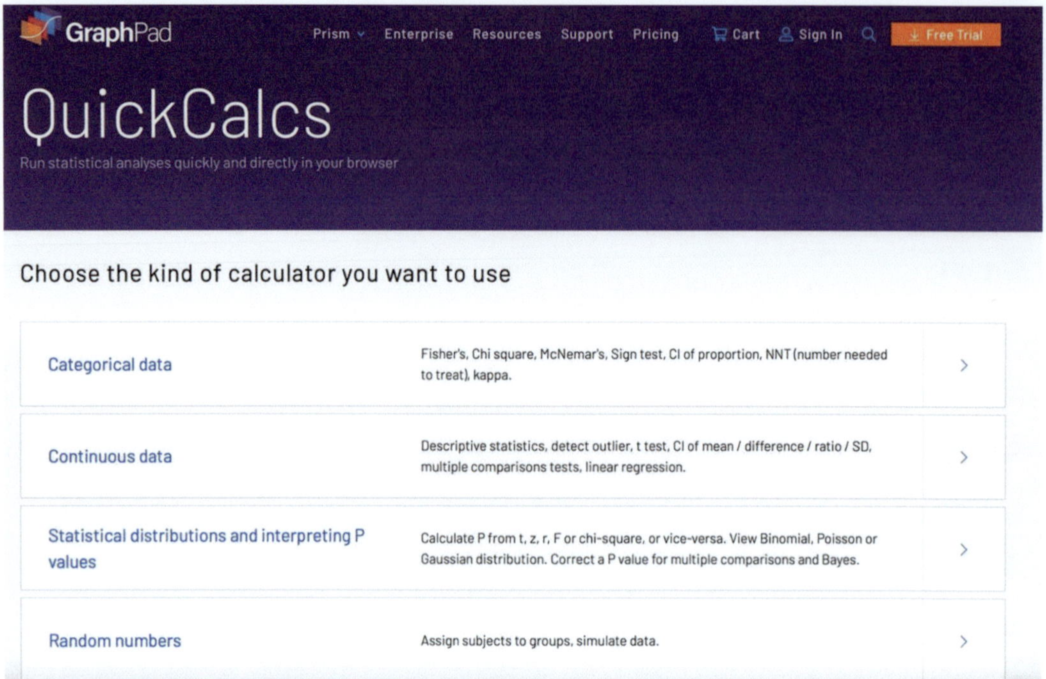

Fig. 3.7 Homepage of the QuickCalcs website

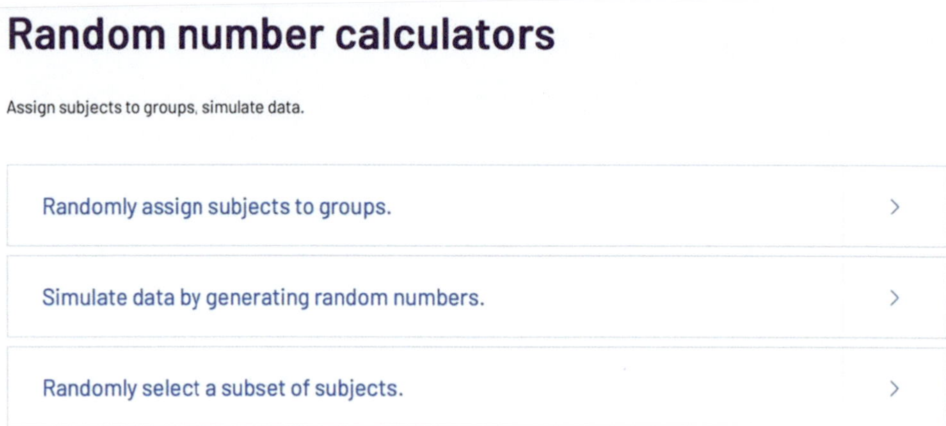

Fig. 3.8 Available options displayed after selecting the "Random Number" function in QuickCalcs

occurs in the control group while a change is observed in the experimental group, it can reasonably be assumed that the treatment caused the change.

If the control group responds similarly to the experimental group, the observed change may be attributed to chance.

In many clinical situations, using a pure experimental or control group is not always feasible due to ethical concerns. As a result, clinical researchers often compare a new treatment with an existing standard treatment. In such designs, the goal is to determine whether the new method is more effective than the current one. However,

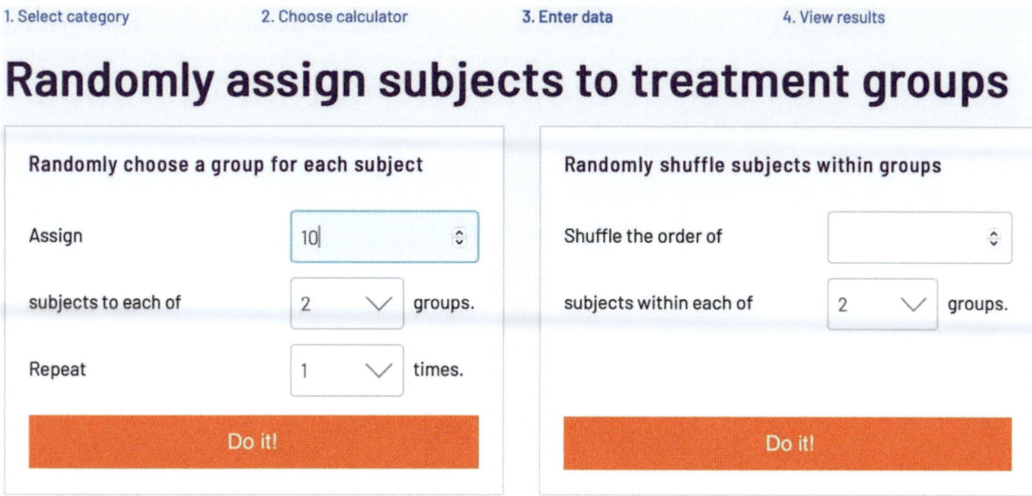

Fig. 3.9 Example setup for allocating 20 participants into two groups of 10 in QuickCalcs

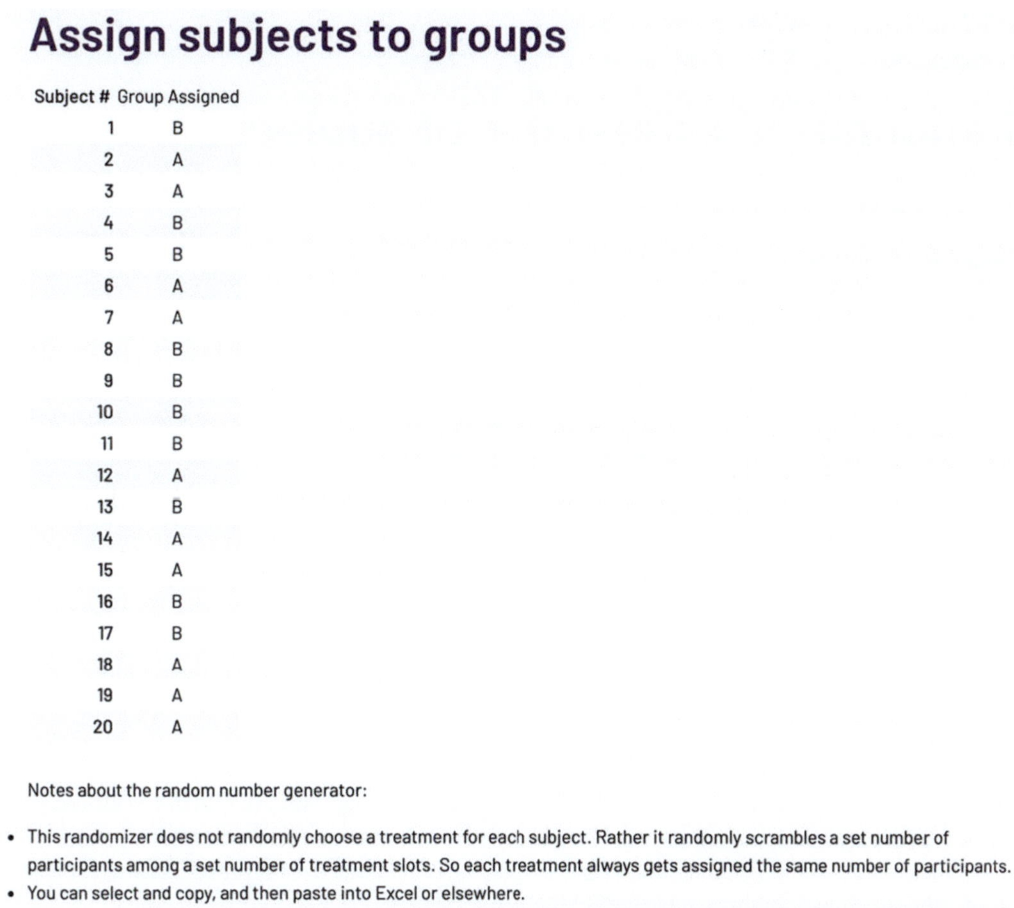

Fig. 3.10 Example of group assignment result from the QuickCalcs randomization tool

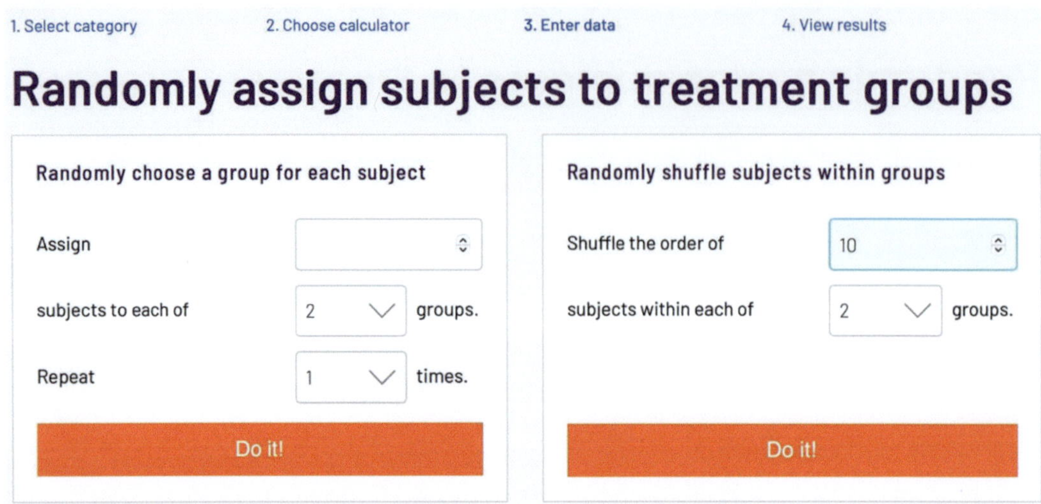

Fig. 3.11 Example of setting up a random arrangement of participant order within each of two groups using a randomization tool

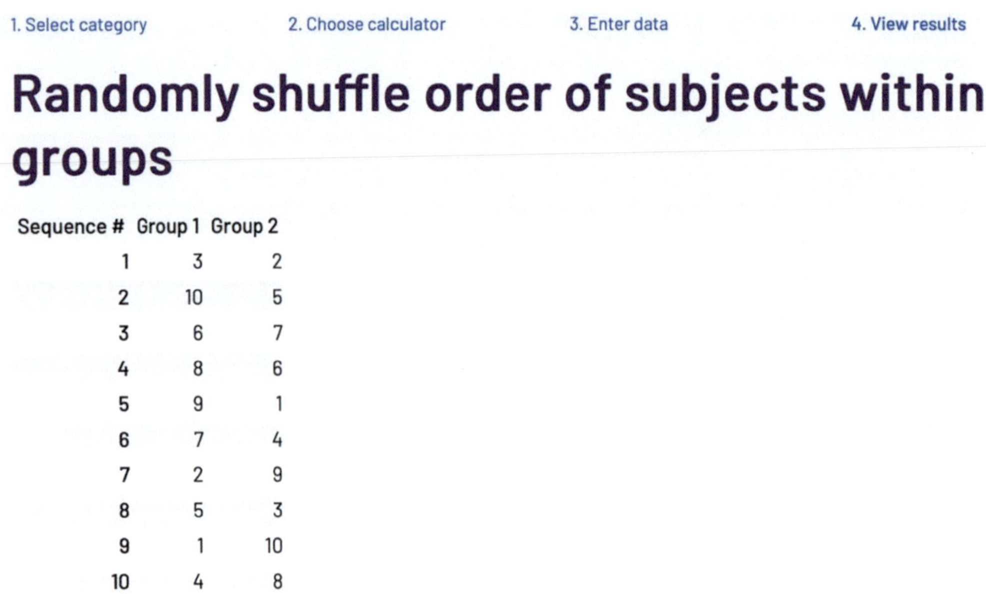

Sequence #	Group 1	Group 2
1	3	2
2	10	5
3	6	7
4	8	6
5	9	1
6	7	4
7	2	9
8	5	3
9	1	10
10	4	8

Fig. 3.12 Output showing randomly arranged participant order within each of the two groups

if the current treatment has not been previously validated through control group studies, it becomes difficult to confirm that the observed improvements are genuinely due to the effectiveness of either treatment. In this case, even if both groups show improvement, one cannot conclude whether both treatments were equally effective, or whether the observed effects occurred by chance without any intervention.

A Randomized Controlled Trial (RCT), also referred to as a Randomized Clinical Trial, is a study design in which participants are randomly assigned to different groups before the treatment begins. The outcome variables are then compared among groups such as treatment, placebo, or control.

3.4 Research Protocol

In order to control the effects of extraneous variables within an experimental setting, researchers must ensure that such variables are applied equally across all groups. This traditional notion of control can only be realistically implemented in laboratory environments, where environmental factors are tightly regulated. However, in clinical settings, achieving such a level of control is much more difficult. One major issue lies in the fact that laboratory conditions do not always mirror clinical conditions, which limits the generalizability of laboratory findings to real-world practice.

Therefore, clinical researchers must identify potential sources of contamination affecting the dependent variables and attempt to minimize their impact. For instance, they should strive to standardize environmental variables such as time of day, room location, lighting, noise, and temperature across all participants. While it is not always possible for every participant to experience identical procedures, clearly written research protocols that are followed consistently can help control the influence of many related extraneous variables. Such protocols ensure consistency in treatment and measurement procedures.

A research protocol must clearly outline the sequence of activities the participant will undergo, specific instructions given to participants, timing of interventions and measurements, measurement devices and methods, and other relevant details. Researchers often read instructions aloud to participants to ensure standardized communication. The criteria used to assess the dependent variable must be clearly defined, and the reliability of measurements must be verified. To enhance reliability, examiners must be properly trained. In some cases, controlling participant behavior before testing is also necessary, such as dietary intake, physical activity, sleep duration, medication use, fatigue, and alcohol consumption. Researchers should observe and evaluate these potential influences throughout the study period.

For example, when measuring facial skin elasticity using a cutometer or similar device, the protocol must be described in sufficient detail to allow replication by other investigators. This helps minimize measurement error. A protocol for such a measurement might include the following:

1. *Preparation Procedure:*

   Was the skin cleansed prior to measurement? How long was the skin allowed to stabilize before testing? Were any skincare products applied beforehand?

2. *Positioning and Stabilization Method:*

   Was the subject seated or lying down during the test? Was the head supported with a chin rest or neck cushion? How was movement minimized during the measurement?

3. *Rest Periods Between Measurements:*

   If multiple measurements were taken, how much rest was allowed between each trial? Was the same site re-measured or were multiple sites involved?

4. *Position of the Subject:*

   What was the posture of the subject (e.g., supine, seated upright)? Was the angle of the head or facial muscles controlled during the test?

5. *Order of Testing:*

   Which facial regions were tested first (e.g., forehead, cheek, jawline)? Was the measurement performed on both sides of the face? Were all measurements completed in a standardized sequence?

6. *Instructions and Encouragement to Subjects:*
   Were standardized instructions read aloud to all subjects? Was any verbal feedback or encouragement provided during the test (e.g., "stay still")?

7. *Measurement Technique:*
   Was the skin elasticity measured via suction (e.g., using a cutometer) or via indentation? Were peak recoil times or viscoelastic parameters recorded?

8. *Device and Settings:*
   What device was used? What were the technical specifications and settings (e.g., probe size, suction pressure, measurement time)? Were calibration checks performed?

3.5 Blinding

In experimental research, the possibility of bias from the observer or assessor is a significant concern. If participants are aware of the experimental setup or the researcher's expectations, consciously or unconsciously, it may influence their behavior or the way results are reported. To prevent such bias, the double-blind study design is often employed. In a double-blind study, neither the participant nor the investigator knows which group the participant has been assigned to until after data collection. The most rigorous form of blinding is a blind design in which the individuals administering the treatment, those assessing the outcome variables, the data analysts, and the participants themselves are all unaware of group assignment.

In some cases, a placebo may be used to prevent the subject from knowing whether they are receiving the real treatment. However, full double blinding is not always feasible. In such cases, a single-blind study may be used, in which only the participants are unaware of the treatment they are receiving. Alternatively, only the investigators or the outcome assessors may be blinded.

A double-blind study ensures that both the patient (or subject) and the investigator or assessor are unaware of whether the participant is in the treatment or control group, or whether they are receiving the actual intervention or a placebo. For example, in a pharmaceutical study, neither the person administering the drug nor the person taking it knows whether the substance is active or inert, and only a third party not involved in the experiment holds the code that matches participants to the treatment groups.

For instance, in a study evaluating the efficacy of topical niacinamide in improving facial skin appearance, a randomized, double-blind, placebo-controlled, split-face design was utilized. Participants applied a 5% niacinamide formulation to one side of the face and a placebo to the other side over 12 weeks. Neither the participants nor the evaluators knew which side received the active treatment. This design ensured that any observed differences in skin appearance could be attributed to the treatment itself rather than to participant or evaluator expectations (Bissett et al. 2005).

3.6 Design Strategies for Controlling Inter-Subject Variability

Among the various strategies to control for inter-subject variability, the most fundamental is random assignment, which aims to evenly distribute subject characteristics across groups. However, random assignment is not a perfect mechanism. Even when implemented properly, it is possible that critical variables may still be unevenly distributed among groups. To ensure that certain variables are more evenly distributed across experimental conditions, several additional techniques can be employed, including selecting a homogeneous group of participants, matching participants, repeated-measures design, blocking, and analysis of covariance (ANCOVA).

1. *Selecting a Homogeneous Group of Participants*

When certain subject characteristics are suspected to influence the dependent variable, the simplest method of control is to limit the study to participants who share similar attributes. For example, if one assumes that males and females may respond differently to a particular intervention, the researcher may choose to include only female participants. If age is believed to be a potential confounding variable, the sample may be further restricted to females between the ages of 20 and 30.

This approach assumes that, by controlling for variables such as age and gender, all other characteristics will be approximately evenly distributed across groups. The major drawback of this method is that the study findings can only be generalized to individuals who fit the criteria of the study sample—for instance, women in their 20s and 30s, as in the example above.

2. *Blocking*

Another strategy for controlling the effects of attribute variables, which function as extraneous variables, is to incorporate them as independent variables within the experimental design. For example, if a researcher is interested in the potential effect of age, participants can be divided into three groups: those in their 20s, 30s, and 40s or older. Each of these age ranges is referred to as a block, and the variable used to create the blocks (in this case, age) is called a blocking variable. Through this process, the researcher can analyze how the treatment effects may vary by age within the context of the experimental design. A block refers to a group of participants who are homogeneous or who share a particular characteristic. When participants within each block are randomly assigned to treatment groups, the design is known as a randomized block design. While this design increases the complexity of data analysis and interpretation, it can be expanded to include multiple blocking variables at the design stage. For instance, one could evaluate the effectiveness of two different topical treatments across various age groups and both sexes by using blocking.

Age group	Topical treatment A	Topical treatment B
Block 1 (20s)	$n_1 = 20$ participants	$n_2 = 20$ participants
Block 2 (30s)	$n_3 = 20$ participants	$n_4 = 20$ participants
Block 3 (40s)	$n_5 = 20$ participants	$n_6 = 20$ participants

3. *Matching*

Another strategy for addressing confounding variables is to use matching based on certain characteristics. For example, if a researcher is concerned that age and sex may influence the dependent variable, participants in the experimental and control groups can be matched to ensure equivalent distributions for these attributes. Matching involves identifying participants who share similar characteristics and then randomly assigning the members of each matched pair to different groups. This approach is known as a matched pairs design.

Matching can be achieved by intentionally selecting pairs of participants from a pool of individuals with similar characteristics. One member of each pair is then randomly assigned to the experimental group, and the other to the control group. To facilitate effective matching, it is often necessary to define acceptable ranges for the variables of interest. For example, when matching participants by age, the researcher might allow a ± 2-year age range. Matching becomes increasingly challenging as the number of variables used for matching increases, making it more difficult to find suitable participants.

In a study by Wall et al. (2023), patients who underwent aesthetic breast surgery were matched based on demographics, comorbidities, type of operation, and incision pattern. The researchers then applied force-modulating tissue bridges to evaluate their effect on postoperative wound formation.

4. *Repeated Measures on the Same Subjects*

One of the most effective strategies to control for inter-subject variability is through self-controlled methods, that is, by applying repeated measures on the same subjects. In this design, a single group is exposed to all levels of the independent variable, and outcomes are compared within each individual depending on the treatment condition. This is referred to as a repeated-measures design, in which each participant is assessed multiple times under different conditions. This approach ensures the highest degree of homogeneity between treatment conditions, since each subject is perfectly matched with themselves. Individual characteristics such as gender, cognitive ability, physical traits, and age are assumed to remain constant across treatments. Therefore, any observed differences are more likely attributable to the treatment itself than to other designs.

Repeated-measures designs are particularly useful when the goal is to observe how individuals respond across time or under different conditions. For example, suppose we want to compare skin hydration levels at three different time points following the application of a hyaluronic acid-based facial serum. Rather than dividing 30 participants into three separate groups of 10, it is more effective to apply all three time-point measurements (e.g., baseline, 2 weeks, 4 weeks) to the same 30 individuals. In this case, sufficient rest intervals between assessments should be allowed, and the order of the conditions should be randomized.

Another example would be comparing facial skin elasticity in various facial regions, such as the forehead, cheeks, and jawline, within the same participant, or evaluating changes in skin pigmentation at different stages after fractional laser treatment (e.g., 1 week, 4 weeks, and 8 weeks post-procedure). These are also instances of repeated-measures design. In such cases, statistical analysis is typically conducted using repeated-measures ANOVA.

In a study by Gold et al. (2018), a novel hyaluronic acid gel was injected into one nasolabial fold, while a comparator gel was injected into the opposite fold of the same participants. This split-face design allowed for direct comparison of the fillers' efficacy within the same individuals, utilizing a repeated-measures design where the type of filler served as the repeated factor.

In repeated-measures designs, the same dependent variable is measured on multiple occasions for each subject. The simplest example is a pre–post design, where the dependent variable is measured twice. These types of data are typically analyzed using paired t-tests.

The advantages of repeated measures are clear: they require fewer subjects and inherently resolve the problem of between-group variability. However, there are several issues to consider with this design, such as carry-over effects, latent effects, and learning effects.

1. Carry-over effect occurs when the effects of a prior treatment persist and influence the response to the next treatment. For example, applying a topical agent that continues to affect skin texture when a second treatment is introduced.
2. Latent effect arises when a later treatment activates or interacts with a dormant effect from an earlier treatment. This is especially important in drug trials, where latent effects may invalidate a repeated-measures design.
3. Learning effect occurs when responses improve merely as a result of repeated exposure to the treatment or task. For example, if participants are repeatedly assessed on their ability to perform facial muscle exercises designed to enhance skin tightness or reduce wrinkles, their scores may improve over time, not necessarily due to the treatment's effectiveness, but simply because they have learned how to perform the exercises more effectively with practice. As a result, even if a treatment applied later has no actual physiological benefit, performance may appear to improve, misleading the interpretation of the treatment's impact.

5. *Analysis of Covariance (ANCOVA)*

The final method for controlling confounding variables is not applied during the design phase, but rather at the analysis stage after data collection is complete. Analysis of covariance

(ANCOVA) is based on the principles of both analysis of variance (ANOVA) and regression analysis. Instead of explaining the detailed statistical procedures here, the concept of ANCOVA will be introduced through a study example.

For example, let us assume that there are two treatment groups, and 40 participants are randomly assigned into each group with 20 individuals. The researcher applies Skin Regeneration Cream A to participants in experimental group 1 and Skin Regeneration Cream B to those in experimental group 2, then compares post-treatment skin elasticity to evaluate the effectiveness of each cream.

If participants using Cream A show higher average skin elasticity than those using Cream B, the researcher may initially attribute the difference to the formulation of the cream. However, an important consideration arises—skin elasticity can also be influenced by individual characteristics such as age, baseline hydration levels, or UV exposure history. If participants in group 1 are generally younger than those in group 2, the observed improvement in skin elasticity may stem from age differences rather than the effect of the cream itself.

ANCOVA allows the researcher to statistically control for the influence of such extraneous variables (e.g., age), thereby clarifying the true effect of the independent variable—in this case, the skincare treatment. In this context, these extraneous variables are referred to as covariates. Conceptually, ANCOVA artificially equalizes groups and evaluates how the dependent variable changes under such equalized conditions by removing the influence of covariates.

In the example above, if it is discovered after the experiment that participants who used Treatment Cream A were, on average, older than those who used Treatment Cream B, ANCOVA allows researchers to analyze how the treatment creams affect outcomes such as wrinkle reduction or skin hydration while statistically equalizing the age factor across both groups.

ANCOVA is particularly useful for adjusting for initial differences between groups. For instance, if there is a difference in pre-test scores between two groups, even if there is a difference in post-test scores after the treatment, it may not necessarily be due to the treatment itself. In such cases, ANCOVA helps control for the pre-treatment score as a covariate, allowing for a more accurate assessment of treatment efficacy.

In summary, when studying the relationship between independent and dependent variables, there are often numerous confounding factors that can influence the results. These confounding variables are factors other than the independent variable of interest that may affect the dependent variable. There are two approaches to controlling confounding variables: one is to address them during the experimental design phase, and the other is to control them statistically after the experiment has been completed.

(1) *Controlling at the Experimental Design Stage*

First, researchers can expose all participants to the confounding variable equally. For example, in a study examining the effects of a new facial filler technique on skin elasticity, if gender is suspected to influence outcomes, the study might include only female participants to eliminate the gender effect.

Second, researchers can randomly assign participants to different treatment conditions. Through randomization, confounding variables are more likely to be evenly distributed across groups.

Third, researchers can include the confounding variable as an experimental factor within the design itself, as seen in blocked designs. For example, participants may be stratified by age group, and equal numbers from each group are assigned to different treatments.

(B) *Controlling at the Statistical Analysis Stage*

A statistical method of controlling confounding variables is to perform an analysis of covariance (ANCOVA) during the data analysis phase in order to eliminate the effects of those variables.

References

Bissett DL, Oblong JE, Berge CA. Niacinamide: A B vitamin that improves aging facial skin appearance. *Dermatol Surg*. 2005;31(7 Pt 2):860–865.

Gold MH, Baumann LS, Clark CP III, Schlessinger J. A Multicenter, Double-Blinded, Randomized, Split-Face Study of the Safety and Efficacy of a Novel Hyaluronic Acid Gel for the Correction of Nasolabial Folds. *J Drugs Dermatol*. 2018;17(1):66–73.

Wall HC, Halani SH, Mosieri C, Daniel C, Gallo L, Eaves FF 3rd, Coroneos CJ. Tension Reduction With Force Modulating Tissue Bridges Reduces Wounds in Breast Surgery. Aesthet Surg J. 2023 Nov 16;43(12):1471–1480

Validity of Experiments

4

For a study to be considered valid, it is essential to assess whether what the researcher intended to measure or observe was, in fact, accurately measured or observed. Validity must be examined from two perspectives: internal validity and external validity. Internal validity concerns the question: "Is the researcher truly observing or measuring what they intended to?" External validity addresses the extent to which the conclusions drawn from the research can be generalized to other populations or settings.

4.1 Internal Validity

Internal validity refers to the question of whether the treatment (independent variable) in an experimental study truly caused the observed change in the dependent variable. In other words, it questions whether other variables may have contributed to the observed change. Extraneous variables, aside from the independent variable, can threaten internal validity and interfere with causal inference. A true experimental design generally has high internal validity because it incorporates randomization and the use of a control group.

Internal validity is a crucial condition to consider when interpreting experimental results. Threats to internal validity include historical events, maturation of subjects during the study period, testing effects on subjects, selection bias, and subject attrition.

History/Events

In experimental research, history refers to events that occur during the course of the study. These are incidents that take place between the pretest and posttest, potentially affecting the dependent variable alongside the independent variable, thereby creating the illusion that any observed change is solely due to the treatment.

This issue becomes more serious as the time interval between pretest and posttest increases, making the control of timing an important consideration. History effects refer to the influence of unexpected or uncontrolled events, not part of the experimental intervention, that occur after the application of the independent variable or between the pretest and posttest. For instance, suppose a researcher is studying the effects of two types of facial treatments on reducing periorbital wrinkles. In this case, the "history" threat may arise if, during the study period, participants engage in additional skin treatments, such as using home-based anti-aging devices or receiving other cosmetic procedures, that could affect the skin's elasticity or wrinkle appearance. Similarly, if a new clinician replaces the original practitioner during the course of the study, differences in technique or communication style may also influ-

K.-H. Yi, *Statistical Research Methods for Dermatologists and Plastic Surgeons*,
https://doi.org/10.1007/978-981-95-5668-7_4

ence the outcomes, thereby introducing bias into the dependent variable.

In some cases, history can also refer to broader life events. For instance, consider a study evaluating the effectiveness of a smoking cessation program. If a participant's spouse becomes pregnant or gives birth during the program, the participant may be more motivated to quit smoking for personal or family reasons—independent of the actual intervention—thus confounding the treatment effect.

In studies involving a single-session intervention where data is collected over a short period of time, the threat of history is generally minimal. For example, if a researcher applies a 10-minute hyaluronic acid mask to improve skin hydration and immediately measures the skin's moisture levels afterward, there is little opportunity for extraneous historical events to influence the dependent variable. However, even in such controlled settings, factors like conversations during the treatment, the participant's movement through different rooms, changes in ambient temperature or humidity, or encounters with other participants could unintentionally influence the outcome. These seemingly minor events can introduce bias and compromise the internal validity of the study.

Maturation

The second factor that threatens internal validity relates to processes that emerge over time. Maturation refers to internal changes that occur within the participant simply due to the passage of time, independent of any external events. These changes can include natural growth and development, aging, wound healing, surgical recovery, cognitive advancement, fatigue, or even hunger. Without a control group, it becomes difficult to determine whether observed improvements are due to the treatment, natural maturation, or an interaction of the two.

Maturation may influence participants to respond differently in subsequent measurements. This could be because they have become older, physically stronger, more skilled, more fatigued, or bored compared to the initial measurement, which in turn affects the experimental outcomes. For instance, when studying the effectiveness of therapy for post-stroke communication disorders, some degree of spontaneous recovery may occur over time, even without any specific intervention, due to the patient's inherent capacity for healing.

This issue is common in clinical studies, especially when there is a long interval between pre- and posttests. In particular, in developmental studies with children, improvements can occur without any therapeutic intervention. Wound healing, reversal of age-related symptoms, neurological regeneration, and post-surgical recovery are all examples of possible maturation effects.

For example, if a group of fifty 5-year-old children shows a 20-point improvement in performance after a year-long early education program, it remains unclear whether the change was due to the program or natural cognitive development over time. Some children may show similar progress even without the program. A control group that does not receive the intervention would allow for a more accurate assessment of how much improvement would have occurred naturally.

In the context of cosmetic dermatology and plastic surgery, a study might aim to determine whether improvements in skin elasticity or facial volume after a treatment are truly attributable to the intervention itself—or whether such changes are partially due to time-dependent recovery processes like natural collagen regeneration or resolution of post-procedural inflammation. Likewise, if the study focuses on delaying the progression of skin laxity, it may be difficult to separate the effects of the treatment from the subject's naturally slowing aging process over the same period.

Testing

Testing effects refer to the influence that taking a test for the first time can have on performance in a subsequent test. When participants are aware that they will be tested again, or if the initial test experience is unique or impactful, this experience may influence their future responses. In other words, the act of data collection itself can alter how participants respond on a dependent variable, independent of any intervention. Testing effects typically arise from increased familiarity with the measurement tool, leading to improved performance or skill development over time. For example, in an educational context, participants may learn actual information during the pretest, which in turn improves their posttest performance independently of any educational intervention.

If a coordination test is administered before and after treatment, patients may score higher on the post-treatment assessment simply because they had the opportunity to practice the coordinated movement during the pretest. Testing effects can also arise in cases where the measurement procedure itself alters the independent variable. For example, suppose a study is evaluating whether a topical tightening serum improves skin elasticity in the lower face. If skin elasticity is repeatedly measured using a suction-based device that stretches the skin, the repeated measurements themselves might stimulate skin tension or blood flow, thereby increasing elasticity regardless of the serum's actual effects.

Another example: in a study evaluating the effectiveness of educational materials on postoperative scar care following cosmetic surgery, patients might first be given a survey to assess their baseline knowledge. If the same questionnaire is used again after the intervention, any improvement may partly be due to the initial survey sparking curiosity—patients may have looked up the information on their own or asked their care provider—resulting in better scores that are not entirely due to the educational program. Meanwhile, a group that only takes the posttest wouldn't be influenced in the same way by the initial measurement.

Instrumentation Issues

The condition of the instruments used in a study can significantly affect measurement outcomes. The device may not be properly calibrated or adjusted, or it may be too old and worn to produce accurate readings. The sensitivity of the instrument also influences the measurement results. Additionally, if the person operating the instrument during the pretest differs from the person operating it during the posttest, variations in measurement scores may occur. Observers may also become more experienced or skilled by the time they conduct the posttest, which could inadvertently influence their measurements.

It also includes cases where the instrument (or assessor) used during the initial measurement differs from the one used later, where the instrument is not appropriate for the participant being measured, or where the assessor fails to perform the measurement accurately. For instance, when assessing facial wrinkle severity, standardized grading scales such as the Fitzpatrick Wrinkle Scale may be used, but scores can vary depending on the subjective judgment of the evaluator. Therefore, clinicians or researchers should undergo sufficient training to ensure a high level of interrater reliability before conducting assessments.

Statistical Regression

There is a tendency of extreme pretest scores (either very low or very high) to regress toward the mean during posttesting, regardless of any treatment effect. Extremely low scores tend to increase, while extremely high scores tend to decrease, resulting in scores that cluster near the average. This effect typically occurs when subjects are selected based on extreme scores. This is referred to as statistical regression. This effect typically occurs when subjects are selected based on extreme scores.

For example, if a study aims to examine how a specific pigmentation-reducing treatment affects patients with either very severe or very mild facial hyperpigmentation, subjects can be divided into two groups based on their pre-treatment assessment scores. A potential regression effect may occur if, in the post-treatment assessment, the scores of both groups move toward the average, even in the absence of any true treatment effect.

For instance, when measuring cognitive development in very young infants, it is expected that their baseline cognitive development scores will be relatively low due to their age. If a cognitive development enhancement program is implemented a few months after the pre-assessment and the level of cognitive development is measured again, significant improvement may be observed. However, this outcome may reflect not only the effect of the program itself but also the effects of natural maturation and statistical regression toward the mean.

In summary, statistical outliers tend to influence the regression line. That is, when participants are selected based on extreme scores, they are likely to show scores closer to the mean at the time of the next test, even in the absence of any real treatment effect. It is necessary to find methods to account for such errors, or at the very least, acknowledge this limitation when interpreting results. One approach to minimize regression effects is to assign subjects with low scores randomly into both the treatment and control groups and compare the outcomes between them.

Selection Bias

Selection bias occurs when a control group is not properly chosen, resulting in a lack of equivalence between the control and experimental groups. Ideally, subjects should be randomly selected from the population and then randomly assigned to each group. However, this is often unrealistic in actual practice. In experimental studies, researchers commonly use convenience sampling to recruit participants, and then randomly assign them to experimental or control groups.

However, if true random assignment is not strictly followed, selection bias can occur. Without random allocation or proper matching procedures, there may be meaningful differences between groups. For instance, a group consisting of volunteers who actively signed up for the study may differ significantly from a group of participants who joined for other reasons, thereby introducing bias. To avoid a sample consisting of participants with characteristics that may distort the results, it is necessary to use random assignment across two or more groups.

For example, in situations where it is difficult to recruit participants, researchers may assign individuals to experimental and control groups based on availability. If a participant assigned to the experimental group is deemed unsuitable or refuses participation, researchers may be tempted to place them in the control group instead. This compromises group equivalence from the beginning, leading to systematic bias. To prevent such issues, random assignment or matching should be performed at the participant allocation stage.

Mortality (Attrition)

Mortality, or attrition, refers to the phenomenon in which participants from either the experimental or control group drop out before the study is completed. Even if both groups were initially equivalent in quality, participant dropout during the study period can affect the experiment or create differences in the results.

In clinical research, it is common to encounter situations where participants withdraw from the study or are excluded before the trial is completed. For example, in a clinical study evaluating the effectiveness of an intensive microneedle radiofrequency treatment for acne scars, participants were randomly assigned to the treatment and control groups. Suppose, however, that those assigned to the treatment group had more severe scarring or lower pain tolerance. These participants might find the procedure more uncomfortable or emotionally distressing, leading to higher dropout rates in the treatment group compared to the control group.

As a result, even if random assignment was properly done at the outset, by the end of the study, the characteristics of the experimental and control groups may no longer be equivalent. If the remaining participants in the experimental group show no improvement, it becomes difficult to determine whether this was due to the treatment's lack of effectiveness or because only a specific subset of participants remained in the group after others had dropped out.

The concern with attrition is not merely about the reduction in sample size—whether 10 or 20 participants out of 50 or 100 drop out—but rather that the individuals who drop out may differ in important ways from those who remain.

For example, in an experimental study designed to compare responses to two levels of pain—low and high—it was hypothesized that men possess higher endogenous pain tolerance than women. Based on this assumption, an equal number of male and female participants were selected and randomly assigned into four groups to receive one of the two pain stimuli. During the pretest, pain was induced, but several female participants, fearing the pain, withdrew before the posttest. As a result, only those women who were less fearful continued with the study, which may have led to findings that do not accurately reflect the overall population.

No matter how well-designed a study is, it is difficult to completely prevent participant attrition. Participants may withdraw due to illness, relocation, or even death-factors often beyond the researcher's control.

Intention-to-treat (ITT) analysis refers to analyzing data based on the original group assignments, assuming that participants received the treatment they were initially allocated to, regardless of whether they completed the treatment. For example, in a clinical trial, participants are randomly assigned to an experimental or control group. However, during the course of the study, some may relocate, pass away, or refuse the assigned intervention. Others may initially receive the assigned treatment but later switch to a different one (crossover). By the final stage of the study, the number of participants in each group may be lower than at the start. At first glance, it might seem reasonable to exclude participants who did not complete the treatment and analyze only the remaining data. However, doing so reduces the sample size and makes it difficult to determine whether the differences between groups are truly due to the treatment or simply because the remaining participants are those who were healthier or more resilient. In such cases, the ITT approach assumes that all participants received their initially assigned treatment and includes them in the final analysis. In other words, even if participants dropped out or did not complete the treatment, they are still counted in the analysis as originally assigned. This method is widely used in controlled clinical trials because it preserves the benefits of randomization and reduces bias. A corresponding approach to ITT is on-protocol analysis, which analyzes participants according to the treatment they actually received. In this approach, if a participant was initially assigned to the experimental group but ended up receiving a different intervention, their data would be analyzed as part of the group corresponding to the treatment they actually completed.

Selection–Maturation Interaction

This threat to internal validity occurs when participants are not randomly assigned to groups, when randomization fails, or when other threats such as maturation, history, or instrumentation affect groups differently. A selection–maturation interaction arises when the experimental group experiences maturational changes at a different rate than the control group. For example, suppose a study compares motor learning outcomes of a therapeutic intervention between 3-year-old and 10-year-old children. Any observed difference may be due not solely to the treatment, but to developmental changes (i.e., maturation), which vary between the two age groups.

If the groups differ initially, changes in the dependent variable may result from both their baseline differences and the interaction between those differences and maturational development. Even if the groups appear similar at baseline, improper selection may result in differing maturation effects that influence the outcome. For example, suppose the experimental group is composed of boys, while the control group consists of girls. Even if the pretest scores are equivalent, the posttest results may be influenced by differences in maturation associated with gender, rather than the treatment itself.

4.2 External Validity

External validity concerns the extent to which the results of a study can be generalized to other populations, settings, treatment variables, or measurement variables. Researchers should not only be attentive to factors that threaten internal validity, but also to those that limit generalizability. The following are factors that can threaten external validity:

Subject Selection

Generalization refers to the degree to which findings from a sample (study participants) can be observed in the larger population. The critical question is whether the sample adequately represents the target population, and to what extent its characteristics align. The more these characteristics diverge, the more difficult it becomes to generalize the findings. For instance, if a study is conducted on individuals within a specific age group, gender, disease condition, or functional status, applying the results to individuals who do not share these characteristics may not be justifiable. Additionally, when study participants are volunteers, generalizing those results to a population that includes non-volunteers can be problematic. Hence, caution is required when interpreting the generalizability of results.

Setting

For example, suppose a study on the effectiveness of laser treatment for skin rejuvenation was conducted in a specialized dermatology clinic. The findings may not be directly generalizable to other settings, such as general dermatology practices or aesthetic spas. To strengthen the external validity of such interventions, replication studies across diverse clinical and nonclinical environments are required.

Time

The timing of a study can also influence its external validity. Results obtained at one point in time may not be applicable to a different temporal context. For instance, suppose a study conducted 20 years ago demonstrated that a specific dietary intervention effectively reduced cholesterol levels. Applying those findings to today's population may not be appropriate, as public awareness regarding the role of diet and exercise in cardiovascular health has significantly increased. In contrast to two decades ago, contemporary society is more informed through mass media and public health initiatives, which could alter the intervention's effectiveness in the present day.

Hawthorne Effect

Between 1924 and 1927, the Western Electric Hawthorne Works in Chicago conducted a series of experiments at its Hawthorne Plant to determine whether adjustments in lighting, temperature, and work hours would improve productivity. Interestingly, regardless of whether lighting was increased or decreased, all participants in the study showed improved performance compared to before. This outcome was attributed not to the experimental conditions themselves, but to the fact that participants were aware they were being observed as part of a study. This phenomenon is referred to as the Hawthorne Effect.

When participants are involved in an experiment, they often receive special attention, which can in turn influence their behavior. This attention may alter participants' attitudes, causing them to perform better than they would under normal conditions. In other words, improvements may be observed regardless of the actual treatment simply because of the participants' awareness of being studied. However, in real-world settings—where such focused attention is absent—results may differ.

Researcher Effect

When all participants in a study are female and the experimenters are male—or vice versa—participants may respond differently. Similarly, the age of the experimenter can influence outcomes; responses may differ when experimenters are in their 20 s versus their 40 s. In other words, the psychosocial characteristics of the experimenter play a significant role. Attitudes such as hostility, authoritarianism, warmth, or kindness toward participants can all affect the results of a study. To minimize such influences, employing a double-blind design is recommended. That is, participants may react differently depending on who is administering the treatment, and results may vary depending on the characteristics of the person conducting the study.

In psychology, this phenomenon—where a researcher's expectations influence outcomes—is referred to as the Rosenthal effect. For example, if an observer believes that a certain intervention is effective, they may unintentionally assign lower scores to the control group that does not align with their expectations. To control for the Rosenthal effect, researchers may employ blinding, where the experimenters are unaware of the study's true purpose, or they may even provide deceptive information. However, the latter approach raises ethical concerns and is generally discouraged. A related concept is the Pygmalion effect, which describes how increased expectations or attention from others can lead to improved performance.

Multitreatments

When a subject in a study receives more than one treatment as an independent variable, the results cannot be generalized to environments in which only a single treatment is administered. The combined or cumulative effects of multiple treatments can influence the outcome. Therefore, the findings from studies involving multiple treatments may differ from those that assess a single intervention, and this difference must be acknowledged.

Although these effects may threaten the external validity of the experiment, researchers usually describe such limitations when reporting their results. In order to make valid generalizations, appropriate experimental designs must be selected, and extraneous variables should be controlled. Choosing a suitable research design that aligns with the purpose of the study is of utmost importance.

In conclusion, researchers should strive to adopt a study design that satisfies both internal and external validity. However, as internal validity increases through strict control of experimental conditions, the study may become more distant from real-life settings, thereby reducing external validity. For this reason, it is important to replicate research with new participants in different contexts.

- Ceiling effect
  The ceiling effect occurs when a measurement tool cannot distinguish differences because subjects score at or near the maximum limit. For example, if a pigmentation severity index is applied to a group of individuals with clear skin and minimal discoloration before undergoing a laser toning procedure, the initial scores might already be very low. In this case, the tool cannot detect meaningful improvements post-treatment, as the scores were already at the best end of the scale, reducing the ability to evaluate the laser's efficacy.
- Floor effect
  A floor effect arises when a task or test is too difficult, resulting in most participants being unable to perform it. In such cases, differences among individuals below a certain ability level cannot be identified. For instance, an assessment tool that effectively discriminates among typical students may result in a floor effect if used with children who have intellectual disabilities.
- Confounding variable
  Some people argue that excessive exercise leads to shorter lifespans, citing early deaths among bodybuilders as evidence. It's true that many Olympic lifters from the former Soviet Union and Eastern Europe died in their 40s. However, it was later revealed that their early deaths were not due to intense exercise itself, but rather the excessive use of anabolic steroids—a classic example of a confounding variable.

5 Validity of Measurement

5.1 Validity

Validity refers to the degree to which a measurement accurately reflects what it is intended to measure. For example, if the Korean-Wechsler Intelligence Scale for Children (K-WISC) is used to assess intelligence in a child with a disability who has significant difficulties in verbal expression, the test might inaccurately yield a low score, even though the child may actually possess high intelligence. In such a case, the validity of using the K-WISC for this particular child would be considered low. A more appropriate tool, such as the Korean-Pictorial Test of Intelligence (K-PTI), which does not rely heavily on verbal communication, would better reflect the child's intellectual ability, thereby offering higher validity.

The validity of a measurement indicates how well the tool captures the construct or concept it aims to measure. More specifically, it includes two key aspects: whether the tool actually measures the intended concept, and whether it does so accurately.

There are multiple ways to classify types of validity. One of the most commonly referenced frameworks is that presented in the guidelines published by the American Psychological Association, which outlines three main types: content validity, criterion-related validity (also called empirical validity), and construct validity (theoretical validity). In this context, construct validity refers to theoretical validity, while empirical validity is considered synonymous with criterion-related validity.

Different researchers have proposed various classifications. For instance, Kidder (1981) categorizes validity into face validity, concurrent validity, predictive validity, and construct validity.

Schuerman (1983) categorized validity into four types: criterion validity, which is based on the *empirical or practical aspects* of measurement, discriminant validity, which is grounded in *theoretical considerations*, and factorial validity.

Bailey (1982) suggests face validity, criterion validity, and construct validity, while Nachmias and Nachmias (1976) classify them into content validity, empirical validity, and construct validity. Campbell and Fiske (1959) refer to construct validity as consisting of discriminant validity and convergent validity.

Types of Validity

When measuring a particular concept, validity concerns both what exactly is being measured and whether the instrument truly captures that intended concept. While scholars have categorized types of validity in various ways, the most commonly accepted categories include content validity, predictive validity, concurrent validity, and construct validity.

K.-H. Yi, *Statistical Research Methods for Dermatologists and Plastic Surgeons*,
https://doi.org/10.1007/978-981-95-5668-7_5

Content Validity

How well does a measurement scale represent the concept it is intended to generalize? Does the scale comprehensively cover the construct it aims to measure? There is no purely objective method to determine whether all appropriate content is included in a measurement tool. One approach is to consult a panel of experts to review and evaluate the content of the scale or questionnaire. Because content validity is typically judged through logical and subjective analysis of the items, it is sometimes referred to as face validity. However, some researchers make a distinction between content validity and face validity.

For example, when developing a scale to assess the clinical competency of dermatologists specializing in aesthetic procedures, the items should be constructed based on the typical range of clinical activities performed by such professionals throughout a working day. If, instead of observing 10 dermatologists over the course of 8 full clinic hours each, the tool were developed by observing 100 dermatologists for only one hour at a fixed time of day, the scale would lack both logical and apparent validity. In such a case, a measurement tool with content validity issues would fail to discriminate between actual differences in dermatological competency among practitioners.

Another example: suppose a researcher defines "aesthetic treatment satisfaction" as a patient's perceived improvement in facial symmetry and skin smoothness. To evaluate this, a questionnaire is developed. However, if the questionnaire includes only items related to skin texture while omitting key aspects such as symmetry, pigmentation, or volume loss, the tool would lack content validity. A content-valid instrument should comprehensively reflect all components relevant to aesthetic satisfaction, as supported by theoretical and clinical frameworks.

Predictive Validity

To assess predictive validity, both the measurement result obtained from the assessment tool and the outcome from an external criterion are required. Predictive validity is then quantified by calculating the correlation coefficient between these two results, which is referred to as the validity coefficient. For example, a university would want to admit students who are likely to become high-achieving graduates in the future. The tools for selecting such students may include high school GPA or national standardized test scores, and the external criterion for "successful student" could be their academic performance after admission.

In other words, by calculating the correlation between admission scores and subsequent academic grades, one can evaluate how valid the admission scores are as a predictive tool. Thus, predictive validity requires the presence of an external criterion, a time interval between the initial test and outcome measurement, and allows for statistical quantification of validity.

For example, using a high-frequency ultrasound device, physicians can measure dermal thickness and density before a skin-tightening procedure. These values can then be used to predict whether a patient is likely to experience significant lifting effects or dermal remodeling after treatment with high-intensity focused ultrasound (HIFU).

Concurrent Validity

Concurrent validity refers to the extent to which a new measurement tool correlates with an already validated tool when both are applied at the same time. This method is particularly useful for evaluating whether a new test is more efficient, easier to use, or more practical than an established one. For instance, skin elasticity is often measured using a cutometer, which is considered a validated standard. If a newly developed portable elasticity probe demonstrates a high correlation (e.g., $r = 0.85$) with cutometer readings when used simultaneously, the new device can be said to possess high concurrent validity.

Another example would be a claim that changes in the real-time ultrasound imaging of dermal layers correlate with the firmness profile assessed by a cutometer. If both measurements reflect the same physiological condition at the same point in time, the ultrasound-based measurement may be said to exhibit concurrent validity. Since this method requires comparison with an external standard, both concurrent validity and predictive validity fall under the broader category of criterion-related validity. Draaijers et al. (2004) evaluated the concurrent validity of the Cutometer by comparing its measurements of scar elasticity with subjective assessments and found statistically significant correlations between the two approaches.

[1]Criterion-Related Validity:
Criterion-related validity refers to the degree of correlation between the values measured by the instrument in use and those obtained from a recognized standard or criterion instrument.

1. Concurrent Validity: A type of measurement validity in which a new test is administered alongside an established test within a similar timeframe, allowing researchers to examine the degree of correlation between the two assessments.
2. Predictive Validity: A form of measurement validity used to determine how well the results of one test can predict future performance or outcomes, based on a time-separated correlation between the test in question and a criterion measure obtained later.

Construct Validity

Concepts such as anxiety, creativity, dependency, authority, self-concept, attitude, intelligence, job satisfaction, achievement motivation, reasoning ability, spatial perception, reading comprehension, sociability, patience, pain, proprioception, muscle strength, and functional level cannot be measured directly like height or weight. Abstract concepts like anxiety are referred to as constructs—concepts that are theoretically constructed to explain human behavior. Construct validity refers to the extent to which a given measurement method accurately reflects such a construct. For example, suppose there exists a measurement tool, "A," that claims to measure anxiety. To evaluate the construct validity of tool A, the following steps are typically taken:

1. Operationally define what is meant by "anxiety"—that is, clearly specify the concept.
2. Formulate theoretical hypotheses regarding the specific behavioral characteristics of individuals who are presumed to have high versus low levels of anxiety.
3. Observe whether individuals who score high or low on the anxiety scale actually exhibit the predicted behavioral traits, based on the hypotheses.
4. If a strong relationship is found, then the measurement tool is considered to have construct validity. If not, the theoretical hypothesis may have been incorrect, or the method of data collection may have been flawed. In such cases, construct validity cannot be claimed.

A commonly used method for assessing construct validity is the group comparison method, where the instrument is applied to groups expected to differ on the construct based on known characteristics. For example, if a new instrument is developed to assess the aesthetic improvement of postoperative scars, and it is administered to two groups, patients who have undergone scar treatment and those who have not, it would be expected that the treated group would score higher in aesthetic outcomes. If, despite this theoretical expectation, the results show minimal difference between the two groups, the instrument would be considered to lack construct validity. Some researchers consider discriminant validity to be a component of or synonymous with construct validity.

Tan and Leoni (2015) conducted a study to determine whether the Patient's Self-Assessment Scale (PSA) for facial erythema in rosacea possesses construct validity in assessing the severity of facial redness. The researchers based their

[1]To ensure a measurement tool is properly applied, it is essential to verify its reliability, including whether it consistently produces the same results over time (stability) and whether all items within the instrument measure the same construct (internal consistency). However, even when standardized tools from other countries are used, researchers often rely solely on the reliability data reported at the time of the original tool's development. They may neglect to assess the reliability of the translated version in the context of their own research. This oversight can ultimately lead to significant problems regarding both the validity and reliability of the instrument.

investigation on the theoretical premise that patients' subjective perception of erythema should correlate with clinical evaluations made by trained dermatologists.

Accordingly, the PSA scale was administered to patients with persistent facial erythema, and their scores were compared with clinician-assessed erythema ratings at the same time point. A statistically significant correlation was found between the two sets of scores, indicating that patients with higher PSA scores were also rated as having more severe erythema by clinicians. The researchers concluded that the PSA scores and clinician assessments showed distinct distribution patterns between patients with mild and severe symptoms, thereby providing evidence that the PSA scale demonstrates construct validity in measuring the severity of facial erythema.

The more abstract a concept is, the more difficult it becomes to validate the construct validity of its corresponding measurement tool. While construct validity can be examined through various methods, the central focus is always on testing relationships that have been theoretically predicted and logically analyzed. Common methods used to assess construct validity include the group comparison method, the multitrait–multimethod matrix method, and factor analysis.

In the fields of cosmetic dermatology and plastic surgery, a common error when using measurement instruments is the use of tools whose validity and reliability have not been sufficiently verified. The instruments employed may not have been standardized within the local clinical context, or they may be tools originally developed overseas and used solely in translation without proper cultural or clinical adaptation. In some cases, researchers may develop their own tools locally, but only partial validation, such as content validity without construct validity, may have been performed. Others may extract and translate only certain items from established foreign instruments and use them in their own studies without full validation. When using such tools, it is essential to critically assess whether the instrument in fact measures what it claims to measure, and to evaluate its validity in the context of the specific study objectives and population.

Bibliography

Bailey KD. Methods of social research. 2nd ed. New York: Free Press; London: Collier Macmillan; 1982.

Campbell, D. T., & Fiske, D. W. (1959). Convergent and discriminant validation by the multitrait-multimethod matrix. *Psychological Bulletin*, 56, 81.

Chen, D.; Yin, S.; Lu, X.; Fu, H.; Gao, H.; Zhang, S. Research on the Correlation Between Skin Elasticity Evaluation Parameters and Age. *Cosmetics* 2024, *11*, 205.

Draaijers LJ, Botman YA, Tempelman FR, Kreis RW, Middelkoop E, van Zuijlen PP. Skin elasticity meter or subjective evaluation in scars: a reliability assessment. *Burns*. 2004;30(2):109–114.

Garg SP, Weissman JP, Chwa ES, Galiano RD. Content Validity of a Novel Scar Assessment Tool Evaluating the Career and Sexual Well-being Impact of Scars. Plast Reconstr Surg Glob Open. 2023 Jul 12;11(7):e5118.

Kidder LH. Selltiz, Wrightsman, and Cook's research methods in social relations. 4th ed. New York: Holt, Rinehart and Winston; 1981.

Nachmias D, Frankfort-Nachmias C. Research methods in the social sciences. New York: St. Martin's Press; 1976.

Schuerman JR. Research and evaluation in the human services. New York: Free Press; London: Collier Macmillan; 1983.

Tan J, Leoni M. Erythema of Rosacea: Validation of Patient's Self-Assessment Grading Scale. *J Drugs Dermatol*. 2015;14(8):841–844.

6 Reliability of Measurement

Reliability refers to the ability of a measurement instrument to consistently measure the same phenomenon across repeated applications (Portney and Watkins 2000). In general, when a researcher seeks to evaluate the similarity of obtained values, reliability is assessed by examining the level of agreement. Types of reliability include test–retest reliability, rater reliability, and internal consistency.

A decrease in reliability may be due to flaws in the measurement instrument itself, inaccuracies or inconsistencies in how the evaluator or examiner administers the test, or instability in the phenomenon being measured.

6.1 Test–Retest Reliability

In dermatology, commonly used measurement tools include the visual analog scale (VAS), elastometers, corneometers, Tewameter, and spectrophotometers or digital skin analyzers. These devices are typically used to take repeated measurements at defined intervals, and the similarity between initial and follow-up values is used to assess the tool's reliability. Specifically, a single measurement instrument is applied to the same subject more than once, and the correlation between the scores obtained at different time points is calculated. If the correlation is high, the instrument is considered to have high reliability. This form of reliability is often referred to as the coefficient of stability, as it reflects how consistently a tool yields similar results over time.

There are two main issues associated with test–retest reliability. First is the matter of determining the appropriate time interval between the two measurement sessions. If the interval is too short, reliability may be artificially inflated due to memory or practice effects. Conversely, if the interval is too long, the subject's characteristics may have changed in the meantime, resulting in decreased reliability. Thus, the appropriate time gap should be chosen based on the nature of the study. The second issue is the difficulty of maintaining consistency in the subject's internal motivation, attitude, and adherence to instructions between sessions. Although measurement assumes a standardized environment, attitude, and method, it is often difficult to ensure that the two measurements are conducted under identical conditions. Because of these challenges, test–retest reliability is not widely used except in cases where the influence of memory and practice effects is minimal.

Test–retest reliability refers to how consistently a single measurement tool can measure a given phenomenon over time, or in other words, its stability. It involves assessing whether a tool produces consistent results across two separate occasions, such as a test and retest, or before and after a treatment. If a measurement tool shows poor test–retest reliability, it becomes unclear whether changes in the measured value are due to

K.-H. Yi, *Statistical Research Methods for Dermatologists and Plastic Surgeons*,
https://doi.org/10.1007/978-981-95-5668-7_6

an actual change in the patient's condition or due to instability in the measurement instrument itself.

For example, consider a case in cosmetic dermatology where the severity of post-treatment erythema is measured using a visual analog scale (VAS). If the erythema scores of 10 patients recorded immediately after a laser treatment were 5, 4, 5, 5, 3, 4, 3, 3, 2, 1, and the scores measured one week later were 5, 4, 3, 3, 2, 4, 3, 2, 2, 1, the degree of agreement between the two sets of measurements would reflect the test–retest reliability of the VAS in this context [4].

6.2 Equivalent-Form Reliability

Equivalent-form reliability refers to a method of reliability assessment in which two tests, designed to be equivalent in content and difficulty but different in form, are administered to the same group of individuals. The correlation between the scores obtained from the two forms is then calculated to yield a reliability coefficient. This is also referred to as the coefficient of equivalence.

For example, when administering a standardized college entrance exam, two versions of the test (e.g., Form A and Form B) that are matched in difficulty may be created. The same group of students takes both versions, and the correlation between their scores is calculated. This correlation reflects how consistently the two test forms measure the same construct. Because the goal is to determine how similarly the two tests assess the same characteristic, the resulting coefficient is termed a coefficient of equivalence or parallel-forms reliability coefficient. For this method to be valid, the two test forms should have an equal number of items and be of similar difficulty. However, one major limitation is the difficulty of constructing two sets of test items that are truly equivalent in difficulty and content coverage.

Whereas test–retest reliability involves administering the same test twice to the same sample at different times, equivalent-form reliability involves administering two different but equivalent tests to the same group at the same time and computing the correlation between the scores.

6.3 Rater Reliability

Rater reliability refers to the degree to which evaluators produce consistent results when using a measurement tool.

Intrarater Reliability (Also Known as Intratester or Intraobserver Reliability)

For example, a cosmetic dermatologist evaluates the severity of nasolabial folds in standardized patient photographs using a validated wrinkle severity grading scale. The same dermatologist rates the images again after one week. The degree of agreement between the first and second ratings represents the intrarater reliability of the evaluator. Because the photographs remain unchanged between sessions, this method allows the rater's internal consistency to be assessed independently of changes in the patient's actual condition.

However, such controlled situations—where the subject's condition remains completely stable between assessments—are rare in clinical settings. Suppose a dermatologist evaluates post-procedure skin redness using a clinical erythema scale across five consecutive measurements. Even if the evaluator applies the same scale consistently, slight variations can arise each time due to differences in lighting, angle, or the evaluator's interpretation of subtle redness. These represent potential sources of intrarater error. Moreover, from the patient's side, the skin condition itself may change between measurements. For instance, mild inflammation might subside slightly by the fifth measurement, leading to improved scores unrelated to the evaluator's consistency. Since observed scores reflect both evaluator-related error and actual variation in the skin condition, it can be difficult to distinguish the exact source of variability.

Interrater Reliability (Also Known as Intertester or Interobserver Reliability)

Interrater reliability refers to the degree to which two or more evaluators assign consistent values when assessing the same subject or patient. For example, in a skin quality assessment setting, two dermatologists might simultaneously evaluate the degree of erythema or wrinkle severity in a patient using a standardized clinical scale. Interrater reliability is concerned with how closely their scoring aligns when observing the same condition under the same circumstances.

This form of reliability is particularly important when multiple evaluators are involved in a research study. If their agreement is poor, the variability in collected scores may not reflect true changes in the patient's skin condition or treatment effects, but rather inconsistency caused by insufficient rater training. Therefore, to ensure measurement accuracy, all evaluators should be properly trained and calibrated in advance to achieve a minimum level of agreement.

One simple method to calculate interrater reliability is to use the percentage agreement formula when the measured variable is binary (e.g., yes/no, normal/abnormal). The formula is:

$$\frac{\text{Number of agreements}}{\text{Number of agreements} + \text{Number of disagreements}} \times 100$$

This method is easy to compute, but it tends to overestimate reliability. For instance, if two observers randomly assign "yes" or "no" labels to skin improvement following a treatment, they may agree on approximately 50% of cases purely by chance. An example of how to calculate percent agreement can be found in studies evaluating irritant skin responses. In such studies, two dermatologists may assess the onset time of erythema following the application of a topical irritant. Suppose that, out of 100 observed cases of skin responses, both Rater A and Rater B agreed on the onset of erythema in 50 cases and disagreed in the remaining 50 cases. The percent agreement would be calculated as: 50/(50 + 50) × 100 = 50%. In addition to percent agreement, other methods to evaluate interrater reliability include Cohen's Kappa, analysis of variance (ANOVA), intraclass correlation coefficient (ICC), and rank-order correlation.

6.4 Internal Consistency

Internal consistency refers to the extent to which the items in a questionnaire consistently measure the same underlying construct. This type of reliability is commonly assessed in studies using survey-based instruments. Two common methods used to evaluate internal consistency are the split-half method and test item reliability.

Split-Half Method

The split-half method is used to determine whether the items in a questionnaire consistently assess a particular construct. For instance, the items can be divided into even-numbered and odd-numbered items, and then the correlation coefficient between the scores of the even-numbered items and the scores of the odd-numbered items can be calculated to determine whether the respondents are answering consistently.

Item Reliability

This refers to comparing the reliability of individual items within a questionnaire by evaluating how each item relates to the other items in the same assessment tool. For a high internal consistency reliability coefficient, the items must be highly interrelated. High inter-item correlation is more likely when a test is designed to measure a single trait or ability—that is, when the test is homogeneous in nature. Therefore, if each item is of similar difficulty and aligned with the same construct, higher reliability is achievable. Internal consistency tends to be higher in homogeneous tests or power tests (where there is no time constraint) and lower or distorted in heterogeneous or speeded tests (which impose time limits). A commonly used measure of internal consistency is Cronbach's alpha (α). For example, one may evaluate the internal consistency of items in a questionnaire assessing post-procedure patient satisfaction in cosmetic dermatology.

Statistical software such as SPSS provides item-total correlations and the overall Cronbach's alpha if an item is deleted, allowing for a practical assessment of internal consistency. When the scale is composed of dichotomous items (e.g., yes/no, true/false), the Kuder–Richardson Formula 20 (KR-20) is used. KR-20 was developed by Kuder and Richardson and is named after their initials.

Example
"I often feel stressed as a caregiver."
A "yes" response is scored as 1, and a "no" response is scored as 0.

KR-20 is essentially Cronbach's alpha adapted for binary (dichotomous) data, and its interpretation is the same. In SPSS, selecting Analyze → Scale → Reliability Analysis → Alpha allows for the calculation of KR-20 when using binary data. When using a questionnaire as a measurement tool, it is recommended to include a mix of positively and negatively worded items. During reliability analysis, negatively worded items should be reverse-coded so that all items are scored in the same direction.

6.5 Intra-Subject Reliability

Another important aspect to consider in relation to reliability is intrasubject reliability. This refers to situations in which the characteristic being measured varies significantly within the same individual over time. For example, when measuring transepidermal water loss (TEWL) in a patient with a compromised skin barrier, TEWL values may fluctuate considerably depending on posture, room temperature, emotional stress, or even slight changes in skin surface condition. Therefore, it would be inappropriate to assume that a single TEWL measurement accurately reflects the patient's overall skin barrier status. Unless the evaluator has access to a highly reliable measurement instrument and is an experienced rater under ideal conditions, it is virtually impossible to isolate subject variability from measurement or rater error. Accordingly, when calculating test–retest reliability, the resulting reliability estimate generally reflects a mixture of instrument error, tester error, and intrasubject variability.

6.6 Measurement Error

Measurement error is an essential factor to consider when discussing the reliability of a measurement. There are two main types of measurement error: random error and nonrandom error. Random error, also referred to as nonsystematic error, occurs unpredictably and unavoidably, even when efforts are made to measure as precisely as possible. Nonrandom error, also known as systematic error or sometimes referred to as bias, occurs when measurement values consistently deviate in one direction. For example, if a skin elasticity measuring device consistently underestimates values by 5% compared to the gold standard, this device would be said to have systematic bias. Suppose the actual elasticity values are 10 units, 20 units, and 30 units, but the device records them as 9.5, 19.0, and 28.5, respectively—this indicates a consistent underestimation.

Another example would be the measurement of facial swelling using a three-dimensional skin imaging system. Suppose a clinician uses a miscalibrated imaging device to quantify changes in facial volume before and after a cosmetic procedure. If the system's software has a scaling error that enlarges all measurements by a small fixed percentage, then the recorded volume for every subject will be consistently overestimated. In this case, although the same measurement tool is used consistently, all values would be shifted in the same direction. This type of error, which arises from incorrectly marked calibration or consistently misread scales, is referred to as nonrandom error or systematic error.

6.7 Standard Error of Measurement (SEM)

The standard error of measurement refers to the degree of error that occurs when estimating a true score based on an observed measurement. For example, let's say a patient undergoes 25 repeated assessments of wrinkle depth using a 3D imaging system, and the average wrinkle depth is 0.34 mm with a standard deviation of 0.05 mm. In this case, the standard deviation of 0.05 mm represents the standard error of measurement (SEM). To calculate the confidence interval in which the true score of this patient's wrinkle depth is likely to lie at a 95% confidence level, the formula would be: 0.34 ± 1.96 × 0.05 (0.242 mm to 0.438 mm).

In cases where measurements are collected from multiple participants, particularly when using a reliability coefficient, the SEM can be calculated using the following formula:

$$\text{SEM} = S_X\sqrt{1 - r_{XX}}$$

Here, S_X is the standard deviation of the observed scores, and r_{XX} is the test–retest reliability coefficient of the measurement method. For instance, if wrinkle depth is measured once per person in a sample of 300 patients and the standard deviation is 0.08 mm with a test–retest reliability of $r_{XX} = 0.85$, then:

$$\text{SEM} = 0.08\sqrt{1 - 0.85} = 0.031(\text{mm}).$$

If the mean wrinkle depth across the sample is 0.30 mm, the 95% confidence interval for the population mean is calculated as: 0.30 ± 1.96 × 0.031 = 0.239 mm to 0.361 mm. Similarly, at a 99% confidence level using $z = 2.58$, the confidence interval would be: 0.30 ± 2.58 × 0.031 = 0.220 mm to 0.380 mm.

6.8 Relationship Between Reliability and Validity

The relationship between reliability and validity can be illustrated as shown in Fig. 6.1. As demonstrated in the figure, Panel A represents a set of scores that are relatively reliable but lack validity, indicating the presence of systematic error. Panel B illustrates a situation in which neither reliability nor validity is sufficient, suggesting the presence of random error. Panel C shows a noticeable improvement in reliability compared to Panel B, but reliability still remains relatively low. However, the level of validity appears to be somewhat acceptable. Panel D depicts high levels of both reliability and validity in the measurements.

As these illustrations suggest, improving reliability is a necessary condition for improving validity, but not a sufficient one. In other words, a measurement tool may be highly reliable yet lack validity; however, it is not possible for a tool to be valid if it lacks reliability.

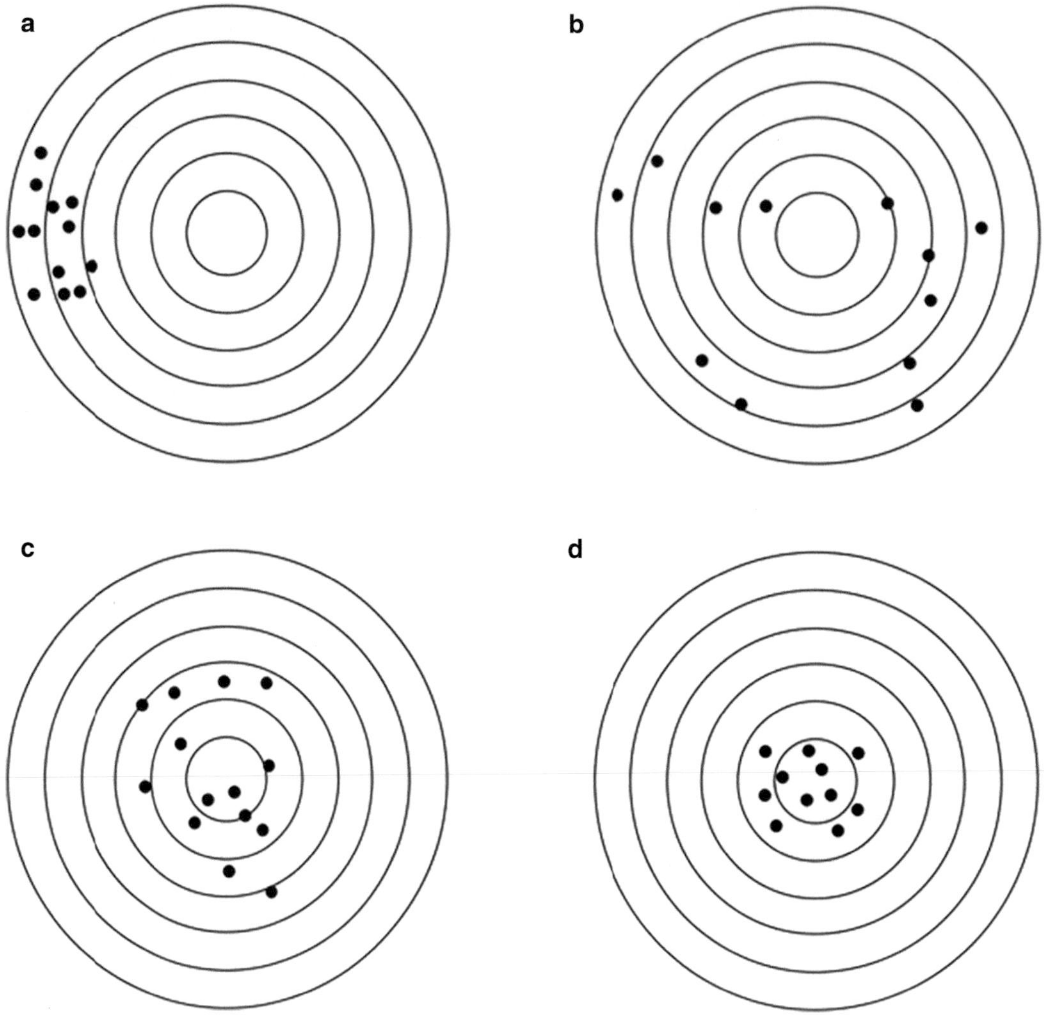

Fig. 6.1 The relationship between reliability and validity

References

1. Aarts P, van Huijstee JC, Ragamin A, et al. *Validity and Reliability of Two Digital Wound Measurement Tools After Surgery in Patients with Hidradenitis Suppurativa.* Dermatology. 2023;239(1):99–108.
2. Cohen JL, Sadick NS, Kirby MT, McLane MP, Lenderking WR, Bender RH, Chen J, Hurley D, Knoble NB, Liu G, Xiang Q, Davidson JA, Goldman MP. *Development and Validation Clinician and Patient Reported Photonumeric Scales to Assess Buttocks Cellulite Severity.* Dermatol Surg. 2020 46(12):1628–1635.
3. Fujimoto Y, Yuri Y, Kato Y, Kinoshita S, Tamiya H. *Intra- and inter-rater reliabilities of skin mechanical properties measured in healthy individuals using skin elasticity meter.* Ann Med. 2023;55(2):2279747.

4. Gallo L, Rae C, Kim PJ, Voineskos SH, Thoma A, Pusic AL, Klassen AF, Cano SJ. *Establishing test-retest reliability and the smallest detectable change of FACE-Q Aesthetic Module scales.* J Plast Reconstr Aesthet Surg. 2024 95:231–238.
5. Huimin K, Rowledge AM, Borzdynski CJ, Miller C, Frescos N, McKenzie G, Perry E, McGuiness W. *Reliability of a Skin Diagnostic Device in Assessing Hydration and Erythema.* Adv Skin Wound Care. 2017 Oct 30(10):452–459.
6. Peperkamp K, Verhulst AC, Tielemans HJP, Winters H, van Dalen D, Ulrich DJO. *The inter-rater and test-retest reliability of skin thickness and skin elasticity measurements by the DermaLab Combo in healthy participants.* Skin Res Technol. 2019;25(6):787–792.
7. Robey C, McCammon K, Perry M, Zagade T, Brugh V, Liu J. *Inter-rater reliability of retrograde urethrograms.* World J Urol. 2023;41(4):1163–1167.
8. Su X, Dong R, Wen Z, Liu Y. *Reliability and Validity of Scoliosis Measurements Obtained with Surface Topography Techniques: A Systematic Review.* J Clin Med. 2022;11(23):6998.
9. Swanson E. *Validity, reliability, and the questionable role of psychometrics in plastic surgery.* Plast Reconstr Surg Glob Open. 2014 2(6):e161.
10. Tian WM, Porras Fimbres DC, Tran MM, Zeng SL, Gnaedinger AG, Kaplan S, Marcus JR, Patel A. *Quality and Reliability of 2D and 3D Clinical Photographs in Plastic Surgery: A Scoping Review.* Aesthetic Plast Surg. 2025 Feb 27.
11. Z Paul Lorenc, Derek Jones, Jeongyun Kim, Hee Min Gwak, Samixa Batham, Ginny Vachon. *Validating a Series of Photonumeric Rating Scales for Use in Facial Aesthetics Using Statistical Analysis of Intra- and Inter-rater Reliability* Aesthetic Surgery Journal Open Forum 2021;3(4).

7 Statistical Analysis and Experimental Design

Statistical analysis plays a crucial role in experimental design. Two main types of statistical methods commonly used for analyzing experimental data are descriptive statistics and inferential statistics. Descriptive statistics are used to describe, organize, and summarize data. This includes measures of central tendency (such as the mean and median) and measures of relative position and variability (such as range, standard deviation, and coefficient of variation). In descriptive statistics, data from all participants in the sample are expressed numerically—for example, by presenting the mean and standard deviation.

Inferential statistics, on the other hand, allow researchers to make conclusions or inferences from sample data and generalize them to the population. Common statistics used in experimental research include t, F, and r. For instance, suppose a researcher is interested in whether the observed difference in means between an experimental group and a control group also exists in the population from which these samples were drawn. In such cases, a t-test is used to draw conclusions. It is generally recommended to present both descriptive and inferential statistics in a research report.

Inferential statistics can be classified into parametric and nonparametric tests. Parametric tests require strict mathematical assumptions to be met, while nonparametric tests do not. The appropriate statistical method should be chosen based on the experimental design and the characteristics of the collected data. A statistical method aligned with the experimental design should be specified from the research planning stage. Statistical analysis is a critical part of research—an inappropriate statistical approach can lead to misunderstanding. If a researcher lacks sufficient understanding of statistics, it is advisable to consult a statistician regarding experimental design and data analysis.

Inferential statistics and significance testing play an important role in experimental design. The purpose of conducting a significance test is to evaluate hypotheses. Table 7.1 summarizes examples of statistical methods used for significance testing and their corresponding purposes. For more detailed statistical methods, refer to Chap. 15 of this book.

K.-H. Yi, *Statistical Research Methods for Dermatologists and Plastic Surgeons*,
https://doi.org/10.1007/978-981-95-5668-7_7

Table 7.1 Inferential statistics for significance testing

Statistical method	Purpose
Parametric tests	
t-test	To determine whether the means of two groups differ significantly
Analysis of variance (ANOVA)	To determine whether the means of three or more groups differ significantly, or to examine interactions among factors
Post-hoc tests	To identify which specific groups differ when the F-value from ANOVA is significant
Nonparametric tests	
Chi-square test	To determine whether two frequency distributions differ significantly
Mann–Whitney U test	To determine whether the medians of two groups differ significantly
Kruskal–Wallis test	To determine whether the medians of three or more groups differ significantly

7.1 Study Designs for Experimental Research

Accurate study design is critical, as poorly structured research can lead to misinterpretation of results. Even when a large amount of data has been collected, significant issues may arise if the study design is flawed. Therefore, the purpose of the research must be clearly defined from the outset. There are many different types of study designs used in research. The most appropriate design for a given study should be selected based on the research objective, available resources, and ethical considerations.

7.2 Experimental Studies and Observational Studies

In experimental studies, the researcher actively intervenes in a way that may influence the outcomes. A common form of experimental research is clinical research, which involves therapeutic interventions introduced by the investigator. Other examples include animal studies and laboratory-based research conducted under controlled conditions. Experimental research is considered to provide the strongest evidence for testing research hypotheses, as it allows for control over variables that could influence the results. However, such studies are not always feasible, particularly when involving humans or animals, due to ethical concerns.

Observational studies are commonly used in epidemiology. For example, in a cohort study (a cohort refers to a specific population group, the development of a particular disease is prospectively followed over time, and the incidence of the disease is compared between a group exposed to a certain factor and a group not exposed), case–control studies are another example, in which the researcher does not take any action that could affect the outcomes but simply observes the results. Unlike interventional studies, researchers in observational studies do not assign participants to exposure or control conditions. Because observational studies cannot fully control for all confounding variables, the evidence they provide may be less robust than that of experimental studies. Nevertheless, in certain contexts, observational research may be the only appropriate or feasible method to achieve a study's objective.

7.3 Cross-Sectional or Longitudinal Studies

A study conducted at a specific point in time is referred to as a cross-sectional study. Examples include surveys and population censuses. Because it is not possible to determine when a disease occurred prior to the study, one can only describe an association between cause and effect, but not establish a causal relationship. Moreover, cross-sectional studies cannot investigate disease incidence, that is, the number of new cases over a given period, nor can they evaluate trends that develop over time. The advantage of cross-sectional studies is that they can generally be conducted in a short period of time and at a relatively low cost, and they are useful for generating research hypotheses.

For example, let us assume a study was conducted in which women were surveyed regarding their current facial wrinkle severity, and then their dietary habits were recorded. Participants who consumed diets rich in fruits and vegetables tended to show fewer facial wrinkles, whereas those with diets high in red meat and snacks had more pronounced wrinkles. Even if a statistically significant difference in wrinkle severity was found between these groups, it would be difficult to determine causality in a cross-sectional study. This is because it remains unclear whether the dietary habits caused the difference in wrinkle formation, or whether individuals with fewer wrinkles were simply more inclined to follow healthier diets. A cross-sectional study design cannot establish temporal precedence, and therefore can only suggest possible hypotheses—not confirm cause-and-effect relationships.

Another example is a study by Shinji Iizaka (2017). Researchers measured the stratum corneum hydration levels of community—dwelling older adults over the age of 65 and examined their relationship with lifestyle—related factors. Suppose that individuals who used moisturizers daily and engaged in regular physical activity showed higher hydration levels compared to those who did not. Even if the two groups exhibited significant differences in skin hydration, it is difficult to establish a causal relationship. That is, it is unclear whether the higher hydration levels were due to the use of moisturizers and exercise, or if individuals with naturally better skin conditions were more likely to maintain such habits. A cross-sectional study does not allow for definitive conclusions about cause and effect; however, it is still valuable in generating hypotheses for future research.

A longitudinal study involves tracking a sample of subjects over a specific period of time. There are two main types of longitudinal studies: prospective and retrospective studies. A prospective study follows participants forward in time from a specific starting point to observe outcomes as they occur. In contrast, a retrospective study begins with groups that have already been classified based on outcomes, and then looks backward to investigate potential contributing factors from the past. Longitudinal studies generally require more time and resources to conduct compared to cross-sectional studies. Additionally, if the study relies on participants' memory or previously recorded medical charts, the data may be subject to bias due to potential inaccuracies or inconsistencies in recall or documentation.

7.4 Bias

Bias is said to occur when there is a systematic error between the research results and the actual circumstances. The major types of bias are as follows:

1. Observer bias: This occurs when an observer consistently overestimates or underestimates the value of a particular variable.
2. Confounding bias: This arises when factors that are associated with both the risk factor and the outcome are not properly controlled, leading to a spurious statistical association.
3. Selection bias: This occurs when individuals included in a study are not representative of the target population, resulting in incorrect generalization of the findings.
4. Information bias: In epidemiology, this refers to errors arising from the incorrect classification of exposure to an etiological agent or misclassification of the variables or outcomes being assessed. In psychology, it refers to cognitive bias, where information is misjudged or interpreted inaccurately due to the evaluator's cognitive tendencies.
5. Publication bias: This occurs when studies with statistically significant or positive findings are more likely to be published, while studies with negative or inconclusive results remain unpublished, thereby skewing the available evidence.

Bias may also arise from other sources such as recall, assessment, or allocation errors, which can distort the validity of research findings.

7.5 Variation

The variation observed in collected data can be divided into two categories: factors that can be explained, such as measurement error, and random factors that reflect unexplained differences between individuals. When a variable exhibits substantial variation during measurement, the accuracy of parameter estimation decreases, and the standard error increases. Therefore, minimizing variation and improving the accuracy of estimation are essential. The following approaches are commonly used to achieve this:

Replication

Replication enhances the precision of estimates. In actual research, individual variables are often measured two or three times under each condition. However, if repeated measurements are not independent, careful consideration must be given when applying statistical methods to analyze such data. A common approach is to use the mean of multiple measurements instead of relying on a single value. In some cases, statistical methods specifically designed for repeated measures must be applied.

Sample Size

Choosing an appropriate sample size is critical in research design. As the sample size increases, the standard error of the estimate decreases, which in turn improves accuracy and increases the statistical power[1] of the study. Ideally, the required sample size should be calculated prior to conducting the study.

Specialized Experimental Designs

Modifying a basic experimental design can lead to more accurate estimations, especially when comparing the effects of one or more treatments applied to experimental subjects. Experimental subjects represent the smallest independent units for analysis (e.g., patients, blood samples, skin patches). When experimental subjects are randomly assigned to treatment groups and no additional design features are included, the study is referred to as a completely randomized design. This type of design is easy to analyze but may be inefficient if there is substantial variability among the study subjects. In such cases, techniques like blocking or crossover designs are used to reduce the impact of variability.

[1] Statistical power ($1—\beta$): the probability of correctly rejecting the null hypothesis when it is false.

Blocking

Blocking refers to the process of grouping similar experimental materials or creating experimental environments that are as uniform as possible. These homogeneous groups or conditions are called blocks. A general principle in blocking is to minimize variability within blocks and maximize variability between blocks.

It is possible to organize experimental subjects who share similar characteristics into homogeneous blocks or strata (e.g., blocking by age group). The variability among individuals within a block will then be less than the variability among individuals across different blocks. Subjects within each block are randomly assigned to treatments, and treatment effects are compared within blocks rather than across the entire population. This approach allows for more precise estimation of treatment effects compared to when blocking is not used.

7.6 One-Group Pretest–Posttest Design

When the conditions of controlling extraneous variables, randomization of samples, and manipulation of treatments are all satisfied, the study is considered a true experimental design. A quasi-experimental design is defined as one where any of these conditions is not met.

In a one-group pretest–posttest design, a single group is studied. The sequence consists of a pretest (O_1), followed by the treatment (X), and then a posttest (O_2). In this notation, "O" represents an observation or measurement, and "X" represents the treatment or intervention. To evaluate the treatment effect, the posttest score (O_2) is compared with the pretest score (O_1). A major limitation of this design is the absence of a control group, which introduces threats to internal validity such as history, maturation, and testing effects. Therefore, it can be difficult to determine whether observed changes are due to the treatment or the interaction of these confounding variables.

This type of design is considered meaningful in cases where the treatment effect is already well established in previous studies, making the inclusion of a control group unnecessary. For example, suppose a study is conducted to determine whether a cryotherapy gel or a cryo roller produces greater skin cooling effects. Since both modalities are already widely known to have skin cooling efficacy, based on previous studies, a control group may not be necessary. When using this design, statistical analysis methods such as the paired t-test can be used if parametric test conditions are satisfied. If the data do not meet parametric assumptions, the Wilcoxon matched-pairs signed-rank test is an appropriate nonparametric alternative.

$$O_1 \quad X \quad O_2$$

7.7 Pretest–Posttest Control Group Design

This design is an extension of the previously discussed one-group pretest–posttest design, with the addition of a control group. Participants are preselected and then randomly assigned to one of two groups. The experimental group undergoes a pretest, receives the treatment or intervention (X), and then takes a posttest. The control group also receives a pretest and posttest but does not receive the treatment. That is, both groups follow the same procedures except that the control group does not receive the intervention.

This is the most commonly used and traditional experimental design, and its use of a control group enhances its validity. In this design, the researcher expects conditions such as: $O_1 = O_3$, $O_3 = O_4$, $O_2 > O_1$ or $O_2 < O_1$, and $O_2 > O_4$. Although the groups are randomized, a pretest is conducted to confirm that the two groups are equivalent at baseline. If the correlation between the pretest and posttest in the control group is close to 1, it suggests that the impact of extraneous variables such as history, maturation, testing, instrumentation, or regression to the mean is minimal. Errors due to selection bias are assumed to be addressed through the randomization process. However, if participants drop out of the study, equivalence between groups may be compromised, which this design does not address.

$$\begin{array}{cccc} R & O_1 & X & O_2 \\ R & O_3 & & O_4 \end{array}$$

This design can be slightly modified by incorporating matching. For example, participants may be matched based on characteristics such as blood pressure, age, or body weight, with one member of each matched pair assigned to the experimental group and the other to the control group. This variant is referred to as a pretest–posttest control group design with matching.

7.8 Two-Group Pretest–Posttest Design

In this design, two experimental groups are used, and both are subjected to randomization. This design is often employed in clinical settings for two main reasons: first, when it is difficult to establish a true control group, and second, when withholding treatment from a group raises ethical concerns.

In such cases, one group receives a new or experimental treatment, while the other group receives a traditional or standard treatment. The purpose is to compare the effectiveness of the two interventions.

$$\begin{array}{cccc} R & O_1 & X_1 & O_2 \\ R & O_3 & X_2 & O_4 \end{array}$$

7.9 Solomon Four-Group Design

The Solomon Four-Group Design was introduced by R. L. Solomon in 1949. Among the experimental designs discussed so far, this is considered the most robust. Although it is more complex, it offers the highest level of internal validity. In this design, participants are randomly assigned to four groups: two experimental groups and two control groups. The first group receives a pretest, treatment, and a posttest. The second group receives both pretest and posttest, but no treatment. The third group receives treatment and a posttest, without a pretest. The fourth group only receives a posttest. This can be illustrated as follows:

$$\begin{array}{cccc} R & O_1 & X & O_2 \\ R & O_3 & & O_4 \\ R & & X & O_5 \\ R & & & O_6 \end{array}$$

This design allows the researcher not only to compare differences between experimental and control groups after the intervention, but also to examine the interaction between the pretest and the treatment. Specifically, the effects of the pretest and its interaction with the treatment can be assessed by comparing O_2 and O_5 (Group 1 vs. Group 3), and by comparing O_4 and O_6 (Group 2 vs. Group 4). The underlying assumptions of this design are as follows:

$$O_1 = O_3, O_4 = O_6, O_2 = O_5$$
$$O_2 > O_1, O_2 > O_4, O_2 > O_6$$
$$O_5 > O_1, O_5 > O_4, O_5 > O_6$$

The primary advantage of this design is its ability to control for pre-experimental influences such as history and maturation. However, its main disadvantage lies in its limited practicality due to the difficulty of simultaneously managing four groups within a single study. Particularly, it requires twice as many participants compared to other designs and demands significantly more time and resources to execute. The appropriate method of statistical analysis for this design is a 2 × 2 factorial analysis of variance (Table 7.2).

Table 7.2 2 × 2 factorial design table

		Pretest	
		Present	Absent
Treatment	*Present*	Experimental group 1	Experimental group 2
	Absent	Control group 1	Control group 2

7.10 Nonequivalent Control Group Design

This is a type of quasi-experimental design that closely resembles the pretest–posttest control group design, but with a fundamental difference: the lack of equivalence between the groups. Therefore, issues related to the selection of participants pose a significant threat to internal validity. However, this issue can be addressed to some extent through statistical methods. For example, conducting an analysis of covariance (ANCOVA) allows researchers to compute adjusted means, and a subsequent test for differences can help determine the effect of the intervention even when the groups are not equivalent.

$$\frac{O \quad X \quad O}{O \qquad\quad O} \leftarrow \text{Randomization}\,\textit{not}\,\text{applied}$$

7.11 Factorial Design

The experimental designs discussed thus far have assumed only one independent variable. However, in practice, researchers often wish to examine the effects of two or more independent variables within a single study. A factorial design is a powerful approach used to investigate both the main effects of each independent variable on the dependent variable, as well as their interaction effects. When a study includes multiple independent variables, investigating each variable separately through individual experiments is inefficient and costly. A factorial design enables simultaneous analysis of multiple variables, which greatly enhances the practicality and richness of experimental results.

The simplest factorial design is a 2 × 2 design, where two independent variables (e.g., two types of treatment) are each studied at two levels. This design is particularly useful when the goal is to examine how more than one independent variable influences a single dependent variable in a single experiment. Consider the following example: research has indicated that individuals' acceptance of cosmetic surgery can be influenced by their partner's perceived attractiveness and the nature of comments received about their appearance. In a study employing a 2 × 2 factorial design, participants were exposed to scenarios varying in partner attractiveness (high vs. low) and partner commentary (positive vs. negative).

The findings revealed that women with highly attractive partners who received negative comments about their appearance exhibited a higher acceptance of cosmetic surgery for social reasons. This interaction effect suggests that the combination of partner attractiveness and negative feedback can significantly impact one's body image and openness to cosmetic procedures.

Factorial designs can accommodate more than two independent variables, and each variable can be studied at more than two levels. The most basic form of factorial design is one in which two independent variables are each studied at two levels, known as a 2 × 2 design. In the example below, "treatment frequency" and "treatment duration" are the two independent variables (factors), and "0.5 MHz vs. 2 MHz" and "5 seconds vs. 20 seconds" represent the levels of each factor. A total of 40 participants were randomly assigned into four groups and received radiofrequency treatment accordingly. The results are summarized in Table 7.3.

In the above example, the research question is, first, does treatment frequency (X_1) affect wrinkle depth reduction (Y)? The answer would be yes, as the wrinkle reduction for the 0.5 MHz group was 11.5%, while for the 2 MHz group it was 18.0%. This suggests that the 2 MHz frequency was more effective, and this is referred to as the main effect of treatment frequency.

The second research question is whether treatment duration (X_2) affects wrinkle reduction. The answer would be that there is little to no effect, since the improvement was 14.0% in the 5-second treatment group and 15.5% in the 20-second group—an insignificant difference.

The third research question is whether treatment frequency and treatment duration interact to affect wrinkle reduction. This is referred to as an interaction effect. If there were a significant interaction, the effect of frequency would vary greatly depending on the duration. However, in this case, there is no meaningful interaction, as both frequencies yielded consistently better outcomes regardless of the duration. The frequency had a notable impact on wrinkle reduction regardless of treatment time.

Table 7.4 presents a hypothetical dataset in which an interaction effect is assumed to exist.

In this case, when observing the wrinkle reduction effect across all groups, the treatment at 2 MHz appears more effective overall than at 0.5 MHz, showing a greater average reduction (15.5% vs. 12.5%). However, when treatment duration is considered, the effect varies: with 5-second treatments, the higher frequency (2 MHz) yields greater improvement (19.0% vs. 9.0%), but with 20-second treatments, the lower frequency (0.5 MHz) results in greater improvement (16.0% vs. 12.0%). This illustrates an interaction effect, in which the effect of one

Table 7.3 Results by treatment duration and treatment frequency

	Treatment frequency				
Treatment duration		0.5 MHz	2 MHz	Mean	Difference
	5 sec	11.0(%)	17.0(%)	14.0(%)	+6.0(%)
	20 sec	12.0(%)	19.0(%)	15.5(%)	+7.0(%)
	Mean	11.5(%)	18.0(%)	14.75(%) (overall mean)	
	Difference	+1.0(%)	+2.0(%)		

Table 7.4 Interaction of treatment duration and treatment frequency

	Treatment frequency				
Treatment duration		0.5 MHz	2 MHz	Mean	Difference
	5 sec	9.0(%)	19.0(%)	14.0(%)	+10.0(%)
	20 sec	16.0(%)	12.0(%)	14.0(%)	−4.0(%)
	Mean	12.5(%)	15.5(%)	14.0(%) (overall mean)	
	Difference	+7.0(%)	−7.0(%)		

independent variable (frequency) depends on the level of another variable (treatment duration).

If another factor, such as gender (male, female), were added to the above design alongside treatment frequency and duration, the result would be a 2 × 2 × 2 factorial design. This would allow for the examination of the main effects of treatment frequency, treatment duration, and gender, as well as the interaction effects between treatment frequency × treatment duration, treatment frequency × gender, treatment duration × gender, and the three-way interaction treatment frequency × treatment duration × gender. The advantage of using a factorial design is that it allows researchers to simultaneously investigate the individual effects of two or more independent variables, as well as their interaction effects.

7.12 Crossover Design

In this type of design, all participants are rotated through every intervention. It is also referred to as a rotation design, counter-balanced design, or switch-over design.

In conventional research designs, comparisons are typically made between individuals belonging to different groups. For example, most clinical studies are between-subject (group comparison) studies, in which each participant receives one or two contrasting treatments. However, within-subject comparisons may be more efficient in certain circumstances, as they tend to involve less measurement variability than comparisons between different individuals. In such cases, each participant can serve as their own control. Within-subject (repeated measures) comparisons allow for more precise estimation of treatment effects and often require a smaller sample size to achieve the same level of statistical precision as between-subject comparisons.

An example of a research design that allows for within-subject comparisons in clinical research is the crossover design. A crossover design involves applying multiple treatments to the same individuals at different time points in a randomized order. When two different treatment methods are administered to the same participant, the sequence of administration is randomized to eliminate potential time-related effects. To prevent carry-over effects from the first treatment influencing the results of the second, a washout period is introduced between treatment phases. This period allows any lingering effects of the first treatment to dissipate. Ultimately, both treatments are administered to each individual, and differences in response are analyzed within the same person.

	1*st* Period	2*nd* Period	
Group A	X_1O		X_2O
Group B	X_2O		X_1O

This experimental design includes two treatment conditions, X1 and X2, both of which are applied to both groups. As such, this design involves three key factors: group, time, and treatment condition. The effects of each treatment can be compared as follows:

$$\text{Effect of X1}: \text{Group A at time point 1} + \text{Group B at time point 2}$$
$$\text{Effect of X2}: \text{Group A at time point 2} + \text{Group B at time point 1}$$

For example, consider a study involving 45 adult participants conducted to evaluate the impact of onabotulinumtoxinA (Botox) treatment on mood and self-perceived appearance. Initially, 30 participants were randomly assigned to the treatment group and received onabotulinumtoxinA injections in the upper facial region, while the remaining 15 participants were placed in the placebo group and received saline injections. After one month, the groups crossed over: those who had received placebo now received the active treatment, and vice versa. Outcome variables such as mood, satisfaction with appearance, and overall quality of life were assessed using standardized self-report questionnaires at each stage. This crossover design allowed the researchers to compare the effects of onabotulinumtoxinA treatment versus placebo within the same individuals, thereby minimizing inter-individual variability and enhancing the precision of the treatment effect estimation.

7.13 Single-Subject Design

In some experimental studies, it is difficult to form a group due to the small number of available cases. Additionally, when it is ethically inappropriate to withhold treatment from a control group, a single-subject design provides a way to evaluate treatment effects without including a control or comparison group. For example, when conducting experimental research with children who have developmental disabilities, it is often nearly impossible to find subjects with comparable abilities. Moreover, assigning a control group that receives no intervention, as in conventional group-comparison studies, may raise ethical concerns.

A single-subject design involves only one participant, with the intervention applied over a substantial period of time. While it shares similarities with time-series design in that repeated measurements are taken over time, the key distinction lies in the number of participants: time-series design typically involves a group, whereas single-subject design involves only one. Likewise, although a single-subject design resembles a case report in having a single individual as the focus, a case report lacks experimental control and simply describes symptoms and treatment processes, making it fundamentally different from a single-subject design.

Three key features of single-subject design are as follows: First, the dependent variable is continuously and repeatedly measured within a single subject. Second, the subject serves as both the control and the experimental unit. Third, multiple measurements are taken to assess the treatment effect. Because this design does not involve a representative sample of the population, generalizing its results is inherently limited.

There are several threats to the validity of single-subject designs. First, the testing effect, where repeated testing may improve or deteriorate performance independently of the intervention. Second, the Hawthorne effect, in which the subject's awareness of being observed may itself alter their behavior. To minimize this, researchers can alternate between baseline and intervention phases. Third, history and maturation effects, which refer to external events or natural development influencing the results. Repeated data collection during both the baseline and intervention phases helps reduce this threat. Fourth, and most critically, is the issue of generalizability. To enhance external validity, replication of the study across multiple participants, settings, and practitioners is necessary.

In a single-subject design, it is essential to clearly operationalize the target behavior or outcome variable and ensure high reliability in data collection. For instance, if the goal is to reduce postoperative periorbital swelling in blepharoplasty patients through manual lymphatic drainage massage, the method of measuring improvement must be precisely defined. Will the outcome be evaluated by photographic swelling grade, ultrasonographic measurement of periorbital thickness, or patient-reported comfort levels? In each phase of the study, inter-rater reliability for the outcome variable must also be evaluated. If "periorbital swelling reduction" is operationally defined as a decrease of more than 20% in ultrasound-measured subcutaneous thickness at the lower eyelid, then pre-training among raters is crucial to ensure consistency in assessment.

For example, suppose two raters independently assess the degree of periorbital swelling reduction following lower eyelid surgery. Based on standardized pre- and post-treatment images, Rater A judges the swelling to have been sufficiently reduced, showing a 1.2 mm decrease in subcutaneous tissue thickness, while Rater B measures a 1.3 mm decrease. In this case, a simple agreement rate may be calculated as 1.2 / 1.3 = 0.92, or 92%. While this method of agreement calculation is straightforward, it has several limitations.

As an alternative method for assessing inter-rater agreement, suppose two raters evaluate the same patient at 8 standardized postoperative time points to judge whether periorbital swelling has been reduced based on clinical photography or ultrasound imaging. At each time point, both raters record whether swelling is "reduced" (+) or "not reduced" (−). If the two raters disagree on a particular time point, this is marked with a * symbol. Table 7.5 illustrates the pattern of agreement and disagreement between the raters.

Table 7.5 Rater agreement on periorbital swelling reduction

Postoperative time point	Rater A	Rater B	Disagreement
1	+	+	
2	+	−	*
3	+	+	
4	+	+	
5	−	−	
6	−	+	*
7	+	+	
8	+	+	

To calculate the percentage agreement between raters, the following formula is used:

$$\frac{Number\ of\ agreements}{(Number\ of\ agreements + Number\ of\ disagreements)} \times 100 = \frac{6}{(6+2)} \times 100 = 75\%$$

In a single-subject design, measurement values are typically displayed graphically, and the resulting patterns are analyzed either visually or statistically. When visual analysis is used, judgments are made based on changes in variability, trend, and level.

One commonly used visual method is the celeration line (also known as the split-middle procedure), which follows a specific set of steps:

1. First, draw a vertical line to divide the data collected during the baseline phase in half.
2. Next, determine the median of each half of the baseline data (to the left and right of the vertical line) and connect the two medians with a straight line.
3. Then, shift the line vertically so that there are an equal number of data points above and below the line.
4. Finally, extend this line into the treatment phase and observe whether the data points during the intervention period fall above or below the extended trend line.

While visual analysis remains a primary approach in single-subject design, the use of conventional statistical methods has been a subject of debate. Some researchers compare the mean values of measurements taken during the baseline and intervention phases using a t-test. When a larger number of data points is available, an analysis of variance (ANOVA) may be conducted. However, before applying such methods, researchers must carefully consider whether the assumptions underlying each statistical test are satisfied (Fig. 7.1).

Common experimental formats used in single-subject research include the A-B design, reversal design, multiple-baseline design, and alternating treatment design (Harris and Riffle 1986; Cuvo et al. 2002). These designs may be represented using a system of coding to indicate the structure of each phase and intervention (Table 7.6).

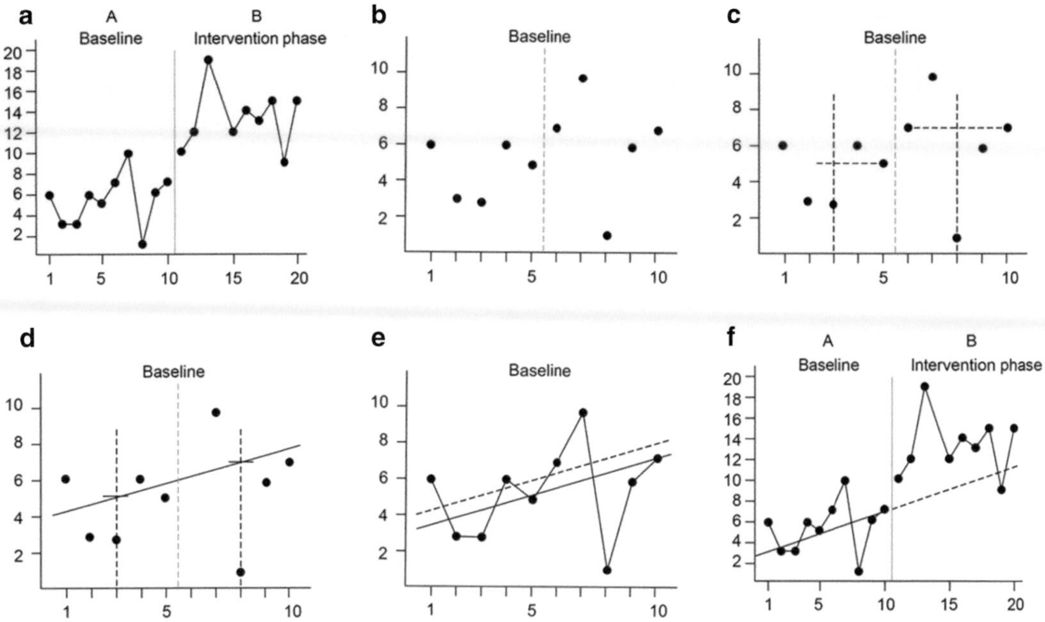

Fig. 7.1 How to draw a celeration line

Table 7.6 Types of single-subject experimental designs

Type	Symbolic notation
A-B design	A-B
Reversal design or withdrawal design	A-B-A, A-B-A-B
Multiple-baseline design	Across subjects
	Across behaviors
	Across conditions(settings)
Alternating treatment design	A-B-A-C-A
Interaction design	A-B-A-C-A-BC-A

A Baseline phase, *B* Intervention phase 1, *C* Intervention phase 2, *BC* Combined intervention

References

Cristel RT, Gandhi ND, Issa TZ, Kola E, Demesh D, Dayan SH. A Randomized, Single-Blind, Crossover Study Evaluating the Impact of OnabotulinumtoxinA Treatment on Mood and Appearance During the COVID-19 Pandemic. *Aesthet Surg J.* 2021;41 (9):NP1199-NP1205.

Cuvo AJ, May ME, Post TM. Effects of living room, Snoezelen room, and outdoor activitieson stereotypic behavior and engagement by adults with profound mental retardation. Research in Developmental Disabilities. 2002;22:183–204.

Harris SR, Riffle K. Effects of inhibitive ankle-foot orthoses on standing balance in a child with cerebral palsy:A single-subject design. Phys Ther. 1986;66:663–667.

Shinji Iizaka. Skin hydration and lifestyle-related factors in community-dwelling older people, *Archives of Gerontology and Geriatrics,* Volume 72, 2017:121–126.

Mekić S, Jacobs LC, Hamer MA, et al. A healthy diet in women is associated with less facial wrinkles in a large Dutch population-based cohort. *J Am Acad Dermatol.* 2019;80 (5):1358–1363.e2.

Bibliography

1. Ai X, Chen L, Lan Y, et al. Efficacy and safety of a non-invasive, home-based radiofrequency device for facial rejuvenation: An open-label, intraindividual controlled trial. *J Cosmet Dermatol.* 2024;23(3):862–868.
2. Alster TS, Doshi SN, Hopping SB. Combination surgical lifting with ablative laser skin resurfacing of facial skin: a retrospective analysis. *Dermatol Surg.* 2004;30(9):1191–1195.
3. Bazargan AS, Tabavar A, Roohaninasab M, et al. Evaluation of the effect of botulinum toxin injection in aggravating or improving seborrheic dermatitis symptoms: A prospective, single-arm clinical trial. *Skin Res Technol.* 2023;29(10):e13478.
4. Cotofana S, Mehta T, Davidovic K, et al. Identifying Levels of Competency in Aesthetic Medicine:

A Questionnaire-based Study. *Aesthet Surg J.* 2024;44(10):1105–1117.
5. DeLozier JB, Holcomb JD. Helium Plasma Dermal Resurfacing With and Without Concurrent Aesthetic Surgery of the Face and Neck: A Retrospective Review. *Aesthet Surg J Open Forum.* 2022;4:ojac061.
6. Fulchiero GJ Jr, Parham-Vetter PC, Obagi S. Subcision and 1320-nm Nd:YAG nonablative laser resurfacing for the treatment of acne scars: a simultaneous split-face single patient trial. *Dermatol Surg.* 2004;30(10):1356–1360.
7. Ghaheri BA, Lincoln D, Mai TNT, Mace JC. Objective Improvement After Frenotomy for Posterior Tongue-Tie: A Prospective Randomized Trial. *Otolaryngol Head Neck Surg.* 2022;166(5):976–984.
8. Hersant B, SidAhmed-Mezi M, Niddam J, et al. Efficacy of autologous platelet-rich plasma combined with hyaluronic acid on skin facial rejuvenation: A prospective study. *J Am Acad Dermatol.* 2017;77(3):584–586.
9. Holcomb JD, Doolabh V, Lin M, Zimmerman E. High energy, double pass helium plasma dermal resurfacing: A prospective, multicenter, single-arm clinical study. *Lasers Surg Med.* 2022;54(5):648–662.
10. Huang YL, Wallace CG, Hsiao YC, et al. Botulinum Toxin to Improve Lower Blepharoplasty Scar: A Double-Blinded, Randomized, Vehicle-Controlled Clinical Trial. *Aesthet Surg J.* 2021;41(9):1003–1010.
11. Zirovich MD, Pangarkar SS, Manh C, et al. Botulinum Toxin Type A for the Treatment of Post-traumatic Headache: A Randomized, Placebo-Controlled, Cross-over Study. *Mil Med.* 2021;186(5-6):493–499.

8 Levels of Measurement

Measurement is the process of assigning values or numerals to represent the actual properties or characteristics of a variable according to a set of defined rules. Simply put, measurement is the act of assigning numbers to specific entities. The term numeral refers to a symbolic or notational representation expressed in the form of a number, but it does not always imply a quantitative meaning. For example, the number printed on a soccer player's jersey or the numerical coding in a questionnaire (e.g., '0' for "No" and '1' for "Yes") are instances of such symbolic numerals.

Variables can be classified into continuous and discrete types. A continuous variable can theoretically take on an infinite number of values within a given range. Although these variables cannot be measured with absolute precision, the degree of detail is limited by the sensitivity and accuracy of the measurement tools. Examples include body weight, skin thickness, or wrinkle depth. A discrete variable (also known as a noncontinuous or categorical variable) can only take on certain distinct values and cannot be subdivided further. Examples include the number of treatment sessions required to achieve a desired effect, the number of complications during postoperative follow-up, or the number of family members under the age of 18.

Precision refers to the exactness of a measurement. For statistical purposes, values may be expressed to several decimal places. The degree of precision depends not only on the sensitivity of the variable itself but also on the measurement instruments and the sensitivity of the data analysis system. For instance, a value such as 1.473826 is considered more precise than 1.47. However, excessive precision is not always useful—for example, blood pressure readings are commonly recorded as whole numbers for practical purposes.

Measurement provides a quantitative expression of certain properties of an object or subject. In most cases, measurement is a form of abstraction or conceptualization, as only a limited number of variables can be directly measured. For example, lesion diameter or periorbital wrinkle depth are among the few characteristics that can be directly and objectively quantified using imaging or measurement devices.

Most human characteristics are difficult to observe and measure directly. As a result, many clinical variables are assessed through indirect means. For example, temperature is inferred through the reading of a thermometer, and heart rate or muscle activity is often measured indirectly using tools such as electrocardiography (ECG) or electromyography (EMG).

The ability to measure a variable—whether directly or indirectly—depends on how well the variable is defined by the person conducting the measurement. Physical and physiological variables such as temperature, body weight, and

K.-H. Yi, *Statistical Research Methods for Dermatologists and Plastic Surgeons*,
https://doi.org/10.1007/978-981-95-5668-7_8

heart rate are relatively straightforward to measure. However, more abstract concepts, such as cognitive ability or muscular strength, are more difficult to quantify, as there are many different ways to define and measure them. A single measurement value cannot be interpreted as an absolute indicator of an individual's strength or capacity.

Measurement involves assigning numbers to objects or individuals according to well-defined rules. These rules reflect the amount and unit of measurement. Some variables, such as length, weight, angle, and grip strength, can be clearly and consistently measured. However, in clinical practice, especially in cosmetic and plastic surgery, there are variables that are more complex and require operational definitions. These include skin firmness, muscle tone around the periorbital region, manual resistance in facial musculature, aesthetic function, or subjective ratings of skin improvement. An operational definition refers to the process of defining a variable in terms of the specific conditions under which it is measured, thereby giving it practical meaning.

Numbers are often used to represent the relative order of variables. However, not all measurement scales are appropriate for this structure. For example, if Patient A's facial muscle strength is rated as "G+" and Patient B's as "G−" using a modified manual muscle testing scale, it does not necessarily imply that Patient A generates greater force than Patient B. The ordinal scoring system may be internally consistent within an individual over time, but its cross-individual comparability is limited. Not all types of measurement data are suitable for arithmetic operations such as multiplication or division. For certain variables, it may be more appropriate to express results in terms of frequencies or proportions.

Depending on the nature of the variable being measured, different rules are applied. To clarify this process, measurements are commonly classified into four levels of measurement: nominal, ordinal, interval, and ratio scales. The level of measurement determines the appropriate statistical methods for data analysis.

8.1 Levels of Measurement

Measurement is a critical component in clinical evaluation, treatment planning, and research for practitioners in cosmetic dermatology and plastic surgery. Most data used in both clinical practice and research are derived through some form of measurement. Measurement can be defined as the process of transforming observations into structured data (Michel 1982). The characteristic or property being measured is referred to as a variable. Variables are generally classified as either qualitative or quantitative, depending on whether they can be quantified. Qualitative variables are those that cannot be measured numerically, such as gender, place of origin, or occupation. In contrast, quantitative variables are those that can be expressed numerically, such as intelligence quotient (IQ), height, or body weight. Some researchers further categorize qualitative variables as discrete variables, and quantitative ones as continuous variables.

In experimental research, variables are also categorized based on their functional roles in the study. A variable that is manipulated or controlled by the researcher, such as a type of treatment applied, is called an independent variable. The outcome that is influenced by this manipulation is referred to as the dependent variable. The characteristics of independent and dependent variables are summarized in Table 8.1.

For example, if the application of fractional CO_2 laser treatment leads to improved skin texture, then the laser treatment is the independent variable, and skin texture improvement is the dependent variable. Likewise, if varying the injection depth of hyaluronic acid filler results in changes in wrinkle depth, then the injection depth

Table 8.1 Characteristics of independent and dependent variables

Independent variable	Dependent variable
Cause	Effect (or result)
Treatment	Physiological response
X-axis (abscissa, X)	Y-axis (ordinate, Y)
Controlled factor	Outcome
Manipulated variable	Measured variable

is the independent variable, and the measured wrinkle depth is the dependent variable.

Before initiating measurement, it is essential to select the relevant variables and clearly define them. In the fields of cosmetic dermatology and plastic surgery, many commonly used variables have been internationally defined and standardized. Examples include skin elasticity, scar thickness, and wrinkle depth-variables that are frequently assessed in both clinical and research contexts. After defining each variable operationally, they are typically categorized into two or more distinct categories. The simplest form involves the presence or absence of a given feature or response. For instance, patients may be classified based on whether post-procedural erythema is present or not. Each patient participating in the study is assigned to one of two mutually exclusive categories. After this classification process, it is necessary to consider the level of measurement applicable to the variable being assessed. The level of measurement of a variable is classified into four distinct types, as described below.

Nominal Scale

Among the four levels of measurement, the nominal scale represents the lowest level. In this scale, the numbers assigned to categories are used solely for identification purposes and have no quantitative meaning. For example, in a study categorizing the site of a procedure, patients who underwent facial procedures may be placed in one category and those who underwent body contouring procedures in another. If the first group is assigned the value "1" and the second "0," this is considered a nominal level of measurement. These categories must be mutually exclusive, meaning each subject can be assigned to only one category. If a participant underwent both facial and body procedures, then a third category must be created and assigned a number distinct from those used for the initial two groups.

There is no limit to the number of categories that can be used in a nominal scale. However, the numbers assigned cannot be mathematically manipulated—they cannot be added, subtracted, multiplied, or divided. When data are measured using a nominal scale, the statistical operations that can be performed include frequencies, percentages, chi-square tests (χ^2), and phi coefficients (φ).

Examples of variables measured on a nominal scale in cosmetic and plastic surgery might include: type of procedure (e.g., filler injection, laser resurfacing, thread lifting), presence or absence of postoperative bruising, laterality of facial asymmetry (left or right), gender of the patient (male, female), dominant hand (right-handed, left-handed), and ability to perform skincare independently (yes/no).

Ordinal Scale

The ordinal scale, also known as a rank-order scale, differs from the nominal scale in that there is a clear order or ranking among the categories. In this scale, the numbers assigned to each category reflect only their relative rank (Fig. 8.1). For example, if a patient's skin elasticity is rated on a scale such that "excellent" is scored as 3, "moderate" as 2, "poor" as 1, and "none" as 0, this represents an ordinal level of measurement.

The numbers used in an ordinal scale differ in meaning from those in a nominal scale. While numbers in a nominal scale do not indicate any order, numbers in an ordinal scale imply that $3 > 2 > 1 > 0$. However, the difference between 3 and 2 is not necessarily equal to the difference between 2 and 1. Thus, while it can be said that a patient rated "3" has better skin elasticity than one rated "2," it is not appropriate to assume that the degree of improvement from "1" to "2" is equivalent to that from "2" to "3."

When data are measured using an ordinal scale, statistical analyses such as medians, percentiles, quartiles, and rank correlation coefficients can be applied. Examples of ordinal-scale variables in cosmetic and plastic surgery include: severity of postoperative edema (e.g., none = 0, mild = 1, moderate = 2, severe = 3), patient satisfaction after facial filler procedures rated as poor (1), fair (2), good (3), or excellent (4), pain inten-

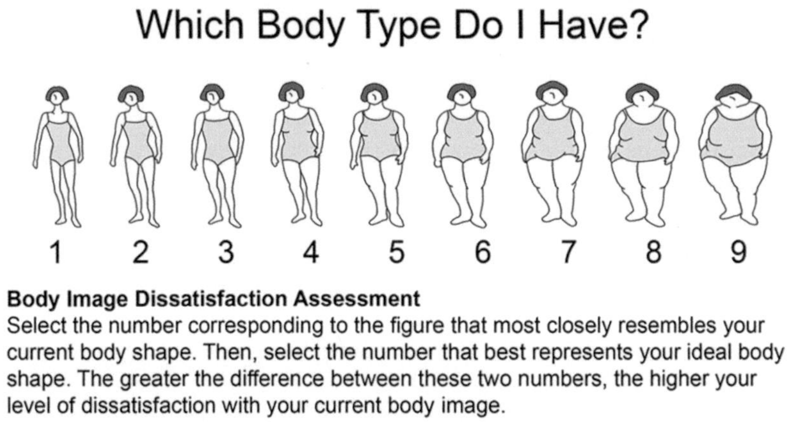

Fig. 8.1 Example of an ordinal scale: the body image dissatisfaction assessment

sity ratings using a 4-point or 5-point scale, and skin laxity grading (e.g., grade 0: no laxity to grade 3: severe laxity). Other examples of ordinal scales include Likert-type scales commonly used in the social sciences to measure attitudes or beliefs.

Interval Scale

The interval scale, also referred to as the equal interval scale, represents a higher level of measurement than both the nominal and ordinal scales discussed previously. In this scale, the intervals between the values are assumed to be equal, meaning that the difference between any two adjacent values is consistent throughout the scale. It is important to note that the zero point on an interval scale is arbitrary and does not indicate a true absence of the quantity being measured. A classic example of an interval scale is temperature measured in degrees Celsius. For instance, the difference between 10 °C and 20 °C is the same as the difference between 20 °C and 30 °C—both have a 10-degree interval. However, it would be incorrect to state that 20 °C is "twice as hot" as 10 °C, because 0 °C does not represent an absence of temperature. It is simply a conventionally defined point—the temperature at which water freezes. Furthermore, the concept of "zero" varies depending on the temperature scale: in Celsius, 0° represents the freezing point of water. In Fahrenheit, 0° corresponds to a much lower temperature (with water freezing at 32 °F and boiling at 212 °F). And in Kelvin (absolute temperature), 0K represents absolute zero, where molecular motion ceases. Other common examples of interval scales include humidity, intelligence quotient (IQ), and body temperature.

Ratio Scale

The ratio scale, also known as the proportional scale, represents the highest level of measurement. Like the interval scale, it maintains equal distances between measurement units, but unlike the interval scale, it also possesses a true, absolute zero point. In other words, a score of zero on a ratio scale indicates a complete absence of the attribute or ability being measured. For example, when measuring joint range of motion, a value of 40 degrees can be interpreted as twice the movement of 20 degrees. This interpretation is possible because the scale has an absolute zero and allows for meaningful ratios to be made. Data measured on a ratio scale can be subjected to all basic arithmetic operations—addition, subtraction, multiplication, and division. Examples of variables measured using a ratio scale include nerve conduction velocity, length of a compression garment or surgical splint, duration of treatment sessions, and number of treatment sessions administered.

8.2 Levels of Measurement and Data Analysis

Researchers should aim to use the highest possible level of measurement when collecting data. Higher-level scales, such as the interval and ratio scales, provide more detailed and nuanced information compared to lower-level scales, such as the nominal scale. Because higher-level measurements retain greater informational richness, they allow for more powerful and sensitive statistical analyses. Conversely, when data collected at a higher measurement level are converted to a lower scale, some information is inevitably lost.

Consider, for example, a dataset of body weights collected from 10 study participants (Table 8.2). When measured using a ratio scale, the data contain complete quantitative information, including exact differences and proportions between individuals. If the same data were converted to an interval scale, this would involve assigning a value of zero arbitrarily to the lightest individual (Participant B), and then adding 5 points for every 5 kg increase in body weight compared to that person. In such a case, differences like 20 − 15 = 40−35 would be valid under the assumption of equal intervals, though the zero point no longer holds absolute meaning.

However, as with interval scales, actual body weight values for each individual cannot be known. For instance, while Participant B may be the lightest, an interval scale does not reveal whether they weigh 10 kg (like an infant) or 110 kg (like an adult). The actual weight remains unknown—only the relative difference in weight is preserved.

Table 8.2 Hypothetical data on body weight of wrestling athletes

Participant	Ratio scale	Interval scale	Ordinal scale	Nominal scale
A	180 kg	70	10	1
B	110 kg	0	1	2
C	165 kg	55	8	1
D	130 kg	20	5	2
E	175 kg	65	9	1
F	115 kg	5	2	2
G	125 kg	15	4	2
H	150 kg	40	7	1
I	145 kg	35	6	2
J	120 kg	10	3	2

When data are measured on an ordinal scale, individuals are ranked in order from lightest to heaviest. The lightest person is assigned a value of 1, and the heaviest a value of 10. In this case, a substantial amount of information is lost compared to ratio scale data. For example, while we know that Person A is heavier than Person B, we do not know by how much. The difference might be 5 kg or 150 kg; this detail is not preserved in ordinal measurement.

Lastly, when body weight is categorized using a nominal scale, the study participants may be arbitrarily divided into lightweight and heavyweight groups. For example, individuals weighing 150 kg or more are assigned to the heavyweight category and coded as "1," while those under 150 kg are coded as "2." This form of measurement provides only minimal information. Within a given category, it is impossible to determine who is heavier or by how much.

As demonstrated, the lower the level of measurement, the less information is retained and available for analysis. Therefore, researchers should strive to use the highest possible level of measurement to minimize information loss. It is also important to understand that when higher-level data are converted to lower levels, some of the original information is inevitably lost. Although numbers across different scales may appear similar, the appropriate statistical methods for analyzing these numbers vary depending on the scale.

The ideal level of measurement among the four is the ratio scale. Accordingly, researchers should always identify which level of measurement their variables fall into—both at the planning stage and during data analysis. This is crucial because certain statistical techniques are only appropriate for specific levels of measurement. Failing to recognize this can lead to serious analytical errors.

Among the four measurement levels, the ratio scale represents the highest level, while the nominal scale is the lowest. Even when a variable is

Table 8.3 Characteristics of different levels of measurement

Scale	Characteristics
Nominal	1. Lowest level of measurement; also known as a *classificatory scale* 2. Objects or phenomena are assigned to categories based on specific criteria 3. Categories must be mutually exclusive; each subject must belong to exactly one group 4. Numbers used in a nominal scale cannot be mathematically calculated; however, since the number of subjects in each group can be identified, relative frequencies or the mode for each group can be calculated
Ordinal	5. Groups are categorized based on operationally defined attributes with a meaningful order 6. Intervals between ranks are not equal, so relative magnitudes cannot be determined Example: Modified Ashworth Scale score 7. It is neither meaningful nor possible to apply basic arithmetic operations such as addition, subtraction, multiplication, or division to variables measured on an ordinal scale 8. Since ranks are assigned discretely, ordinal scores are fundamentally similar in form to nominal scores. Ordinal values do not represent quantity, but only indicate relative position within a distribution 9. It is possible to calculate the median, quartiles, percentiles, and rank correlation coefficients for variables measured on an ordinal scale
Interval	10. Contains all properties of an ordinal scale, plus equal distances between values 11. The zero point is arbitrary, not absolute 12. In terms of temperature, 0 °C does not mean the absence of heat, but rather serves as a reference point between positive and negative temperatures 13. If the actual numerical values are not the same across two interval scales, one cannot be directly converted into another form. For example, 100 °F and 100 °C are not comparable. To make a meaningful comparison, they must be converted using a common ratio 14. It is possible to calculate the arithmetic mean, and operations such as addition and subtraction can be performed; however, multiplication and division are not permitted on interval scale data
Ratio	15. Highest level of measurement 16. Equal intervals and absolute zero point 17. Scores represent true quantities and allow full arithmetic operations Example: weight, height, range of motion, time, force 18. Measurements can be converted between units (e.g., inches to cm)

optimally defined at a specific level, it can still be redefined operationally at a lower level. Therefore, it is best practice for researchers to measure variables at the highest level possible, as this allows for more powerful and precise analytical procedures.

Finally, when discussing results or interpreting data, researchers must ensure that their conclusions are consistent with the level of measurement used during data collection. For example, if ordinal-scale data are mistakenly analyzed or interpreted as though they were measured on a ratio scale, this represents a serious methodological flaw. A clear understanding of measurement levels is essential for drawing valid and meaningful conclusions from the collected data (Table 8.3) (Svensson 2000; Merbitz et al. 1989; Claesson and Svensson 2001).

References

Svensson E. Comparison of assessment in using continuous and discrete ordinal rating scales. Biometrical J. 2000;42:417–434.

Merbitz C, Morris J, Grip JC. Ordinal scales and foundations of misinference. Arch Phys Med Rehabil. 1989;70:308–312.

Claesson L, Svensson E. Measures of order consistency between paired ordinal data: Application to the Functional Independence Measure and Sunnaas Index of ADL. J Rehab Med. 2001;33:137–144

9 Survey Research

Survey research is one of the most widely used methods for collecting descriptive data. It is typically conducted with the intention of inferring the characteristics of a population based on sample responses. In survey research, probability-based sampling methods should be used whenever possible, and the target population must be clearly defined.

Surveys are frequently used to examine levels of attitudes, values, knowledge, or experience. For example, a survey may be conducted to examine aesthetic practitioners' attitudes toward aging and end-of-life appearance-related care. Other examples of survey topics include how clinicians determine the appropriate intensity settings for energy-based devices (e.g., radiofrequency or laser systems), how frequently occlusive dressings or silicone scar sheets are used in postoperative care, or what kinds of ethical dilemmas cosmetic dermatologists and plastic surgeons face in clinical practice. The aim of this chapter is to explore the various instruments used in survey research.

Advantages and Disadvantages of Telephone Surveys

Advantages

1. It is relatively easy to obtain a representative sample.
2. On-site data collection is unnecessary.
3. Interviewing costs are relatively low.
4. Data collection is quick.
5. The interview process is simple and cost-effective.

Disadvantages

1. Interviews must be brief.
2. Questions need to be short, and follow-up probing is difficult.
3. It is hard to assess the respondent's environment or context.
4. The survey is limited to individuals with telephone access.

In addition to live telephone interviews conducted by trained interviewers, automated response systems (ARS) offer the benefit of anonymity, which may encourage more candid responses—although response rates tend to be lower. A major limitation of ARS is that it connects only to numbers listed in telephone directories, reducing sample representativeness. To address this, random digit dialing (RDD) is used, which generates the final four digits of phone numbers by computer while fixing the area and exchange codes. This method allows researchers to reach unlisted numbers. However, RDD still excludes individuals who use only mobile or internet-based phones. To address such limitations, the mixed-mode survey (MMS)—which combines landline and mobile sampling—is sometimes employed.

Advantages and Disadvantages of Mail Surveys

K.-H. Yi, *Statistical Research Methods for Dermatologists and Plastic Surgeons*,
https://doi.org/10.1007/978-981-95-5668-7_9

Advantages
1. Suitable for large populations.
2. Relatively low cost.
3. No need for local field researchers.
4. May yield more honest responses for sensitive topics.
5. Avoids interviewer bias present in face-to-face interviews.
6. Respondents have sufficient time, which may promote more thoughtful answers.

Disadvantages
1. Nonresponses to specific items may be difficult to handle.
2. It is challenging to supplement incomplete responses.
3. Low response rates may limit generalizability.
4. Limited control over the administration of the questionnaire.

Advantages and Disadvantages of Internet Surveys (e.g., member surveys, portal-based surveys, email surveys)

Advantages
1. Faster than telephone or mail surveys.
2. More economical than in-person interviews, particularly for data analysis.
3. Can reach expert populations or international respondents that are otherwise difficult to survey.
4. Allows for easy restructuring or reordering of questionnaire items.
5. Accessible 24/7, removing time constraints.
6. Multimedia (video, audio, image files) can be integrated.
7. Can automatically prompt for unanswered items.

Disadvantages
1. Lack of sample representativeness.
2. Generally difficult to prevent duplicate responses.
3. When using email, responses may significantly decrease if surveys are marked as spam.

9.1 Interviews and Questionnaires

In survey research, data are typically collected through either oral interviews or written questionnaires. Both methods are forms of self-reporting, in which the researcher does not directly observe the behavior or attitudes of the respondents, but rather records what the respondents report themselves. When using self-administered formats, particularly for questions involving personal or sensitive topics, responses may be subject to bias or inaccuracy. Nevertheless, when it comes to measuring psychological variables such as perception, fear, motivation, or attitude, few methods are more effective than interviews or questionnaires.

During an interview, the researcher asks the respondent specific questions and records their answers for later analysis. Interviews may be conducted in person or over the phone. When asking personal questions, establishing rapport between the interviewer and the respondent is essential to eliciting honest responses.

Most questions used in interviews are structured, meaning they are standardized and applied uniformly to all respondents. In this format, every participant is exposed to the same questions, in the same sequence, with the same response options. In contrast, unstructured interviews do not follow a fixed agenda. Interviewers are free to ask open-ended questions and explore topics of interest in a conversational manner. This style is commonly used in qualitative studies for collecting rich, in-depth data.

The primary disadvantage of interviews is that they are time-consuming and costly, particularly when researchers must travel to participants' homes or workplaces, especially across large geographic areas. However, interviews provide a valuable opportunity for in-depth analysis of both behaviors and opinions, as researchers can observe respondents directly and probe their reactions.

The use of questionnaires typically involves self-administered, structured instruments completed on paper with a writing tool. This method is generally more efficient than interviews because participants can complete the questionnaire at their convenience, and the written format allows for standardization, ensuring that all respondents are exposed to the same questions in the same way. Furthermore, using a written questionnaire reduces the potential for interviewer bias that may arise from interpersonal interactions.

Questionnaires can promote honest responses by offering anonymity, making them particularly useful for assessing phenomena that are internally observable, such as attitudes, values, or beliefs. However, questionnaires are less suitable for studies requiring objective observation of behavior, such as the performance of specific treatment skills. One major drawback of written questionnaires is the risk of misinterpretation; respondents may choose incorrect answers due to misunderstanding the question. In contrast, in interviews, clarification can be provided through follow-up questions.

The most common method of distributing questionnaires is by mail. Mail surveys are economical and can reach a wide population within a relatively short time. However, a major limitation is their typically low response rate. A response rate of 60–80% is generally considered excellent, though in practice, researchers often achieve 30–60%. Moreover, even among the returned questionnaires, some may be incomplete or inappropriately filled out, further reducing the effective response rate. A low response rate can severely affect the external validity of the study's findings. Therefore, researchers conducting survey studies must make every effort to ensure a sufficiently high response rate.

9.2 Designing Survey Research

Developing a survey instrument is often challenging and time-consuming. It typically requires multiple revisions as well as a certain level of specialized knowledge in measurement development.

Formulating Survey Questions

When designing a questionnaire, the first consideration should be validity—that is, the instrument must measure what it is intended to measure. For example, in a study investigating burnout among cosmetic dermatologists or aesthetic clinicians, several guiding questions might include:

1. How widespread is the experience of burnout among practitioners?
2. What are the symptoms of burnout in this population?
3. Are there specific occupational stressors that trigger burnout in clinical settings?

Once such broad content areas are clearly defined, more specific survey items can be developed to target them effectively. In addition, it is essential to gather background information such as the respondent's age, years of clinical experience, and duration of employment in their current role, as these variables may be related to burnout and its behavioral characteristics.

Reviewing Existing Questionnaires

The second step in questionnaire development involves reviewing instruments that have been used in previous studies. Numerous researchers have already developed a wide range of survey tools for various purposes, and many of these instruments have been evaluated for their validity. For instance, there are many established tools for measuring attitudes, health behaviors, and functional status. By reviewing and adapting these pre-developed instruments, researchers can save a significant amount of time while also designing a questionnaire that is well-suited to the specific needs of their own study. However, it is unwise to adopt previously used questionnaires indiscriminately without carefully considering whether the instrument's original purpose and target population align with the current research context.

Preliminary Drafts

The process of designing a questionnaire typically begins with the researcher drafting a series of questions aimed at identifying specific behaviors, knowledge, skills, or attitudes. These items are grouped into categories that reflect key aspects of the research topic. The flow of the questionnaire should be natural and coherent, enabling the respondent to follow a logical sequence of thought rather than jumping from one idea to another.

Survey instruments often begin with questions about general demographic characteristics, such as age, sex, level of education, occupation, and length of employment. This background information helps researchers compare sample characteristics across groups and assess the generalizability of the findings. Such demographic variables are also necessary for interpreting whether individual characteristics are related to specific response patterns. These general characteristics should be selected carefully to serve the research objectives and should not include irrelevant or unnecessary items that do not contribute to the purpose of the study.

The preliminary draft of the questionnaire should be reviewed by peers or experts, who can provide feedback and suggest modifications regarding content, wording, and structure. This review process helps identify vague, poorly phrased, or overly abstract questions and enables the researcher to make ongoing revisions based on external input. The questionnaire should be refined repeatedly until the researcher is confident that the instrument is clear and aligned with the intended research goals. Although this process can be time-consuming, it is essential for improving the content validity of the survey tool.

Pilot Testing

After revisions have been made, the questionnaire should be pilot tested with a small number of respondents who are representative of the target population. Typically, a pilot group of about 5 to 10 participants is sufficient. The purpose of this step is to identify any items that are unclear or prone to misinterpretation. It is also useful to measure the amount of time it takes for respondents to complete the questionnaire.

Revision

Based on the results of the pilot testing, the questionnaire should be revised and retested as needed. All ambiguities and inconsistencies must be eliminated until the questionnaire achieves an acceptable level of validity. One of the primary concerns in this stage is often the length of the questionnaire. Initial drafts are usually too long. Lengthy questionnaires tend to reduce respondents' motivation to complete them. In the case of mail surveys, long forms can lead to higher rates of nonresponse and yield unreliable data. Therefore, any items that are not directly related to the research objectives should be eliminated without hesitation. Streamlining the questionnaire not only improves its usability but also increases the likelihood of collecting accurate and complete responses.

Finalizing the Questionnaire

To save time, researchers should not simply skim through the questionnaire before distribution. Even if the final version has been tested in a previous sample or with another representative group, its validity must still be verified. The finalized questionnaire should be presented in a format that is user-friendly and easy to follow. Each page must be well-organized, with clearly printed text and adequate spacing between questions to avoid eye fatigue.

The cover page of the questionnaire should include key information such as the purpose of the study, instructions for responding, how and why the respondent was selected, how anonymity will be protected, the estimated time required to complete the questionnaire, and contact information for the researcher. Respondents should also be clearly informed how and by when to return the completed survey. In mail-based surveys, a pre-addressed return envelope must be enclosed, and a clear deadline for return should be specified.

Conducting the Survey

Due to the typically low response rates associated with mail surveys, researchers should plan in advance to use follow-up reminders, such as postcards, letters, or phone calls. About two weeks after the initial mailing, many potential respondents may misplace the questionnaire or forget to complete it. In such cases, a follow-up mailing that includes a duplicate copy of the questionnaire can be helpful, as some respondents may have lost or discarded the original.

9.3 Writing Survey Items

In survey research, questions can generally be categorized into two types: open-ended questions and closed-ended questions. Open-ended questions require respondents to provide free-text answers, while closed-ended questions present a set of predefined response options.

Open-Ended Questions

Open-ended questions do not provide the respondent with a list of options. Instead, the respondent is asked to answer freely in their own words. This format is most effective when respondents are highly engaged and motivated. Open-ended questions are particularly useful during pilot studies, where responses can help identify common themes that may later be organized into fixed categories. They are also effective in capturing personal feelings and opinions.

For example, a question like, *"What aspect of your profession do you find most satisfying?"* may yield a wide variety of responses. However, this makes it difficult to code and analyze due to the diversity and complexity of the answers. Furthermore, because open-ended questions often require more effort and time, they may result in a higher rate of nonresponse or refusal.

Respondents may be reluctant to spend time writing out complete answers, and their responses may be vague, ambiguous, or incomplete—even if they believe their answers are clear. For instance, if asked, *"What types of exercise do you engage in regularly?"* a respondent might list a variety of specific or general activities. If the researcher's goal is to determine what types of physical activity the respondent participates in, it may be more effective to present a predefined list of exercise options to choose from.

Open-ended questions tend to be more effective in interview settings, where the interviewer can probe further for clarification if an answer is unclear. However, they may not be suitable for respondents who dislike reflective thinking or are unwilling to spend time crafting detailed responses.

The advantages of open-ended questions include: the potential to yield more sincere and in-depth responses, a greater ability to assess respondents' attitudes, motivations, and beliefs, and the possibility of uncovering new or unexpected findings.

The disadvantages include the subjectivity involved in interpreting responses and the psychological burden placed on respondents, who must actively think through their answers.

Closed-Ended Questions

Closed-ended questions are designed so that responses are categorized in advance, and the respondent is asked to choose an answer from the provided options.

For example:

Which aspect of your work as a cosmetic practitioner do you find most satisfying?

___ Interaction with patients

___ Solving intellectually challenging problems

___ Collaboration with other healthcare professionals

___ Opportunities for professional growth

This type of question reduces the cognitive burden on respondents, is easily codable, and allows for straightforward interpretation. However, a major limitation of closed-ended questions is that they restrict the respondent's ability to express personal views, which may make it difficult to capture their true opinions.

There are two basic principles to keep in mind when constructing closed-ended items. First, the response categories should be exhaustive—they must cover all plausible options. In the above example, respondents may have additional reasons for job satisfaction that are not represented in the list. Second, the response options must be mutually exclusive—each choice should clearly represent a unique response. For example, "solving intellectually challenging problems" and "opportunities for professional growth" may overlap conceptually. If the researcher wants the respondent to choose only one option, it is helpful to include an instruction such as: *"Please select the one most important reason."*

The simplest form of closed-ended questions provides only two response options, such as:

Are you currently enrolled in a degree program?

___ Yes ___ No

When measuring attitudes or opinions, it is often more effective to offer a range of responses rather than a simple agree/disagree dichotomy. This allows respondents to indicate the degree of their opinion. Typically, 3 to 5 graded choices are provided.

For example:

How important do you believe it is to include a course on research methodology in your area of specialization?

___ Very important
___ Important
___ Somewhat important
___ Not important
___ Unsure

A variation of the closed-ended format is the ranking question, in which respondents are asked to rank a list of options in order of importance.

Below are several factors that might influence your decision to apply to a particular institution. Please rank them in order of importance from 1 to 5 (1 = most important, 5 = least important).

___ Location of the institution
___ Reputation of faculty
___ Academic curriculum
___ Affiliated hospital
___ Research opportunities

Another format occasionally used is branching, which directs respondents to different follow-up questions based on their initial answers. This helps respondents skip irrelevant items and saves time.

Example:

1. *Do you provide consultation services for clinical therapists?*
   ___ No → Skip to Question 3
   ___ Yes
2. *If yes, how many hours per week do you engage in consultation activities?*
   ____ hours/week

Coding of Responses

Responses to closed-ended questions are typically coded, meaning that numerical values are assigned to each possible answer. For example, in the case of gender, males may be coded as "0" and females as "1." For hospital size, facilities with fewer than 50 beds may be coded as "1," those with 50 to 100 beds as "2," and those with more than 100 beds as "3." Coding allows researchers to easily identify how many respondents selected each option and to calculate the frequencies and percentages for each response category. In some studies, cross-tabulation is used to explore relationships between variables. For instance, to examine whether males or females are more likely to work in small versus large medical facilities, researchers can create a cross-tabulation table comparing gender and hospital size.

Wording

Survey questions must be concise and grammatically correct. Respondents tend to avoid engaging deeply with questions that are long or open to multiple interpretations. Therefore, questionnaire designers should ensure that questions are written in a way that can be read quickly and understood at a glance. The wording should be simple enough for even respondents with the lowest level of education to comprehend. In general, shorter questions are easier for respondents to understand and are more likely to capture their attention. However, over-simplifying a question for the sake of brevity may lead to ambiguity. In some cases, a longer question may be necessary to elicit an appropriate response.

Avoid combining two concepts in a single question using "and" or "or." For example, a question such as, *"How many times a week do you ride a bicycle or take a slow walk?"* should be split into two separate questions for clarity.

Researchers often seek to measure the frequency and timing of specific behaviors. For example: *"How many times per week do you drink alcohol?"* and *"How many patients do you treat in a day?"* From the respondent's perspective, such questions can be difficult to answer accurately, as the frequency of behavior may vary significantly day to day, monthly, or seasonally. Therefore, it is helpful to provide a specific time frame. A better alternative might be: *"What was the highest number of patients you treated in a single day last week?"*

Surveys may also include sensitive or personal topics that could make respondents uncomfortable. Some individuals may hesitate to respond until they are assured of anonymity. Questions related to smoking, sexual behavior, alcohol use, substance abuse, or sexual orientation require careful handling. In these cases, it is essential to guarantee anonymity and to clearly inform respondents that they have the right to skip any question or discontinue the survey at any time.

Scales

A scale refers to the numerical values assigned to each response when measuring a respondent's specific attitudes, values, or characteristics. The following are commonly used scales in survey questionnaires:

1. Likert Scales

   The Likert scale was developed by Rensis Likert and is typically presented in the form of five response options: *"Strongly agree," "Agree," "Neutral," "Disagree,"* and *"Strongly disagree."* This scale provides a clearly ordered set of response categories. Likert's item construction generally follows a 5-point format, which remains one of the most widely used methods in modern questionnaire design.

2. Guttman Scales

   The Guttman scale, devised by Louis Guttman, is also widely utilized. This scale is based on the assumption that a person who agrees with a strongly worded statement will also agree with less extreme statements expressing the same attitude. For an example of the Guttman scale format, please refer to the Appendix.

References

1. Bork CE, Francis JB. Developing effective questionnaire. Phys Ther. 1985;907–911.
2. Collen FM, Wade DT, Robb GF, et al. The Rivermead Mobility Index: A further development of the Rivermead Motor Assessment. Int Disabil Stud. 1991:13:50–54.
3. Wang CH, Hsieh CL, Dai MH, et al. Inter-rater reliability and validity of the stroke rehabilitation assessment of movement (STREAM) instrument. J Rehabil Med.2002;34:20–24.

10 Sampling

One of the primary purposes of clinical research is to generalize findings from a study to similar situations or populations. This chapter explores how responses obtained from a small, representative group (sample) can be applied to a larger context (population).

10.1 Population and Sampling

A population refers to the larger group to which specific research findings are intended to be generalized. It is defined as a set of individuals, events, or entities that share specific criteria. For example, if a study is designed to investigate the effectiveness of various nonsurgical treatments for facial wrinkles, the relevant population would include all individuals seeking aesthetic procedures for wrinkle reduction. However, it is generally impractical to examine every individual within a population. Conducting research on a small group is not only more economical and time-efficient, but can also be more accurate, as smaller groups allow for greater control over research procedures and more precise measurements.

Through the process of sampling, researchers select a subgroup of the population, known as a sample. This sample serves as a reference group for drawing conclusions about the larger population.

Importantly, populations are not limited to human subjects. In studies assessing reliability, the population may refer to an infinite series of measurements. In industrial quality control research, a sample may be selected from the stock of products shipped from a specific manufacturing region. In survey research, households may be sampled from a residential population unit. In essence, the population may include any group of interest, such as individuals, locations, organizations, items, animals, or even time points.

Defining the Population

To generalize research findings, it is essential to clearly define the boundaries of the target population. For example, if the study targets individuals undergoing nonsurgical facial rejuvenation procedures, the definition of that population must be explicitly stated. Researchers must establish clear inclusion and exclusion criteria, both internal and external, that precisely define the characteristics of the population. This enables a consistent determination of who should be included or excluded from the study.

Sampling Bias or Error

When estimating population parameters from a sample, some degree of error is inevitable. These errors can be classified into two categories: sam-

K.-H. Yi, *Statistical Research Methods for Dermatologists and Plastic Surgeons*,
https://doi.org/10.1007/978-981-95-5668-7_10

pling error, which arises from the failure to select a sample that accurately reflects the characteristics of the population, and non-sampling error, which occurs during the actual data collection process, such as misreporting or interviewer bias. In a census, where every member of the population is surveyed, only non-sampling error is present; sampling error does not exist.

To generalize results from a sample to the population, researchers must assume that members of the population would respond similarly under similar conditions. However, because human populations are inherently heterogeneous, exhibiting a wide range of behavioral, psychological, and physical traits, a sample can never fully represent the entire population. Nevertheless, proper sampling procedures can be used to minimize sampling error. Sample size is not the only important factor. A small but representative sample of 50 individuals is far more valuable than a nonrepresentative sample of 1000.

Sampling bias[1] occurs when the individuals selected in the sample overrepresent or underrepresent certain characteristics of the population that are related to the subject of study. Bias can be either intentional or unintentional. For example, intentional bias may occur if a clinician excludes individuals who show no treatment response in order to make the intervention appear more effective. Unintentional bias may arise when a researcher studying public attitudes toward cosmetic procedures conducts interviews only in a high-end shopping district, thereby unintentionally approaching individuals who are more image-conscious or socioeconomically advantaged. Furthermore, an interviewer may unconsciously approach individuals who appear more cooperative based on physical appearance, gender, or demeanor. This kind of bias compromises the representativeness of the sample, making the findings inappropriate for generalizing to the broader population.

[1] Bias refers to the difference between the expected value of a sample statistic, which is used to estimate a population parameter, and the true value of that parameter.

Target Population and Sampling Frame

A sampling frame refers to a list or record of all sampling units, and the term is sometimes used interchangeably with sampling list, roster, or sample population (e.g., a patient registry or appointment schedule).

The first step in research planning is to define the total group to which the researcher intends to generalize the study findings. For instance, in a study examining the effectiveness of a new skin rejuvenation protocol, the target population might be defined as adults aged 40–65 who seek nonsurgical facial cosmetic treatments. Because it is not feasible to collect data from every member of this target group, researchers must restrict their investigation to a subset of the population that is accessible for data collection.

This subset is referred to as the accessible population or experimental population. For example, if the accessible population is defined as patients attending a dermatology clinic, then all individuals at that clinic who meet the eligibility criteria (e.g., undergoing facial rejuvenation procedures) would be considered potential participants. The individual patients serve as the basic sampling units, and the research sample is drawn from this accessible population.

Ideally, the accessible population should be representative of the target population. However, this is not always the case in practice, as the accessible population may be biased or exclude certain subgroups. For instance, some eligible patients may not appear on the clinic's appointment list if they are new to the area or recently transferred from another provider. These omissions can introduce bias into the study and potentially affect the results. Because the validity of the accessible population is not guaranteed, researchers must assess how closely it matches the target population. Strictly speaking, a sample drawn from the accessible population is not equivalent to one drawn from the target population itself.

If the differences between the target and accessible populations are too great, it may be preferable to narrow the target population. For example, the target group could be limited to patients who have received at least one year of consistent cosmetic treatment for skin aging. In such cases, the study results should only be generalized to individuals who meet those criteria. Once the accessible population is established, the researcher should create a clear recruitment plan, identifying how to approach potential participants. Not all individuals will agree to take part in the study—some may be uninterested or unwilling to participate. As a result, the final sample may be even smaller than initially expected.

In survey-based research, it is common for many individuals to decline participation. In experimental studies, participants may drop out before data collection is complete. In every type of study, researchers must also be prepared to exclude data from certain individuals due to procedural errors or nonresponse.

10.2 Sampling Techniques

Sampling techniques are broadly classified into probability and nonprobability methods. Probability sampling involves a random selection process in which every element of the population has an equal chance of being selected. When researchers employ random sampling, the resulting sample is generally considered to be representative of the population from which it was drawn. However, because chance is inherently involved in the selection process, it is always possible that the characteristics of the sample may differ from those of the population.

The mean obtained from the sample is subject to randomness and will almost certainly differ—at least slightly—from the true population mean. The difference between a sample statistic and a population parameter is referred to as sampling error or sampling variability. A key strength of random sampling is that such discrepancies are the result of chance alone, rather than systematic bias caused by the researcher's intentions—whether conscious or unconscious. Although random sampling is not perfect, it is generally regarded as the most reliable method for producing samples that accurately reflect the characteristics of the population.

In contrast, the use of nonprobability sampling imposes clear limitations on the generalizability of the findings. If nonprobability sampling methods must be used due to practical constraints, researchers should exercise particular caution when interpreting and applying the results.

10.3 Probability Sampling

The most fundamental method of probability sampling is simple random selection, in which each member of the population has an equal chance of being selected. However, this method is rarely used in practice because it is often impractical to access the entire population. Therefore, clinical research typically employs modified techniques such as systematic sampling or stratified sampling.

Simple Random Sampling

A random sample ensures that each selection is independent and free from bias. In most cases, random samples are drawn from an accessible population based on available records, such as membership rosters or institutional directories (e.g., a national hospital association list). The accessible population is often defined by the availability of such lists. The accessible population is often defined based on the availability of such lists. For instance, if we attempt to draw a sample of cosmetic dermatologists or plastic surgeons using the membership list of a national aesthetic medical society, the population is thereby defined as those professionals who are registered members of that society. Since not all specialists in the field are necessarily affiliated with such associations, it would be inappropriate to generalize the results to all practitioners in cosmetic dermatology or plastic surgery. In clinical research, it is also possible to draw random samples from available patient lists, provided a comprehensive list exists. If such a list is available, simple random selection can be implemented.

Let's take a basic example of simple random sampling: Suppose we want to gather opinions from a sample of 100 students out of a campus population of 1000. The simplest approach is to write each student's name on an identical slip of paper, mix all the slips thoroughly in a box, and draw out 100 of them. All slips should be of identical size and shape, thoroughly mixed, and drawn without visual bias—this constitutes a proper random selection process.

Another common method is to use a table of random numbers, such as the one provided in Table 10.1. These tables are found in most statis-

Table 10.1 Table of random numbers

03	47	43	73	86	36	96	47	36	61	46	98	63	71	62	33	26	16	80	45	60	11	14	10	95
97	74	24	67	62	42	81	14	57	20	42	53	32	37	32	27	07	36	07	51	24	51	79	89	73
16	76	62	27	66	56	50	26	71	07	32	90	79	78	53	13	55	38	58	59	88	97	54	14	10
12	56	85	99	26	96	96	68	27	31	05	03	72	93	15	57	12	10	14	21	88	26	49	81	76
55	59	56	35	64	38	54	82	46	22	31	62	43	09	90	06	18	44	32	53	23	83	01	30	30
16	22	77	94	39	49	54	43	54	82	17	37	93	23	78	87	35	20	96	43	84	26	34	91	64
84	42	17	53	31	57	24	55	06	88	77	04	74	47	67	21	76	33	50	25	83	92	12	06	76
63	01	63	78	59	16	95	55	67	19	98	10	50	71	75	12	86	73	58	07	44	39	52	38	79
33	21	12	34	29	78	64	56	07	82	52	42	07	44	38	15	51	00	13	42	99	66	02	79	54
57	60	86	32	44	09	47	27	96	54	49	17	46	09	62	90	52	84	77	27	08	02	73	43	28
18	18	07	92	46	44	17	16	58	09	79	83	86	19	62	06	76	50	03	10	55	23	64	05	05
26	62	38	97	75	84	16	07	44	99	83	11	46	32	24	20	14	85	88	45	10	93	72	88	71
23	42	40	64	74	82	97	77	77	81	07	45	32	14	08	32	98	94	07	72	93	85	79	10	75
52	36	28	19	95	50	92	26	11	97	00	56	76	31	38	80	22	02	53	53	86	60	42	04	53
37	85	94	35	12	83	39	50	08	30	42	34	07	96	88	54	42	06	87	98	35	85	29	48	39
70	29	17	12	13	40	33	20	38	26	13	89	51	03	74	17	76	37	13	04	07	74	21	19	30
56	62	18	37	35	96	83	50	87	75	97	12	25	93	47	70	33	24	03	54	97	77	46	44	80
99	49	57	22	77	88	42	95	45	72	16	64	36	16	00	04	43	18	66	79	94	77	24	21	90
16	08	15	04	72	33	27	14	34	09	45	59	34	68	49	12	72	07	34	45	99	27	72	95	14
31	16	93	32	43	50	27	89	87	19	20	15	37	00	49	52	85	66	60	44	38	68	88	11	80
68	34	30	13	70	55	74	30	77	40	44	22	78	84	26	04	33	46	09	52	68	07	97	06	57
74	57	25	65	76	59	29	97	68	60	71	91	38	67	54	13	58	18	24	76	15	54	55	95	52
27	42	37	86	53	48	55	90	65	72	96	57	69	36	10	96	46	92	42	45	97	60	49	04	91
00	39	68	29	61	66	37	32	20	30	77	84	57	03	29	10	45	65	04	26	11	04	96	67	24
29	94	98	94	24	68	49	69	10	82	53	75	91	93	30	34	25	20	57	27	40	48	73	51	92
16	90	82	66	59	83	62	64	11	12	67	19	00	71	74	60	47	21	29	68	02	02	37	03	31
11	27	94	75	06	06	09	19	74	66	02	94	37	34	02	76	70	90	30	86	38	45	94	30	38
35	24	10	16	20	33	32	51	26	38	79	78	45	04	91	16	92	53	56	16	02	75	50	95	98
38	23	16	86	38	42	38	97	01	50	87	75	66	81	41	40	01	74	91	62	48	51	84	08	32
31	96	25	91	47	96	44	33	49	13	34	86	82	53	91	00	52	43	48	85	27	55	26	89	62
56	67	40	67	14	64	05	71	95	86	11	05	65	09	68	76	83	20	37	90	57	16	00	11	66
14	90	84	45	11	75	73	88	05	90	52	27	41	14	86	22	98	12	22	08	07	52	74	95	80
68	05	51	18	00	33	96	02	75	19	07	60	62	93	55	59	33	82	43	90	49	37	38	44	59
20	46	78	73	90	97	51	40	14	02	04	02	33	31	08	39	54	16	49	36	47	95	93	13	30
64	19	58	97	79	15	06	15	93	20	01	90	10	75	06	40	78	78	89	62	02	67	74	17	33
05	26	93	70	60	22	35	85	15	13	92	03	51	59	77	59	56	78	06	83	52	91	05	70	74
07	97	10	88	23	09	98	42	99	64	61	71	62	99	15	06	51	29	16	93	58	05	77	09	51
68	71	86	85	85	54	87	66	47	54	73	32	08	11	12	44	95	92	63	16	29	56	24	29	48
26	99	61	65	53	58	37	78	80	70	42	10	50	67	42	32	17	55	85	74	94	44	67	16	94
14	65	52	68	75	87	59	36	22	41	26	78	63	06	55	13	08	27	01	50	15	29	39	39	43
17	53	77	58	71	71	41	61	50	72	12	41	94	96	26	44	95	27	36	99	02	96	74	30	83
90	26	59	21	19	23	52	23	33	12	96	93	02	18	39	07	02	18	36	07	25	99	32	70	23
41	23	52	55	99	31	04	49	69	96	10	47	48	45	88	13	41	43	89	20	97	17	14	49	17
60	20	50	81	69	31	99	73	68	68	35	81	33	03	76	24	30	12	48	60	18	99	10	72	34
91	25	38	05	90	94	58	28	41	36	45	37	59	03	09	90	35	57	29	12	82	62	54	65	60
34	50	57	74	37	98	80	33	00	91	09	77	93	19	82	74	94	80	04	04	45	07	31	66	49
85	22	04	39	43	73	81	53	94	79	33	62	46	86	28	08	31	54	46	31	53	94	13	38	47
09	79	13	77	48	73	82	97	22	21	05	03	27	24	83	72	89	44	05	60	35	80	39	94	88
88	75	80	18	14	22	95	75	42	49	39	32	82	22	49	02	48	07	70	37	16	04	61	67	87
90	96	23	70	00	39	00	03	06	90	55	85	78	38	36	94	37	30	69	32	90	89	00	76	33

tics textbooks. By assigning each of the 1000 students a unique number, one can move sequentially through the random number table, selecting values until 100 individuals have been chosen.

Alternatively, statistical software such as SPSS can generate random samples (Fig. 10.1). For instance:

1. Enter serial numbers from 1 to 1000 in the data sheet.
2. Select: Data → Select Cases → Random sample of cases (Figs. 10.2 and 10.3).
3. Choose the sample size by entering the number of cases or a percentage (Fig. 10.4).
4. Click Continue, then OK to complete the selection.

To select 10% of the subjects as the sample, enter 10 into the designated field. Click Continue, then OK. The cases not selected as part of the sample will be marked with a slash, while the selected cases will be clearly displayed. In this example, the cases numbered 9, 12, 20, and 29 were randomly selected into the sample (Fig. 10.5).

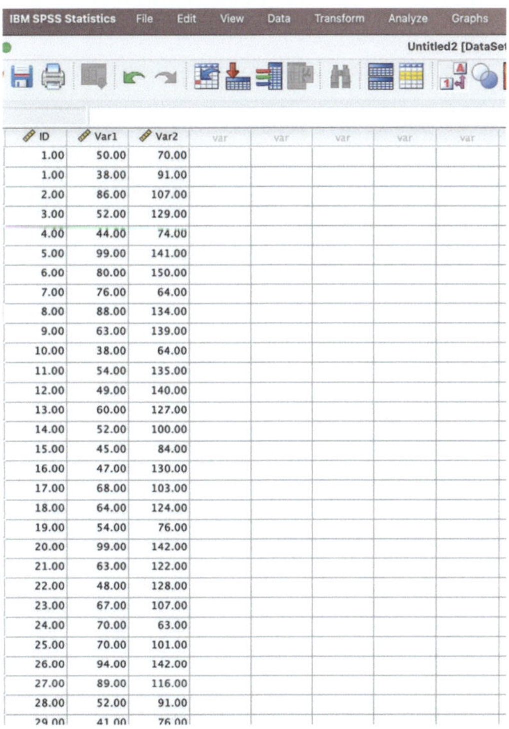

ID	Var1	Var2	var	var	var	var	var
1.00	50.00	70.00					
1.00	38.00	91.00					
2.00	86.00	107.00					
3.00	52.00	129.00					
4.00	44.00	74.00					
5.00	99.00	141.00					
6.00	80.00	150.00					
7.00	76.00	64.00					
8.00	88.00	134.00					
9.00	63.00	139.00					
10.00	38.00	64.00					
11.00	54.00	135.00					
12.00	49.00	140.00					
13.00	60.00	127.00					
14.00	52.00	100.00					
15.00	45.00	84.00					
16.00	47.00	130.00					
17.00	68.00	103.00					
18.00	64.00	124.00					
19.00	54.00	76.00					
20.00	99.00	142.00					
21.00	63.00	122.00					
22.00	48.00	128.00					
23.00	67.00	107.00					
24.00	70.00	63.00					
25.00	70.00	101.00					
26.00	94.00	142.00					
27.00	89.00	116.00					
28.00	52.00	91.00					
29.00	41.00	76.00					

Fig. 10.1 Example dataset loaded in SPSS for demonstrating random sampling procedures

Let us consider an example using a table of random numbers. Suppose the total population consists of 985 individuals, each of whom is assigned a three-digit number ranging from 001 to 985. The researcher selects a starting point arbitrarily, such as by randomly placing a pen on the table or choosing a number at a specific row and column—for instance, beginning at the 12th row, 7th digit. In many random number tables, numbers are separated into groups of two or three digits for ease of reading, but this formatting does not affect the randomness. If the researcher is using three-digit numbers, and the first number at the selected starting point is 977, then subject number 977 is chosen as the first sample. The researcher may then proceed in any consistent direction—downward, upward, or across the table. For example, moving across the row might yield the following sample numbers: 584, 160, 744, and so on. If a number like 998 appears—which exceeds the defined range (001–985)—it is discarded, and the researcher moves on to the next three-digit number. Likewise, if a number is repeated, it is skipped, and the next unique number is selected. This process is called simple random sampling without replacement.

Now, consider using Microsoft Excel to perform random sampling. Begin by launching Excel and assigning serial numbers (1 to 100) to all potential subjects. To randomly select 10 individuals from the list, place the cursor in any cell and enter the following function = RANDBETWEEN(1100) (Fig. 10.6). Press Enter, and Excel will generate a single random number between 1 and 100 (Fig. 10.7). To generate the remaining nine numbers, drag the fill handle (a small cross that appears in the lower-right corner of the cell) either downward or to the right for nine additional cells (Fig. 10.8). Each number corresponds to one of the selected participants in the sample.

Systematic Sampling

To implement systematic sampling, the researcher divides the total number of individuals in the accessible population by the desired sample size. For example, if the list includes 1000 clients, and the goal is to select a sample of 100, every 10th individual on the list would be chosen. The start-

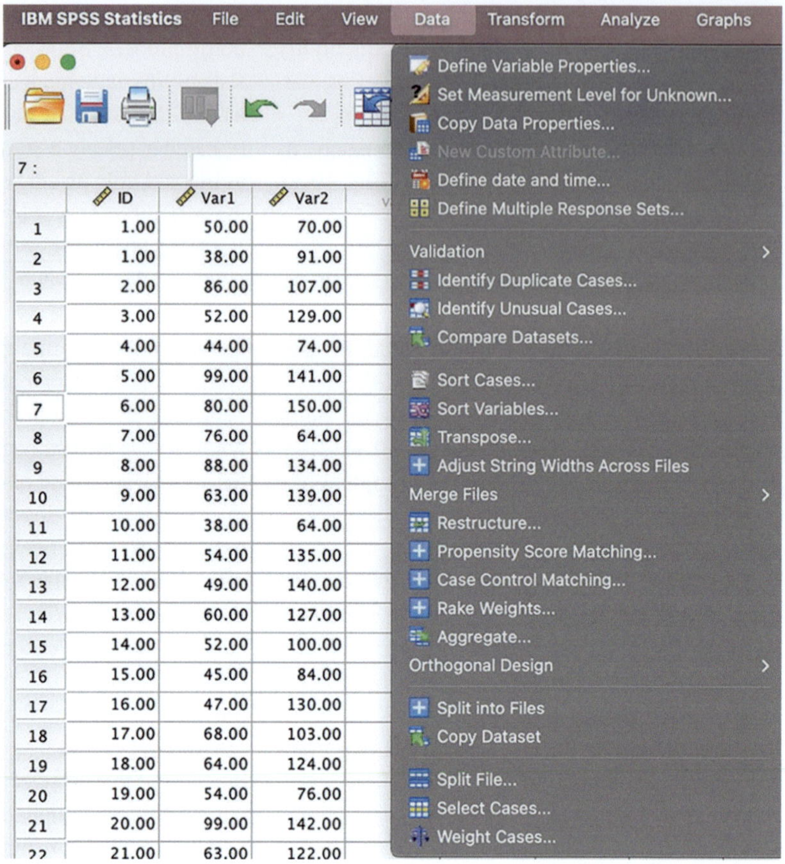

Fig. 10.2 Dropdown menu displayed after selecting the "Data" tab in SPSS, showing available data management options

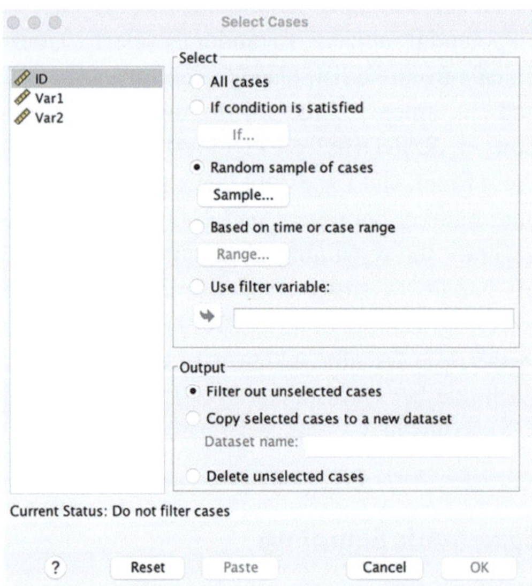

Fig. 10.3 "Select Cases" dialog box in SPSS used for filtering or sampling data

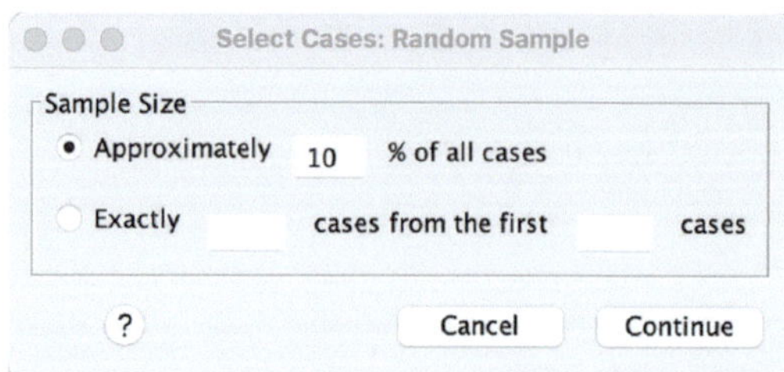

Fig. 10.4 Sampling settings panel displayed after clicking the "Sample" button within the "Select Cases" dialog

ing point is determined at random, often using a table of random numbers to ensure fairness. This method is generally more time-efficient than simple random sampling. Systematic sampling is considered statistically equivalent to random sampling as long as there is no inherent order or cyclical pattern in the list from which the sample is drawn.

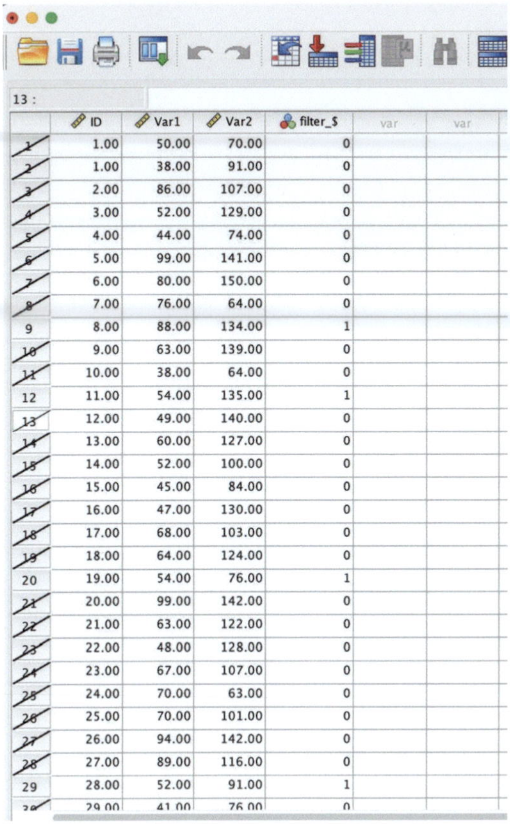

	ID	Var1	Var2	filter_$	var	var
1	1.00	50.00	70.00	0		
2	1.00	38.00	91.00	0		
3	2.00	86.00	107.00	0		
4	3.00	52.00	129.00	0		
5	4.00	44.00	74.00	0		
6	5.00	99.00	141.00	0		
7	6.00	80.00	150.00	0		
8	7.00	76.00	64.00	0		
9	8.00	88.00	134.00	1		
10	9.00	63.00	139.00	0		
11	10.00	38.00	64.00	0		
12	11.00	54.00	135.00	1		
13	12.00	49.00	140.00	0		
14	13.00	60.00	127.00	0		
15	14.00	52.00	100.00	0		
16	15.00	45.00	84.00	0		
17	16.00	47.00	130.00	0		
18	17.00	68.00	103.00	0		
19	18.00	64.00	124.00	0		
20	19.00	54.00	76.00	1		
21	20.00	99.00	142.00	0		
22	21.00	63.00	122.00	0		
23	22.00	48.00	128.00	0		
24	23.00	67.00	107.00	0		
25	24.00	70.00	63.00	0		
26	25.00	70.00	101.00	0		
27	26.00	94.00	142.00	0		
28	27.00	89.00	116.00	0		
29	28.00	52.00	91.00	1		
30	29.00	41.00	76.00	0		

Fig. 10.5 Output in SPSS after randomly selecting 10% of the dataset

Stratified Random Sampling

There are instances in which the characteristics of a sample selected through simple random or systematic sampling do not accurately reflect those of the population. In such cases, stratification can be applied to enhance the representativeness of the sample. Stratified random sampling involves classifying members of the population into homogeneous subgroups (strata). For example, suppose the population consists of 300 first-year students, 300 second-year students, 200 third-year students, and 200 fourth-year students. A random sample drawn from the list of 1000 students may not preserve this distribution.

To control for such imbalances, the population can be divided into four strata, and sampling can then be carried out within each stratum either randomly or using systematic proportional stratified sampling. To obtain a sample of 100 students, the researcher might select: 30 first-year students, 30 second-year students, 20 third-year students, and 20 fourth-year students.

The final sample would better reflect the distribution of the population compared to a simple random sample. Although stratified sampling

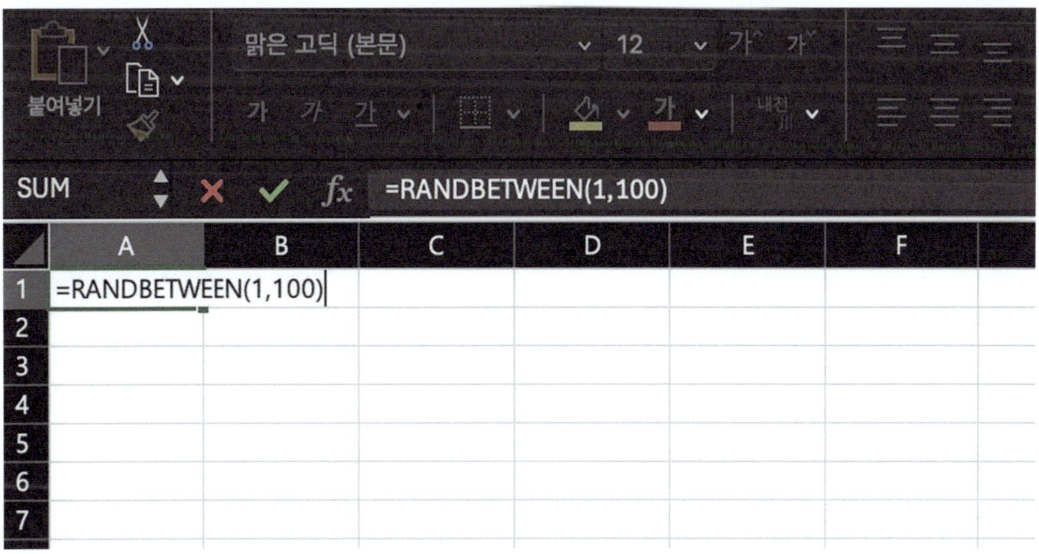

Fig. 10.6 Example of performing random sampling in Excel

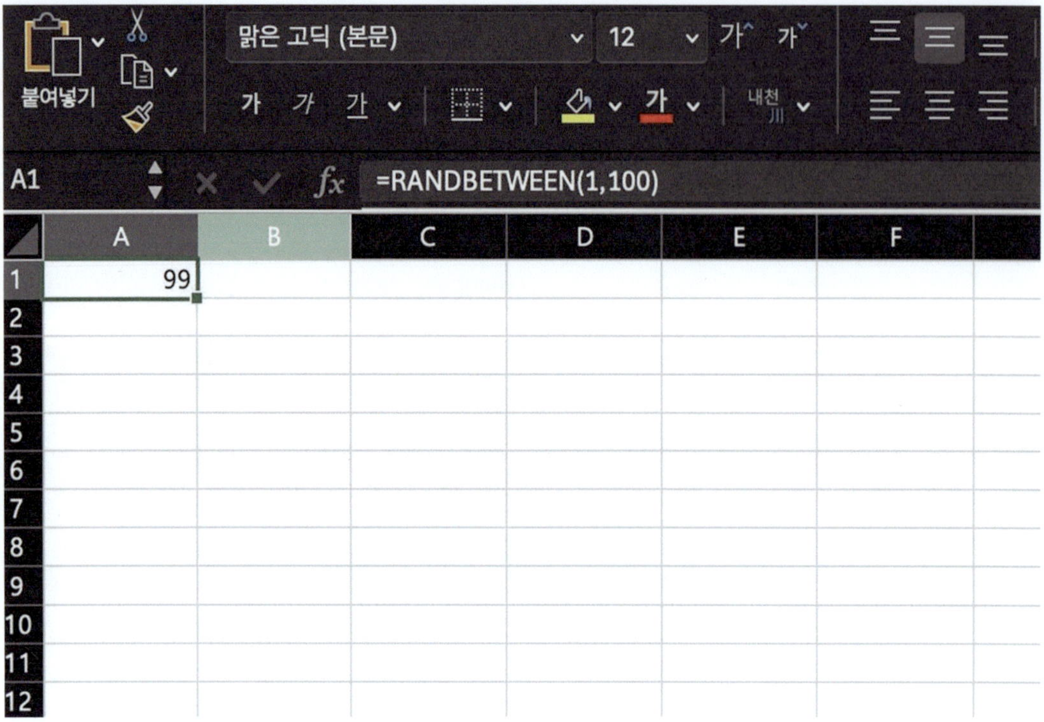

Fig. 10.7 Result of random sample selection in Excel

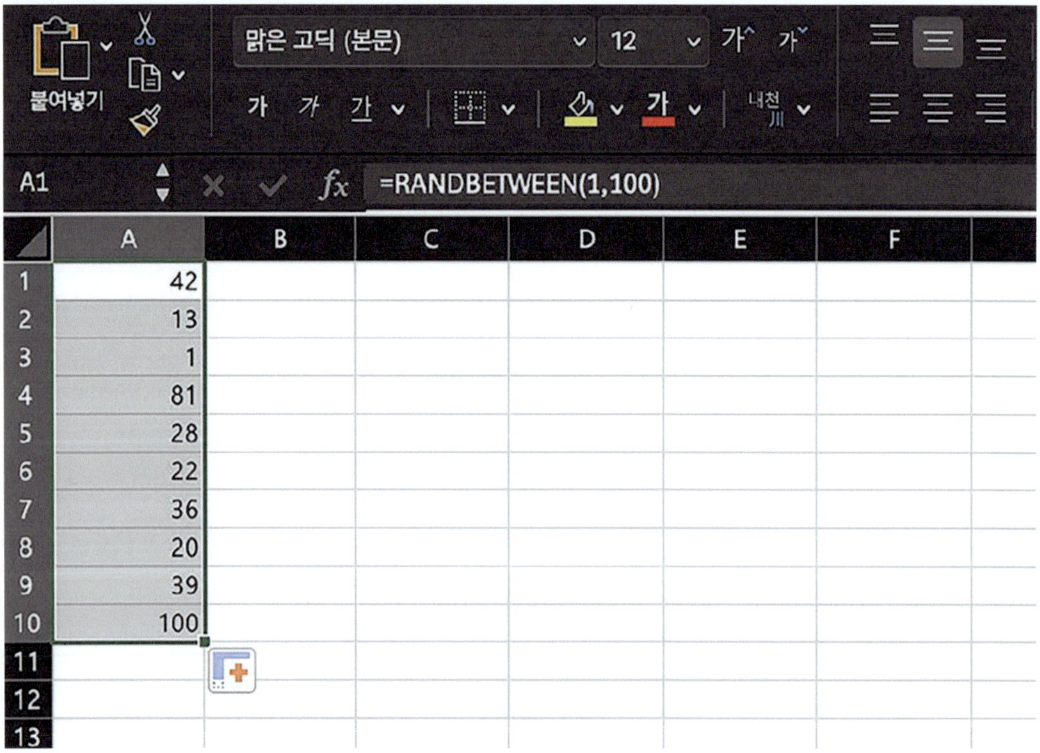

Fig. 10.8 Example of extending random number generation in Excel using the fill handle to create 10 total samples

typically requires more time than other methods, it provides a sample that is more representative and offers more precise population estimates.

Cluster Sampling

When the elements of a population are geographically dispersed, obtaining a complete and accurate list of all members may be impractical or impossible. For example, if a researcher wishes to obtain a sample of aesthetic medicine practitioners working in cosmetic dermatology or plastic surgery clinics across the country, it would be difficult to compile a full national registry of all eligible providers. In such situations, a useful approach is to employ cluster sampling or multistage sampling.[2] Cluster sampling involves selecting a series of cluster units within the population in a stepwise manner.

For instance, suppose we aim to randomly sample 500 practitioners. In the first stage, five regions (e.g., provinces or metropolitan areas) are randomly selected from across the country. In the second stage, 50 dermatology and plastic surgery clinics are randomly selected from within those five regions. In the third stage, all aesthetic practitioners working in the selected clinics are included in the study. The advantage of cluster sampling lies in its efficiency and practicality, especially when managing large, regionally distributed populations. However, it is important to note that this method tends to increase the risk of sampling error compared to other approaches. Researchers frequently use multistage sampling to further refine the process—for example, when randomly selecting households for aesthetic consumer surveys within specific urban districts.

[2]In the first stage, a cluster sampling approach is used to select a number of clusters. In the second stage, subjects are selected from within each cluster using either simple random sampling or proportional stratified sampling methods.

10.4 Nonprobability Sampling

Nonprobability sampling methods are often used when creating a sampling frame or a complete list of the population is impractical or overly complicated, or when the parameter to be estimated is not highly sensitive to whether the sample is probabilistic. In other words, nonprobability sampling is applied in situations where random sampling is not feasible, where the population is not clearly defined, or where sampling error is not a critical concern and probability-based methods are not essential. Compared to probability sampling, nonprobability sampling is generally simpler and more cost-effective, making it attractive for practical research settings. However, it is considered inappropriate for use in statistical hypothesis testing due to its lack of randomization and representativeness.

Convenience Sampling (Availability Sampling)

The most common form of nonprobability sampling is convenience sampling, also known as accidental or incidental sampling. This method involves selecting only those subjects who are easily accessible to the researcher. For instance, if a clinical researcher wishes to examine the effectiveness of fractional radiofrequency treatment on reducing facial pore size, and includes only those patients who happen to visit their own dermatology clinic for the procedure, or selects clients from among regular attendees who are easiest to follow up with, then this sample is based on the convenience of the researcher rather than systematic selection. Similarly, conducting surveys among attendees at a cosmetic exhibition, readers of an online skincare blog, or walk-in customers at a beauty center also constitutes convenience sampling. The major limitation of this method is its restricted generalizability. Individuals who choose to participate may differ significantly from nonparticipants in terms of age, skin condition severity, prior treatment experience, or cosmetic awareness. As such, generalizing the results to a broader population of aesthetic patients may not be appropriate. In practice, a degree of convenience bias may be present in many sampling methods, even those considered more structured.

Snowball Sampling (Chain Referral or Word-of-Mouth Sampling)

Snowball sampling is a method in which subjects are identified through referrals, gradually expanding the sample size as if a snowball were rolling and accumulating more snow. Its use has grown in recent years. While similar to convenience sampling, it differs in that participants who are already enrolled in the study are asked to identify others with similar characteristics who may also be eligible and willing to participate. This method is particularly useful when the target population is difficult to locate or identify, especially when the group possesses specific or uncommon characteristics. In social science research, snowball sampling is frequently used when the population is not well-defined or when traditional sampling methods are not feasible—such as studies involving sex workers, individuals with substance use disorders, or members of sexual minority groups.

The procedure typically involves the following steps:

In the first stage, the researcher identifies initial participants who meet the inclusion criteria and conducts assessments or interviews with them. In the second stage, these participants are asked to refer others who share the same key characteristics. This process of chain referral continues until an adequate sample size is achieved.

For example, a researcher studying the psychosocial impact of laser treatments for visible facial birthmarks (e.g., nevus of Ota or port-wine stains) might begin with a few known patients at a university hospital's dermatology department. These initial participants may then refer others with similar conditions—individuals who may not regularly seek aesthetic care or who are hesitant to come forward on their own. The recruitment continues through this referral process until a sufficient sample is obtained. This technique is also referred to as chain referral sampling.

Quota Sampling (Proportions-Based Sampling)

Quota sampling is a nonprobability sampling method in which the sample is structured to reflect known proportions of a population—for example, based on gender or education level. Suppose it is known that the gender distribution among certified aesthetic practitioners in South Korea is 30% male and 70% female, and the researcher assumes that gender may influence responses. In this case, participants are selected according to the predefined proportions until the target number of responses for each group is met. Although this approach allows researchers to obtain a sample that mirrors specific characteristics of the population, it has limitations. Not all individuals in the population have an equal chance of being selected, and the final sample may not accurately represent the broader attitudes or experiences of the entire population.

Purposive Sampling (Also Known as Purposeful, Judgmental, or Hand-Picked Sampling)

Purposive sampling, also known as judgmental sampling, is used when it is nearly impossible to identify the entire population, although some members can be readily identified. In this method, the researcher or domain expert selects participants based on prior knowledge and professional judgment about their suitability for the study.

For instance, in the field of aesthetic dermatology, a researcher investigating the effects of a multi-session microneedling program on skin texture may review medical charts or conduct interviews to identify patients with specific characteristics, such as mild to moderate atrophic acne scarring. From these, the researcher may intentionally select individuals who are likely to follow treatment protocols consistently over the study period. While purposive sampling shares some similarities with convenience sampling, it differs in that participants are selected based on predefined inclusion criteria rather than mere accessibility. However, as with convenience sampling, the generalizability of findings is limited, since the sample is not randomly selected.

This method is particularly useful in the early phases of research, for example, when evaluating the feasibility of survey instruments or assessing the face validity of a new questionnaire.

References

Greenfield MLVH, Kuhn JE, Wojtys EM. A statistics primer. *Am J Sports Med.* 1996;24:393–395.

Portney LG, Watkins MP. Foundations of clinical research: applications to practice. *Upper Saddle River*, NJ, Prentice Hall, 2000.

Roach KE. A clinician's guide to specification and sampling. *J Orthop Sports Phys Ther.* 2001;31(12):753–758.

11 Basic Statistics (1)

When we measure something—such as muscle tone, rate of recovery, pulmonary capacity, or number of patients—those measurements are referred to as data. For research to hold value, the researcher must present these data in a way that conveys meaning to others. For instance, if a study compares two different facial rejuvenation protocols in patients with photoaged skin and only presents raw numerical values without interpretation, the results lack scientific significance. The researcher must present findings in a meaningful and interpretable manner.

Statistics is a field concerned with the collection, organization, and summarization of data, as well as with making inferences about a population based on a subset of that data. Statistics is broadly categorized into two branches: descriptive statistics and inferential statistics. Descriptive statistics can be subdivided as follows:

1. Measures of Central Tendency
   - (i) Mean (including arithmetic mean, geometric mean, harmonic mean)
   - (ii) Median
   - (iii) Mode
2. Measures of Variation
   - (i) Range
   - (ii) Standard Deviation (SD)
   - (iii) Coefficient of Variation (CV)
   - (iv) Percentiles and Quartiles

Descriptive statistics involves organizing and summarizing a set of data through tables, charts, or summary statistics such as central tendency and variation. This branch is frequently used to present results from survey-based research. Common tools in descriptive statistics include graphs, measures of central tendency, and measures of dispersion. However, descriptive statistics only describe the characteristics of the specific group that was studied, and cannot be generalized to other populations. For example, suppose a study evaluates skin elasticity, dermal thickness, and recovery time after fractional laser treatment in patients with moderate skin laxity. The findings are specific only to the participants in that study, and do not necessarily reflect the characteristics of all patients undergoing the same procedure. To generalize the results, inferential statistics must be employed.

Inferential statistics, in contrast, involves analyzing data to draw conclusions about uncertain or unknown phenomena. It includes methods such as point estimation, interval estimation, and hypothesis testing. This branch of statistics involves formulating models, testing the appropriateness of those models, and using the results to draw conclusions and make predictions. In summary:

1. Descriptive Statistics: Concerned with collecting, organizing, and summarizing data.
2. Inferential Statistics: Concerned with analyzing data to draw conclusions, make decisions, and generate predictions.

K.-H. Yi, *Statistical Research Methods for Dermatologists and Plastic Surgeons*,
https://doi.org/10.1007/978-981-95-5668-7_11

In most contexts, inferential statistics is also referred to as statistical inference, and it is generally divided into estimation (point and interval) and hypothesis testing.

11.1 Descriptive Statistics

Descriptive statistics are used to describe the shape, central tendency, and variability within a set of data. A parameter refers to a measure that describes a characteristic of a population, while a statistic is a numerical value calculated from a sample, used to describe a characteristic of that sample. Common sample statistics include the sample mean ($\bar{x}$) and sample variance (s^2). When researchers aim to generalize from a sample to a population, statistical methods are used to estimate the population parameters.

Frequency Distribution

Methods of displaying descriptive statistics often include frequency distributions, percentages (%), and cumulative percentages. Data can also be presented visually using bar charts, histograms, pie charts, frequency polygons, or stem-and-leaf plots. While similar to bar charts, histograms differ in that the x-axis represents a continuous variable, so there are no gaps between bars. Stem-and-leaf plots are particularly useful for visualizing the shape of a distribution for continuous variables. For instance, let us consider a hypothetical dataset such as that shown in Table 11.1.

When data are listed in the manner shown above, it can be difficult to grasp the overall characteristics at a glance. Let us now organize the data as follows to improve clarity.

Table 11.1 Hypothetical data

60	80	90	94	100	112
68	82	91	95	102	115
72	84	92	95	105	125
77	85	93	96	108	130
77	86	94	98	110	132

In the stem-and-leaf plot shown in Table 11.2, the stem represents the leading digit(s) of the scores, while the leaf corresponds to the final digit. For instance, the values in the first row indicate scores of 60 and 68, whereas the fourth row includes scores of 90, 91, 92, 93, 94, 94, 95, 95, 96, and 98. From this plot, it is evident at a glance that many participants scored in the 90s, and the distribution appears to follow a normal pattern. This method offers the advantage of concisely summarizing the data while retaining the original values in their entirety.

Shape of Distribution

When data are presented in terms of frequency, some distributions appear symmetrical, meaning one half of the data is a mirror image of the other. In Fig. 11.1, examples A and B illustrate symmetrical distributions. In statistical terms, a normal distribution or Gaussian distribution refers to a bell-shaped curve in which most values cluster around the center of the scale, with fewer scores appearing as one moves toward either extreme.

In contrast, a skewed distribution is asymmetrical. The degree to which a distribution deviates from symmetry is called its skewness. In Fig. 11.1, distribution C is positively skewed or skewed to the right, indicating a longer tail on the right side. Distribution D is negatively skewed or skewed to the left, indicating a longer tail on the left side.

Table 11.2 Stem-and-leaf plots

Stem	Leaf
6	08
7	277
8	02456
9	0123445568
10	0258
11	025
12	5
13	02

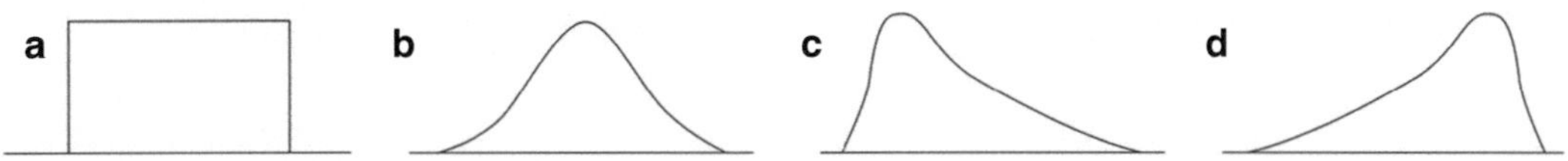

Fig. 11.1 Type of distributions

Skewness and Kurtosis

- *Skewness*: Skewness is a measure of the degree to which a distribution deviates from symmetry. When a distribution is perfectly symmetrical, the skewness (S) equals 0. As shown in Fig. 11.1c, if the distribution is skewed to the right, $S > 0$.
- *Kurtosis*: Kurtosis is a measure that describes the sharpness or peakedness of a distribution. A normal distribution has a kurtosis value (K) of 0. When $K > 0$, the distribution is more peaked than a normal distribution.

Skewness quantifies how much a distribution deviates from being symmetrical around its center.

1. A distribution skewed to the right has $S > 0$
2. A distribution skewed to the left has $S < 0$

Kurtosis indicates how sharply peaked a distribution is. A normal distribution has a kurtosis of 0.

1. If $K > 0$, the distribution is more peaked than normal.
2. If $K < 0$, the distribution is flatter than normal.

Measures of Central Tendency

Mean (Average)

When summarizing a specific characteristic of a group with a single numerical value, the mean is most commonly used. Several types of means exist, including the arithmetic mean, harmonic mean, geometric mean, and trimmed mean. However, the arithmetic mean is the most widely used and understood. The arithmetic mean is calculated by dividing the sum of all measurements or scores within a group by the total number of scores (n).

In a perfectly symmetrical distribution, the mean lies at the center of the distribution, with half of the values above the mean and the other half below it. In statistical notation, the population mean is denoted by the Greek letter μ (mu). The sample mean is represented as $\bar{x}$ (x-bar). It is important to note that the mean does not necessarily represent the "normal" or "healthy" range in clinical interpretation. This is because a value below the mean may still fall within a clinically acceptable range.

The mean[1] is a useful indicator of the overall distribution. However, it often fails to fully represent the data on its own. Specifically, the mean does not account for how individual values differ from each other within a group, nor does it explain the degree of spread or dispersion among the data. For example, suppose Group A and Group B both have an average body weight of 60 kg. While their means are identical, it would be incorrect to conclude that the weight distributions of the two groups are the same. Without examining the distribution shape and spread—specifically variance or standard deviation—one cannot claim that the groups are equivalent. These supplemental statistics are therefore essential in interpreting the mean appropriately.

Median

The median is the value that divides a dataset into two equal halves when the values are arranged in order. For example, in an odd-numbered dataset such as 4, 5, 6, 7, and 8, the middle value—6—is the median. In an even-numbered dataset such as 4, 5, 6, 7, 8, and 9, the median is the arithmetic mean of the two central values (6 and 7), which is 6.5.

[1] It has been said that a fellow with one leg frozen in ice and the other leg in boiling water is comfortable—on average (Yancy 1990).

One key advantage of using the median as a measure of central tendency is that it is not affected by extreme values. Unlike the mean, which reflects the magnitude of values, the median represents their position within the distribution. For this reason, it is especially useful in describing distributions that are skewed or nonnormally distributed.

Summary

When arranging n data values in order of magnitude

1. If n is odd: the median is the value at the $(n + 1)/2$ position
2. If n is even: the median is the average of the values at the $n/2$ and $(n/2) + 1$ positions

Mode

The mode refers to the value that occurs most frequently in a distribution. It can be easily identified by constructing and reviewing a frequency distribution table. When more than one value shares the highest frequency, the distribution is referred to as bimodal (two modes) or multimodal (three or more modes).

While the mode is rarely used to describe central tendency in continuous data, it can be useful when dealing with categorical variables. For example, if one is interested in identifying the most commonly treated type of facial skin concern—such as melasma, post-inflammatory hyperpigmentation, or acne scars—among patients visiting a dermatology clinic over a certain period, analyzing the mode would be a valuable approach.

Comparison of Mean, Median, and Mode

To determine which measure of central tendency is most appropriate for describing a distribution, several factors should be considered (Fig. 11.2). One of the key factors is the level of measurement of the variable. Although the mean is generally the most useful measure, all three measures of central tendency—mean, median, and mode—can be applied when the data are measured on an interval or ratio scale. For data measured on a nominal scale, only the mode is meaningful. When the data are at the ordinal level, both the median and mode may be used.

When presenting results, researchers should consider which measure is the most statistically meaningful. Among the three, the mean is regarded as the most stable measure. That is, if we repeatedly draw random samples from a population, the sample means will vary less than the medians or modes. Only the mean offers a reasonable estimate of the population parameter. For this reason, the mean is more frequently used in statistical analysis for interval and ratio data than the median or mode.

When the data are normally distributed, the mean, median, and mode are all useful. However, for skewed distributions, the mean may have limitations, as it is more susceptible to the influence of extreme values compared to the median or mode. For instance, if a group of exam scores is 78, 80, 82, 85, 85, 85, 86, and 88, and the first score of 78 is replaced by an extreme value of 50, the mean would drop from 83.6 to 80.1. However, the median and mode would remain relatively unaffected. Thus, when dealing with skewed

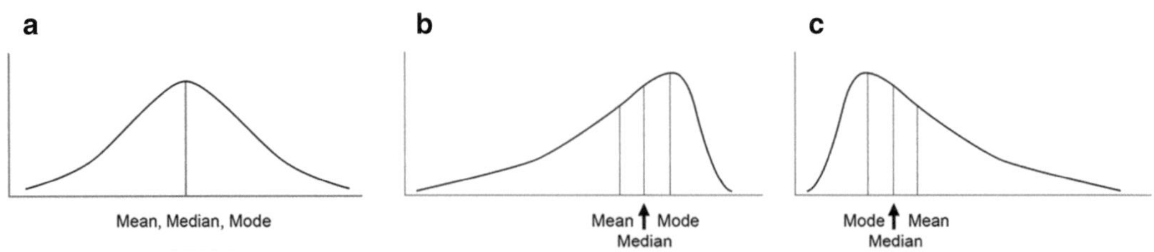

Fig. 11.2 Relationship among the mean, median, and mode depending on the shape of the distribution

data, it is often advisable to report all three—mean, median, and mode—to more accurately describe the characteristics of the distribution.

Measures of Dispersion (Variability)

Dispersion is an important metric that, along with measures of central tendency, describes the shape of a distribution. It indicates how much the values are spread out around a central value.

Range

The simplest way to understand dispersion is by calculating the range. The range is the difference between the highest (maximum) and lowest (minimum) values in a distribution. For example, suppose the distribution of test scores in Group A is: 78, 80, 82, 85, 85, 85, 86, 88. Then the range is: 88–78 = 10. Now suppose Group B has the following scores: 65, 69, 78, 85, 85, 93, 96, 98. The range here is: 98–65 = 33. These results indicate that Group A is more homogeneous, while Group B shows a higher degree of variation.

Although the range is easy to calculate, it only reflects the two extreme values and does not take into account the values that lie between them. Additionally, when comparing two groups with different sample sizes, using the range becomes less effective. Therefore, while the range is useful as a rough descriptive statistic, it is usually presented alongside other measures of dispersion in actual research analyses.

Percentiles and Quartiles

Percentiles are used to describe the relative position of a particular score within a distribution. For example, if a student's score on a university entrance exam is at the 92nd percentile, it means that 92% of the students scored below that student.

Table 11.3 presents glossiness scores measured in 20 patients following a noninvasive facial lifting procedure. Each recorded value represents a score within a ±0.05 range due to the precision of the measuring device. For example, a score of 3.3 indicates an actual range between 3.25 and 3.35. To calculate the 30th percentile, multiply 0.30 × 20 = 6, identifying the 6th score. In Table 11.3, the 6th score is 3.3, and its upper bound is interpreted as 3.35. This means that 30% of the patients scored below 3.35 in skin glossiness after the procedure. Therefore, P_{30} = 3.35. Other percentiles can be calculated using the same method.

Table 11.3 Glossiness scores following a noninvasive facial lifting procedure in 20 patients

Participant	Glossiness score	Participant	Glossiness score
1	2.5	11	3.6
2	2.7	12	3.7
3	2.9	13	3.8
4	3.0	14	3.9
5	3.1	15	4.0
6	3.3	16	4.0
7	3.4	17	4.1
8	3.4	18	4.2
9	3.5	19	4.3
10	3.5	20	4.5

One way to summarize the shape of a data distribution is to present its quartiles. In some cases, the maximum and minimum values may also be reported. The interquartile range (IQR), which is the difference between the third quartile (Q3) and the first quartile (Q1), is often used to describe the degree of dispersion in the data. The IQR represents the range that contains the middle 50% of the observations.

Quartiles divide the data into four equal parts based on percentiles:

1. The first quartile (Q1) corresponds to the 25th percentile.
2. The second quartile (Q2) corresponds to the 50th percentile, which is also the median.
3. The third quartile (Q3) corresponds to the 75th percentile.

In other words, when the data are arranged in ascending order, the quartiles are the values that divide the ordered dataset into four equal parts (Table 11.4). For example, the 25th percentile

Table 11.4 Relationship between quartiles and percentiles

Term	Ascending order position	Descending order position
First quartile (25th percentile)	$(n + 1)/4$	$3(n + 1)/4$
Second quartile (50th percentile, Median)	$(n + 1)/2$	$(n + 1)/2$
Third quartile (75th percentile)	$3(n + 1)/4$	$(n + 1)/4$

(Q1) is the value below which at least 25% of the observations fall, and at least 75% of the observations are greater than or equal to that value.

The first quantile = 25th percentile
The second quantile = 50th percentile (median)
The third quantile = 75th percentile

The quartile deviation is calculated using the following formula.

$$Q = \frac{Q^3 - Q^1}{2}$$

$Q^3 - Q^1$ is referred to as the interquartile range. In the example shown in Table 11.3, the 25th percentile value ($Q1$) is 3.35 (derived by taking the 6th value, 3.3, and adding the upper bound of 0.05), and the 75th percentile value ($Q3$) is 4.05 (the 15th value, 4.0, plus 0.05). Therefore, the quartile deviation Q is calculated as follows:

$$Q = \frac{4.05 - 3.35}{2} = \frac{0.7}{2} = 0.35.$$

Variance

Variance refers to the average of the squared deviations of each measurement from the arithmetic mean. Individual characteristics such as age, body weight, heart rate, nerve conduction velocity, range of motion, muscle strength, and vital capacity naturally vary from person to person. Variance indicates the extent to which each measurement deviates from the mean. A small variance suggests that the data points are closely clustered around the mean, whereas a large variance implies that the measurements are widely dispersed around the mean. Variance is calculated using the following formula (Table 11.5).

Table 11.5 Calculation of variance

x	$(x - \underline{x})$	$(x - \underline{x})^2$
2	−2	4
3	−1	1
$4 = \underline{x}$	0	0
5	+1	1
6	+2	4
$\Sigma = 20/5 = \underline{x} = 4$	$\Sigma = 0$	$\Sigma = 10$

In a population dataset, variance is denoted by σ^2. When the population mean is known, the deviation scores are calculated as $x - \mu$, and the population variance is defined as:

$$\sigma^2 = \frac{\Sigma(x - \mu)^2}{N}.$$

In the case of sample data, the deviation scores are calculated using the sample mean $\underline{x}$ instead of the population mean μ, since the sample does not include all observations from the population. As a result, the sample variance tends to underestimate the actual population variance. To compensate for this bias, the denominator in the sample variance formula is adjusted to $n-1$. Sample variance is denoted by s^2 and is calculated as follows:

$$s^2 = \frac{\Sigma(x - \underline{x})^2}{n - 1}.$$

In the example above, the sample variance is calculated as 10/4 = 2.5.

When dealing with large sample sizes, calculating the variance using deviation scores can be time-consuming due to repeated subtraction and rounding. For this reason, formulas that use raw scores directly are often preferred for calculating variance.

$$s^2 = \frac{\Sigma x^2 - \frac{(\Sigma x)^2}{n}}{n - 1}.$$

The term $\sum x^2$ refers to the sum of the squared raw scores. The numerator of this formula represents the computational expression of the sum of squares (SS).

Table 11.6 A diameter of hypertrophic scars (unit: cm²)

X (cm)	x^2
5	25
2	4
10	100
7	49
6	36
5	25
4	16
8	64
7	49
6	36
$\sum x = 60$	$\sum x^2 = 404$

Table 11.6 presents data on the diameter of hypertrophic scars prior to fractional laser treatment.

$$\underline{x} = 6\text{cm} \qquad \text{n} = 10$$

$$s^2 = \frac{\sum x^2 - \frac{(\sum x)^2}{n}}{n-1} = \frac{404 - \frac{(60)^2}{10}}{10-1}$$
$$= \frac{404-360}{9} = \frac{44}{9} = 4.89\text{cm}^2$$

Since variance is expressed in the squared unit of measurement, it can be difficult to interpret. In the above example, a variance of 4.89 would be presented in cm², but this does not represent an area. This is because the original data—the size of the scar—was measured in centimeters as the diameter. From a research perspective, it is often preferable to report variability using a statistic that is expressed in the same unit as the original measurement. Therefore, in descriptive statistics, variance is not commonly used as a standalone measure; instead, it is mainly applied in analysis of variance (ANOVA) procedures.

Standard Deviation (SD)

Because variance is expressed in squared units of measurement, it is not an appropriate index when one wishes to describe variability using the same unit as the original data. The standard deviation (SD), on the other hand, expresses the dispersion of the data in the same unit as the original measurements. In essence, the standard deviation is the square root of the variance.

$$s = \sqrt{s^2} = \sqrt{\frac{\sum(x-\underline{x})^2}{n-1}}$$

It is commonly denoted by the letter s, and often abbreviated as *SD* in research literature. In sample data, the standard deviation is typically presented alongside the mean to illustrate both central tendency and variability. For example, if Group A has a mean score of 65 with an SD of 6.06, and Group B also has a mean of 65 but an SD of 3.10, this indicates that the measurements in Group B are more tightly clustered around the mean than those in Group A. A larger standard deviation suggests greater variability among measurements within a sample, whereas a smaller standard deviation indicates that the values are more consistent and closer to the mean.

Standard Deviation and Standard Error

The standard deviation (SD) refers to the extent to which individual measurements deviate from the mean—it quantifies the amount of variation or dispersion of a dataset. In the context of a population, this measure is typically expressed as the deviation of each score (X) from the population mean (μ), denoted as ($X - \mu$). When evaluating the distribution of observed values, the standard deviation indicates how closely the data cluster around the mean and therefore serves as a measure of spread. In contrast, the standard error (SE) represents the standard deviation of the sampling distribution of the sample mean. It indicates the precision of the estimated population mean, not the variability of the sample itself. Unlike standard deviation, standard error is not a descriptive statistic and should not be used for descriptive purposes. Nonetheless, in many research reports, standard error is mistakenly reported alongside the mean in place of standard deviation, often as "mean ± SE." This is inappropriate. Researchers sometimes present the SE instead of the SD in order to make the variability appear smaller, as the numerical value of SE is generally less than that of SD. This discrepancy arises because the formula for calculating SE is:

$$\text{standard error} = \sigma_x = \frac{\sigma}{\sqrt{n}}$$

where n is the sample size. Naturally, as n increases, the SE decreases. Thus, SE is intended for inferential statistics, specifically to express the precision of the estimated mean. However, even for that purpose, it is often preferable to report confidence intervals (e.g., 95% CI) rather than the standard error alone, as confidence intervals provide more intuitive insight for readers.

Coefficient of Variation (CV)

When comparing the dispersion between two groups with different means, it is not appropriate to rely solely on the standard deviation. In such cases, the coefficient of variation (CV) can be used. The CV is calculated by dividing the standard deviation by the mean and multiplying the result by 100 to express it as a percentage:

$$CV = \frac{s}{\underline{x}} \times 100$$

By expressing the result in this way, the measurement unit is eliminated. The coefficient of variation is particularly useful for comparing the variability of two datasets when the measurement units differ or when there is a large difference in central tendency. The CV can be used for data measured at the interval scale or higher. A high CV indicates greater variability in the data, while a low CV indicates less variability.

For example, suppose we are evaluating two different tools that measure skin elasticity following facial rejuvenation procedures. With Assessment Tool A, the average elasticity score is 5.0 with a standard deviation of 0.25. With Assessment Tool B, the average elasticity score is 50.0 and the standard deviation is 5.0.

The coefficients of variation for each tool would be:

$$\text{Assessment Tool}\,A = \frac{0.25}{5.0} \times 100 = 5\%$$

$$\text{Assessment Tool}\,B = \frac{5.00}{50.0} \times 100 = 10\%$$

From these results, we can see that Tool B yields greater variability in elasticity scores than Tool A. This demonstrates how the coefficient of variation allows us to meaningfully compare the spread of data between tools, even when the means differ significantly.

In dermatology and cosmetic science, the coefficient of variation is employed to assess the consistency and reliability of various measurement techniques. For instance, studies have utilized CV to evaluate the variability in skin elasticity measurements using optical coherence elastography, as well as in assessing transepidermal water loss (TEWL) to determine skin barrier function. By calculating the coefficient of variation (CV), it is possible to determine which assessment method shows the greatest variability in measurement.

Measures of Dispersion

1. *Range*: The difference between the maximum and minimum values.
2. *Variance* (S^2): $\Sigma\left(X_i - \underline{X}\right)^2 /(n-1)$, where n is the sample size.
3. *Standard Deviation* (SD): The square root of the variance.
4. *Interquartile Range* (IQR): After arranging the data in ascending or descending order, the values are divided into 100 equal parts, known as percentiles. The 25th, 50th, and 75th percentiles are referred to as the first, second (median), and third quartiles, respectively. The interquartile range is calculated by subtracting the first quartile (Q1) from the third quartile (Q3).
5. *Coefficient of Variation* (CV): Used to compare the relative variability between two sample groups. $CV = \left(S / \underline{X}\right) \times 100$, where S is the standard deviation and $\underline{X}$ is the mean.
   - *Random Variable*: When every member of a population has a known and nonzero chance of being selected into a sample, the sampling is called probability sampling. A sample drawn through this method is referred to as a probability sample, and any variable measured from it is termed a random variable. Random variables are typically denoted using specific symbols (Table 11.7).

Table 11.7 Notation of random variables

	Parameter	Statistic
Mean	μ	$\bar{x}$
Variance	σ^2	s^2
Standard deviation	σ	s
Proportion	π	p
Correlation coefficient	ρ	r

11.2 Example of Descriptive Statistics Using SPSS

Launch SPSS and enter the data as shown below. The dataset shown in Fig. 11.3 is a hypothetical example measuring skin hydration scores after two different moisturizing treatments. Group 1 represents the scores after Treatment A, and Group 2 represents the scores after Treatment B. The researcher aims to understand the descriptive statistics related to the skin hydration improvement.

After entering the data, go to Analyze → Descriptive Statistics → Descriptives (Fig. 11.4).

The screen will display the list of variables on the left. Select "score," click the arrow button to move it to the right window, and then click Options (Fig. 11.5).

A new screen will appear showing various statistical options. Select the desired statistics (such as mean, standard deviation, minimum, and maximum), click Continue, and then click OK to view the results (Figs. 11.6 and 11.7).

The following results table will appear. The number of subjects is 16, the range is 32, the mean is 45.63, the standard deviation is 9.06, and the variance is 82.12. The output also provides information on kurtosis and skewness.

Now, let's further explore the same dataset. After the data has been entered, go to Analyze → Descriptive Statistics → Explore (Fig. 11.8).

When the "Explore" window appears, click on "score," then click the arrow button at the top center to move the variable into the right-hand box. Next, click Statistics (Fig. 11.9).

In the Explore: when the "Statistics" appears, select both Descriptives and Percentiles options.

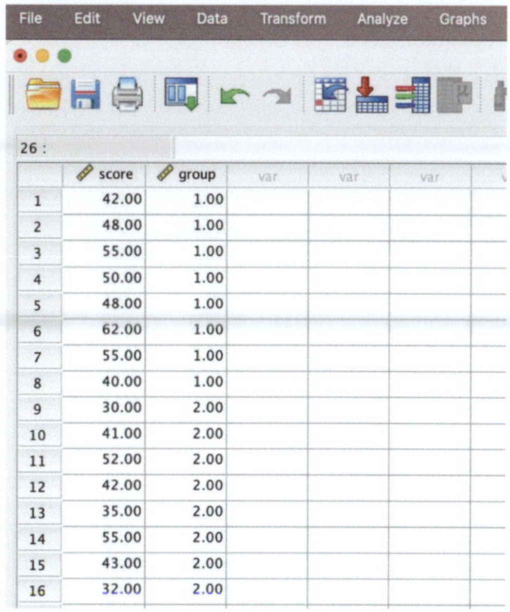

	score	group	var	var	var
1	42.00	1.00			
2	48.00	1.00			
3	55.00	1.00			
4	50.00	1.00			
5	48.00	1.00			
6	62.00	1.00			
7	55.00	1.00			
8	40.00	1.00			
9	30.00	2.00			
10	41.00	2.00			
11	52.00	2.00			
12	42.00	2.00			
13	35.00	2.00			
14	55.00	2.00			
15	43.00	2.00			
16	32.00	2.00			

Fig. 11.3 SPSS Data View showing hypothetical scores used for skin hydration analysis across two treatment groups

After selecting the options, close the window and click Continue (Fig. 11.10).

In the Explore: when the "Plots" appears, select Stem-and-leaf and Histogram under the plots section. Click Continue and then OK to display the results (Fig. 11.11).

The descriptive statistics table will show the information displayed in Fig. 11.12.

The 95% confidence interval for the mean indicates that there is a 95% probability that the true population mean lies between 40.7963 and 50.4537. This interval is calculated assuming a normal distribution, using the z-score of 1.96 and applying the formula: 45.6250 ± 1.96 × standard error. Additional statistics such as the median, 5% trimmed mean (mean calculated after excluding the lowest and highest 5% of data), and quartiles are also provided.

The results also include a separate table for percentiles, making it easy to identify the first quartile ($Q1$) and third quartile ($Q3$) (Fig. 11.13).

The following figures are generated. A histogram illustrating the distribution of skin hydration scores is shown in Fig. 11.14.

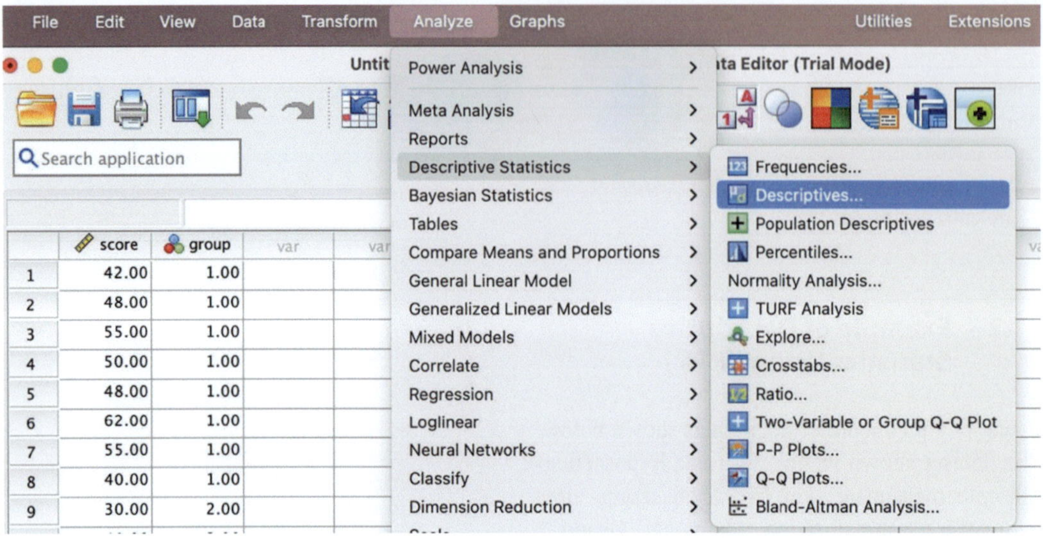

Fig. 11.4 Interface view showing how to navigate to the "Descriptives" tool from the Analyze menu in SPSS

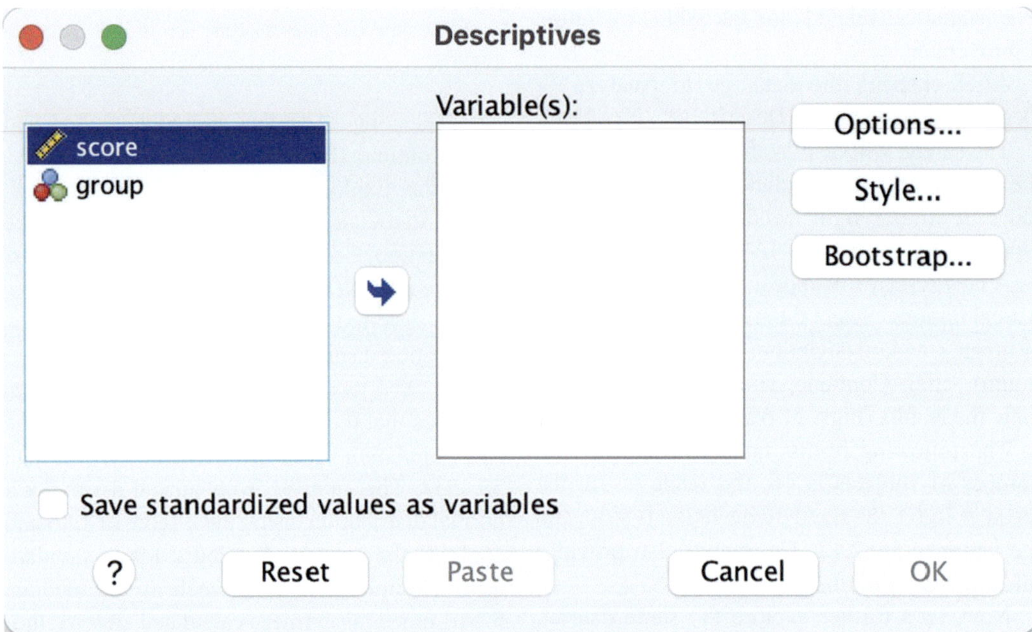

Fig. 11.5 "Descriptives" dialog box in SPSS for selecting variables and summary statistics to compute

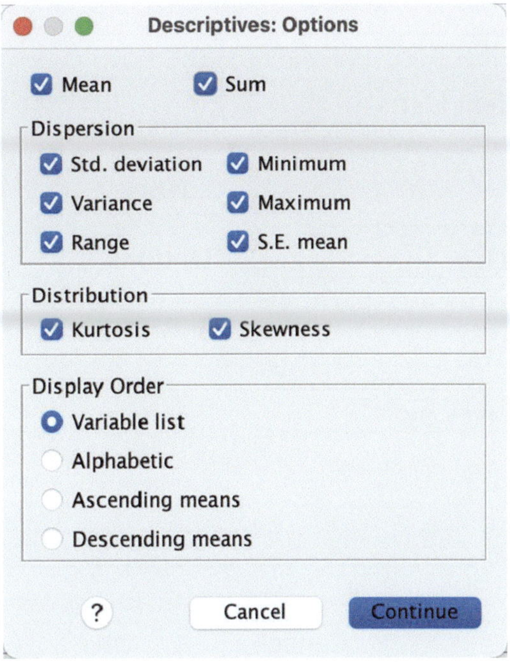

Fig. 11.6 "Options" dialog box within the Descriptives function in SPSS

A stem-and-leaf plot shows the detailed distribution of the data (Fig. 11.15).

A box plot (box-and-whisker plot) visually summarizes the data distribution. In the box plot, the top of the box represents the third quartile ($Q3$), the bottom of the box represents the first quartile ($Q1$), and the line inside the box indicates the median (Fig. 11.16). If the median is centered within the box, it suggests that the distribution is approximately symmetrical. If the whiskers (lines extending from the box) are much longer on one side, it indicates that the data density on that side is much lower. Typically, the whiskers represent either the maximum and minimum values or, in some cases, the 5th and 95th percentiles.

Descriptive Statistics

	N	Range	Minimum	Maximum	Sum	Mean		Std. Deviation	Variance	Skewness		Kurtosis	
	Statistic	Statistic	Statistic	Statistic	Statistic	Statistic	Std. Error	Statistic	Statistic	Statistic	Std. Error	Statistic	Std. Error
score	16	32.00	30.00	62.00	730.00	45.6250	2.26546	9.06182	82.117	-.072	.564	-.668	1.091
Valid N (listwise)	16												

Fig. 11.7 SPSS output from Descriptive Statistics analysis displaying key summary measures

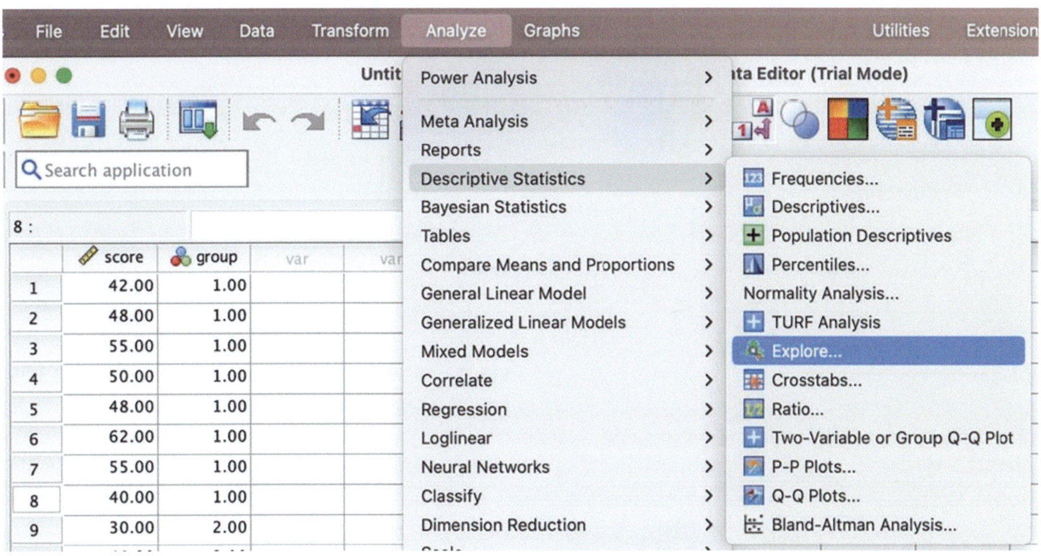

Fig. 11.8 Navigation path to the "Explore" function via Analyze → Descriptive Statistics in SPSS for further exploratory analysis

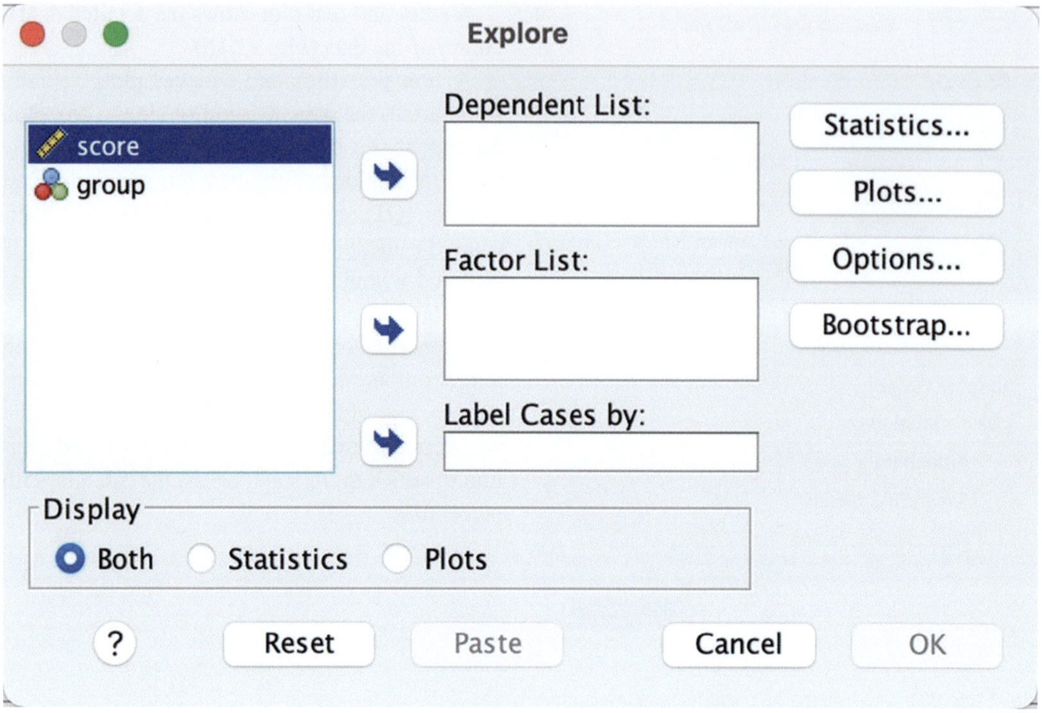

Fig. 11.9 SPSS interface displaying the "Explore" procedure

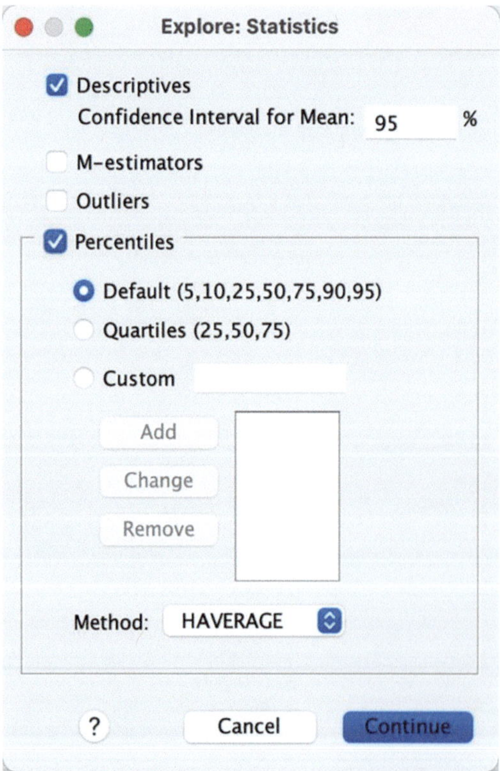

Fig. 11.10 "Statistics" dialog box within the Explore procedure in SPSS

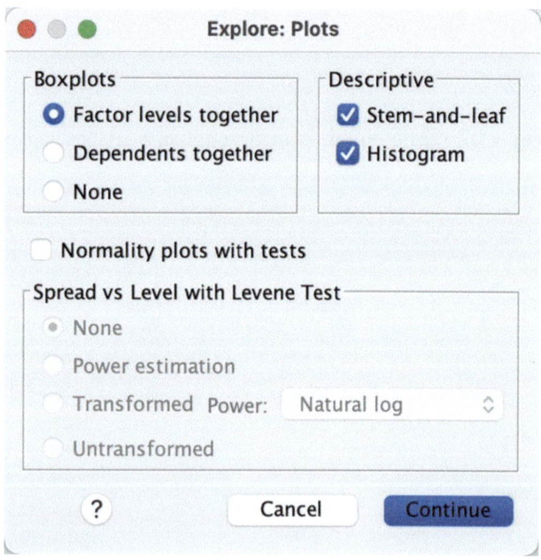

Fig. 11.11 "Plots" dialog box within the Explore procedure in SPSS

Case Processing Summary

	Cases					
	Valid		Missing		Total	
	N	Percent	N	Percent	N	Percent
score	16	100.0%	0	0.0%	16	100.0%

Descriptives

			Statistic	Std. Error
score	Mean		45.6250	2.26546
	95% Confidence Interval for Mean	Lower Bound	40.7963	
		Upper Bound	50.4537	
	5% Trimmed Mean		45.5833	
	Median		45.5000	
	Variance		82.117	
	Std. Deviation		9.06182	
	Minimum		30.00	
	Maximum		62.00	
	Range		32.00	
	Interquartile Range		14.00	
	Skewness		-.072	.564
	Kurtosis		-.668	1.091

Fig. 11.12 Descriptive statistics table generated from the Explore procedure in SPSS

Percentiles

		Percentiles						
		5	10	25	50	75	90	95
Weighted Average (Definition 1)	score	30.0000	31.4000	40.2500	45.5000	54.2500	57.1000	.
Tukey's Hinges	score			40.5000	45.5000	53.5000		

Fig. 11.13 Percentiles table from the Explore procedure in SPSS

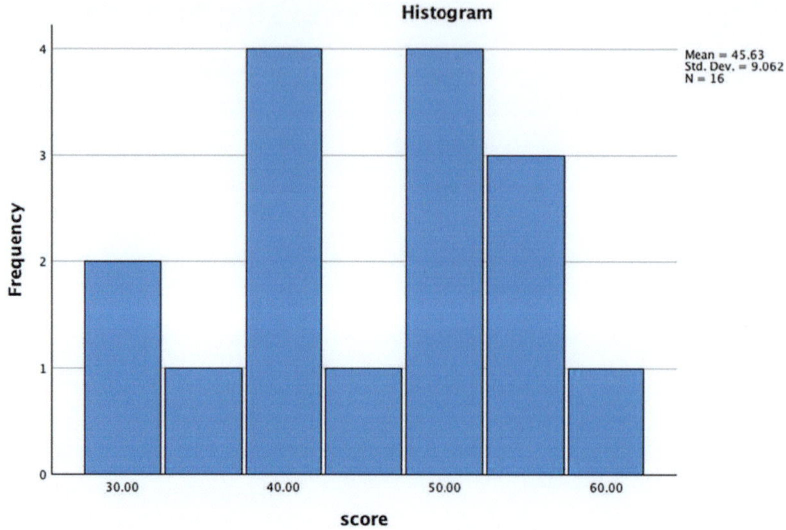

Fig. 11.14 Histogram generated from the Explore procedure in SPSS

```
score Stem-and-Leaf Plot

 Frequency    Stem &  Leaf

     2.00        3 .  02
     1.00        3 .  5
     5.00        4 .  01223
     2.00        4 .  88
     2.00        5 .  02
     3.00        5 .  555
     1.00        6 .  2

 Stem width:     10.00
 Each leaf:        1 case(s)
```

Fig. 11.15 Stem-and-leaf plot generated from the Explore procedure in SPSS

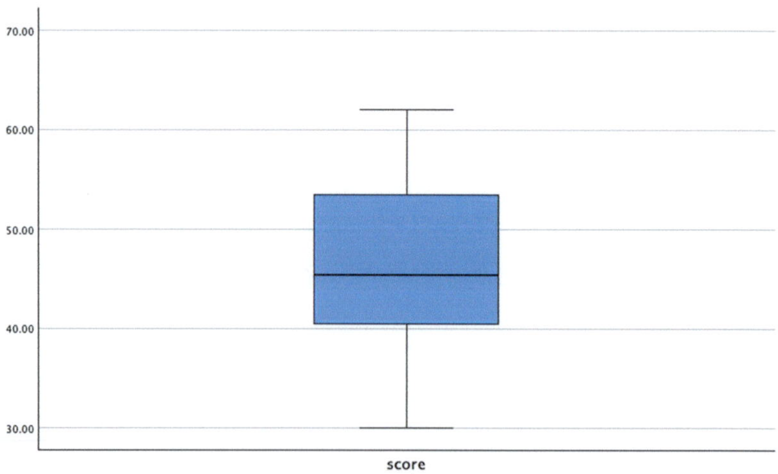

Fig. 11.16 Box plot generated from the Explore procedure in SPSS

11.3 Frequency Analysis of Multiple Responses Using SPSS

Let us explore how to perform a frequency analysis when multiple responses are recorded in a survey. For example, consider the following question:

During the past year, what methods have you used to improve or maintain your skin health? (*Please mark all that apply.*)
① Regular moisturizing
② Professional skincare treatments (e.g., chemical peels, laser therapy)
③ Oral supplements for skin health (e.g., collagen, vitamins)
④ Sun protection (e.g., sunscreen, wearing hats)
⑤ Home-use beauty devices (e.g., LED masks, RF devices)

In this case, if the respondent selected option ①, it is coded as 1, and if not selected, it is coded as 0.

The same coding method is applied from ② to ⑤. For instance, if the first respondent selected ① and ③, and the second respondent selected ①, ②, and ⑤, the data would be entered as follows:

Respondent 1	10100
Respondent 2	11001

Next, proceed to the Variable View to define the variables. In the Variable Label, name the variable appropriately (e.g., "Regular moisturizing"), and in Value Labels, define 0 as "Not selected" and 1 as "Selected," pressing "Add" after each definition. After completing these settings, move on to Defining the Multiple Response Set:

1. Navigate to "Analyze" → "Multiple Response" → "Define Sets."
2. Select and move the variables ("Regular moisturizing," "Professional skincare treatments," "Oral supplements," "Sun protection," "Home-use beauty devices") into the analysis window.
3. Choose "Dichotomies" under "Variables Are Coded As," and set the "Counted Value" as 1 (for selection).
4. Enter an appropriate "Set Name" and "Set Label," then click "Add" and "Close."
   To conduct the frequency analysis:

1. Go to "Analyze" → "Multiple Response" → "Frequencies."
2. In the dialog box, move the newly created multiple response set into the analysis window and click "OK."

Please mark all the cosmetic procedures you have received in the past year:
_____Botulinum toxin injection _____Filler injection
_____Laser resurfacing _____Thread lifting
_____Skin booster treatment _____Microneedling
_____Chemical peeling _____Intense Pulsed Light

Enter the data as described in Fig. 11.17.

Click "Analyze" → "Multiple Response" → "Define Variable Sets" (Fig. 11.18).

Move all the variables listed on the left into the "Variables in Set" box (Fig. 11.19). Confirm that Dichotomies is selected under Variable Coding Format.

Enter 1 for the Counted Value, assign a Name such as *CosmeticProcedures*, and provide a Label describing the variable set (e.g., *Cosmetic Procedures Received*). Then click Add (Fig. 11.20).

You will see that a new multiple response set named $CosmeticProcedures has been created. Click "Close" (Fig. 11.21).

Next, go to "Analyze" → "Multiple Response" → "Frequencies" (Fig. 11.22). Move the $CosmeticProcedures variable into the Table(s) for box (Fig. 11.23).

Click "OK" to proceed (Fig. 11.24).

The output will display the frequency table (Fig. 11.25).

Since multiple responses were allowed, the total number of responses exceeded the number of respondents, resulting in an overall count (e.g., 39). The table also shows the percentage for each cosmetic procedure selected.

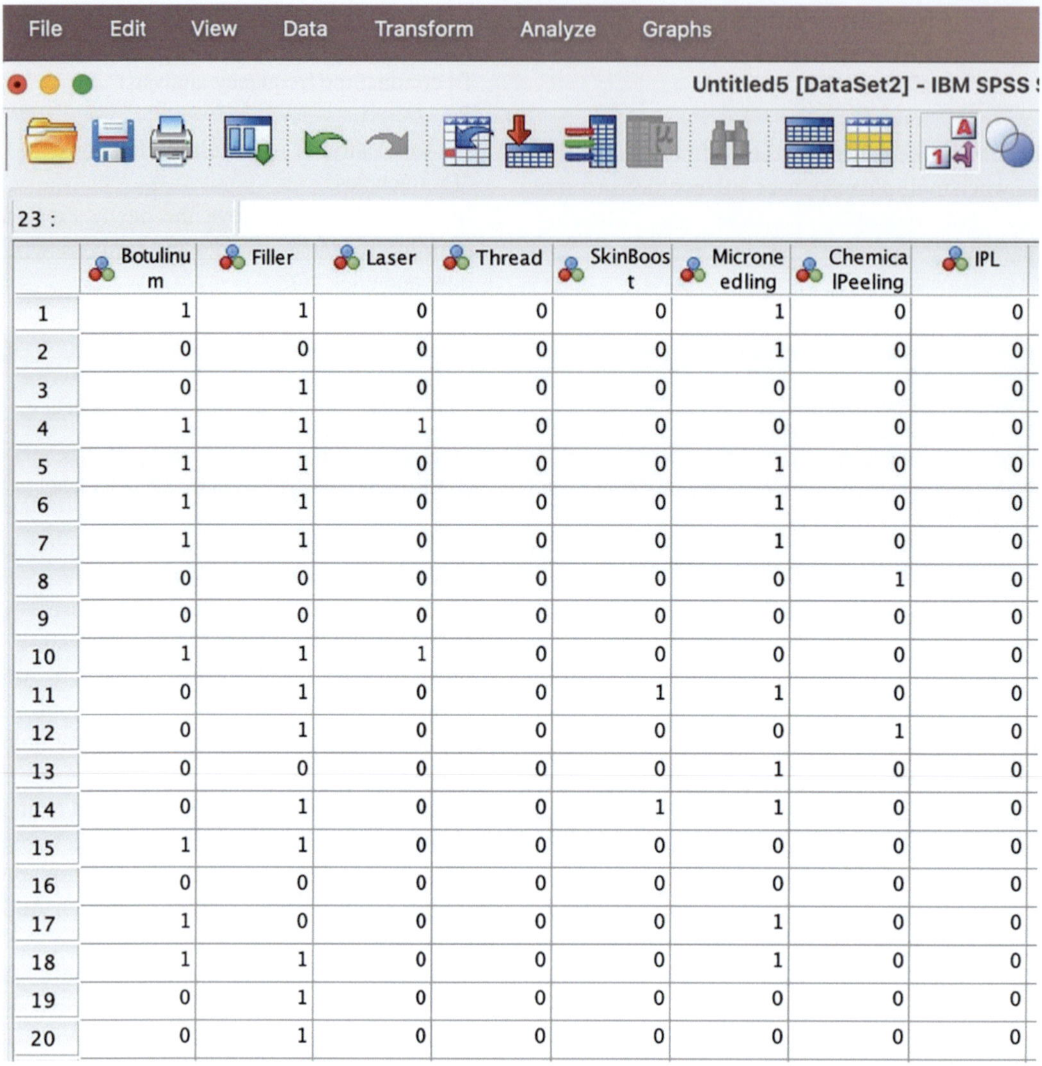

	Botulinum	Filler	Laser	Thread	SkinBoost	Microneedling	ChemicalPeeling	IPL
1	1	1	0	0	0	1	0	0
2	0	0	0	0	0	1	0	0
3	0	1	0	0	0	0	0	0
4	1	1	1	0	0	0	0	0
5	1	1	0	0	0	1	0	0
6	1	1	0	0	0	1	0	0
7	1	1	0	0	0	1	0	0
8	0	0	0	0	0	0	1	0
9	0	0	0	0	0	0	0	0
10	1	1	1	0	0	0	0	0
11	0	1	0	0	1	1	0	0
12	0	1	0	0	0	0	1	0
13	0	0	0	0	0	1	0	0
14	0	1	0	0	1	1	0	0
15	1	1	0	0	0	0	0	0
16	0	0	0	0	0	0	0	0
17	1	0	0	0	0	1	0	0
18	1	1	0	0	0	1	0	0
19	0	1	0	0	0	0	0	0
20	0	1	0	0	0	0	0	0

Fig. 11.17 Example of survey data with multiple response entries prepared for frequency analysis in SPSS

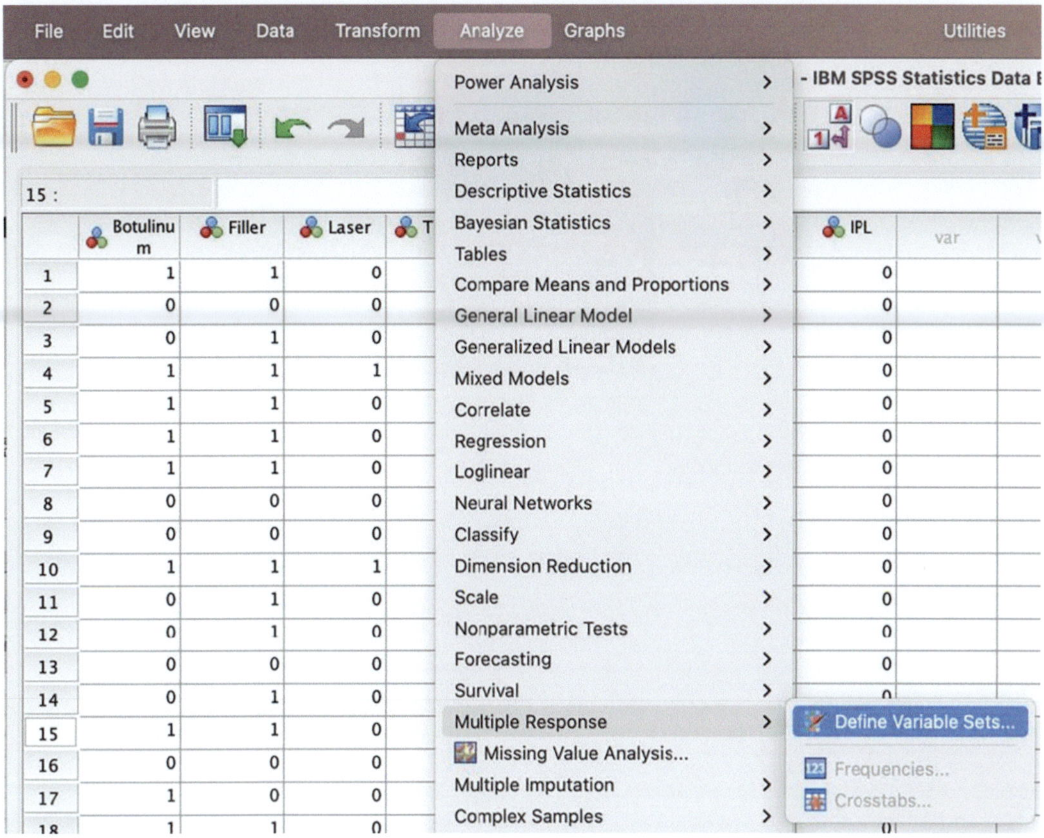

Fig. 11.18 Navigation path to "Define Variable Sets" for multiple response analysis via Analyze → Multiple Response in SPSS

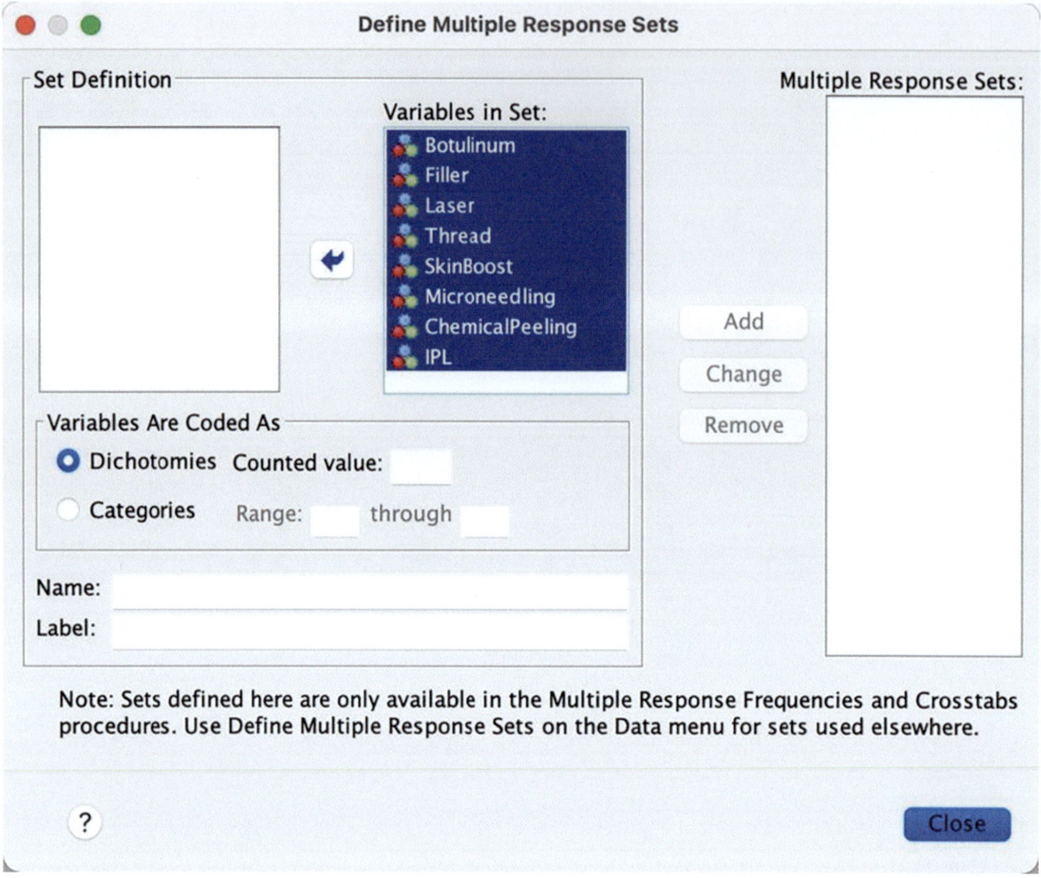

Fig. 11.19 Selecting variables to define a multiple response set in SPSS by moving them into the "Variables in Set" box

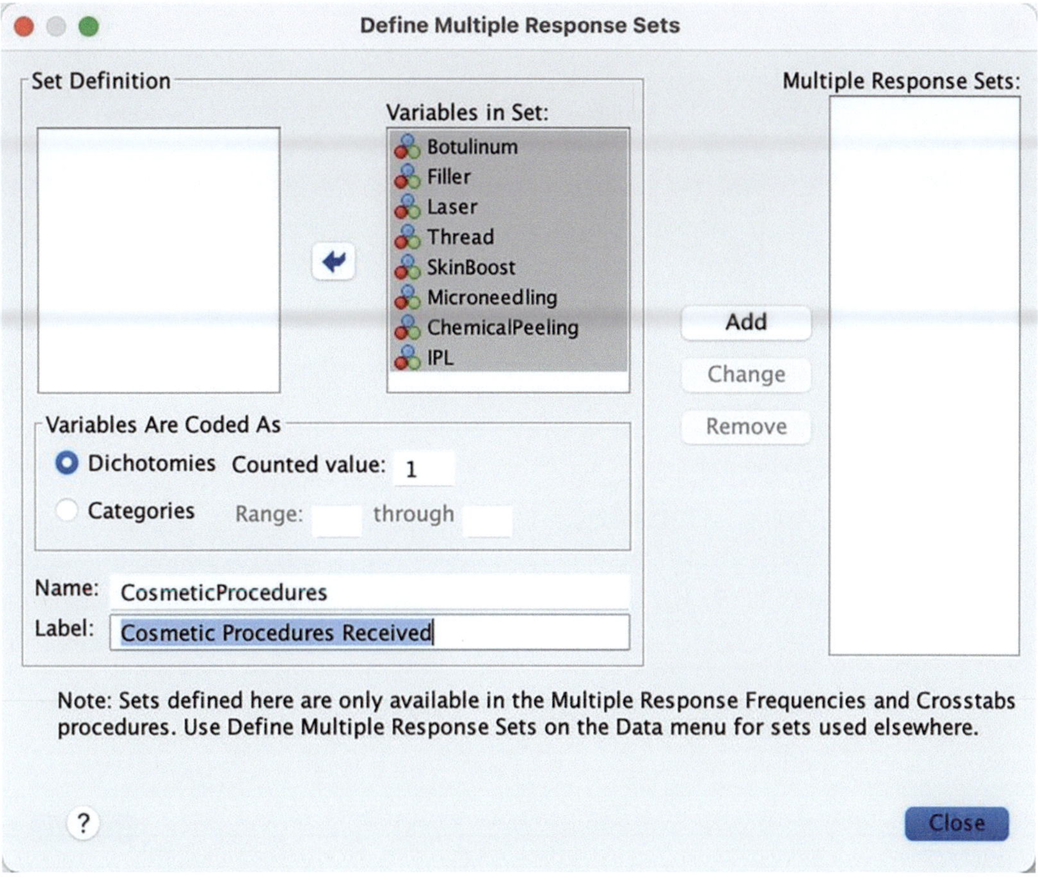

Fig. 11.20 Defining a multiple response set in SPSS by entering the counted value, set name (e.g., CosmeticProcedures), and descriptive label

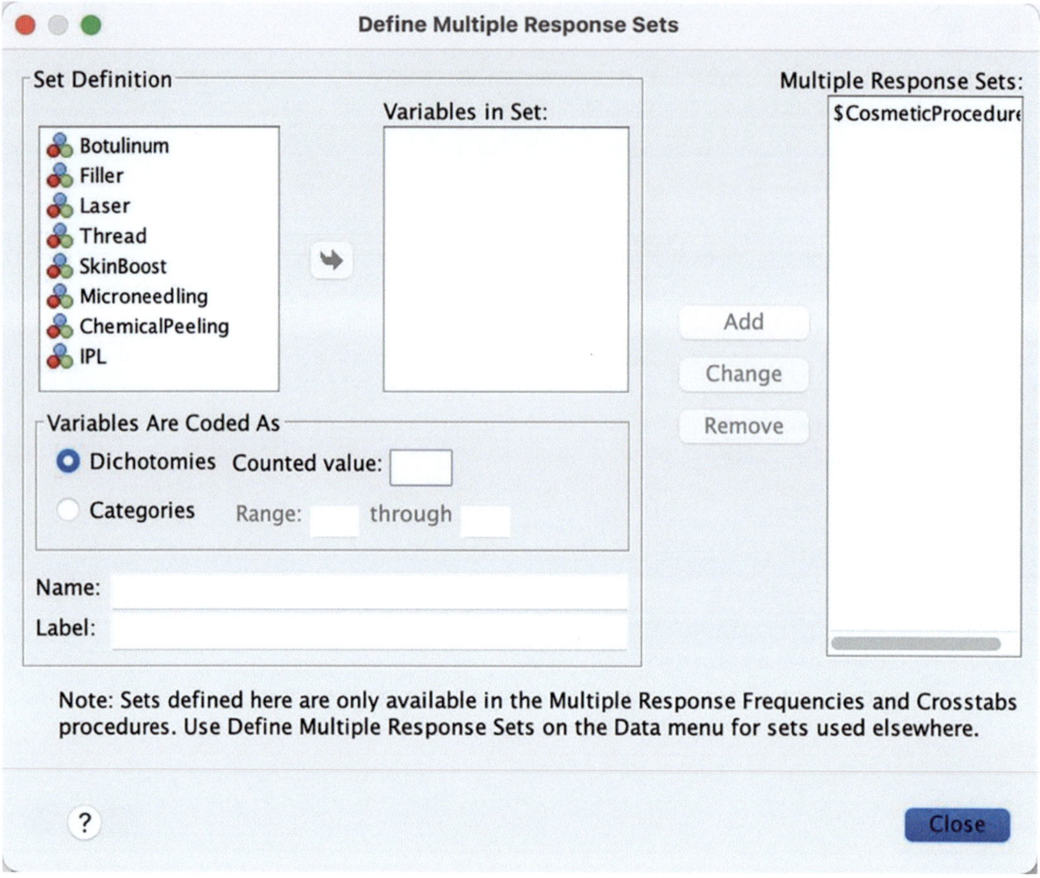

Fig. 11.21 Newly defined multiple response set "CosmeticProcedures" added to the list in SPSS after clicking "Add"

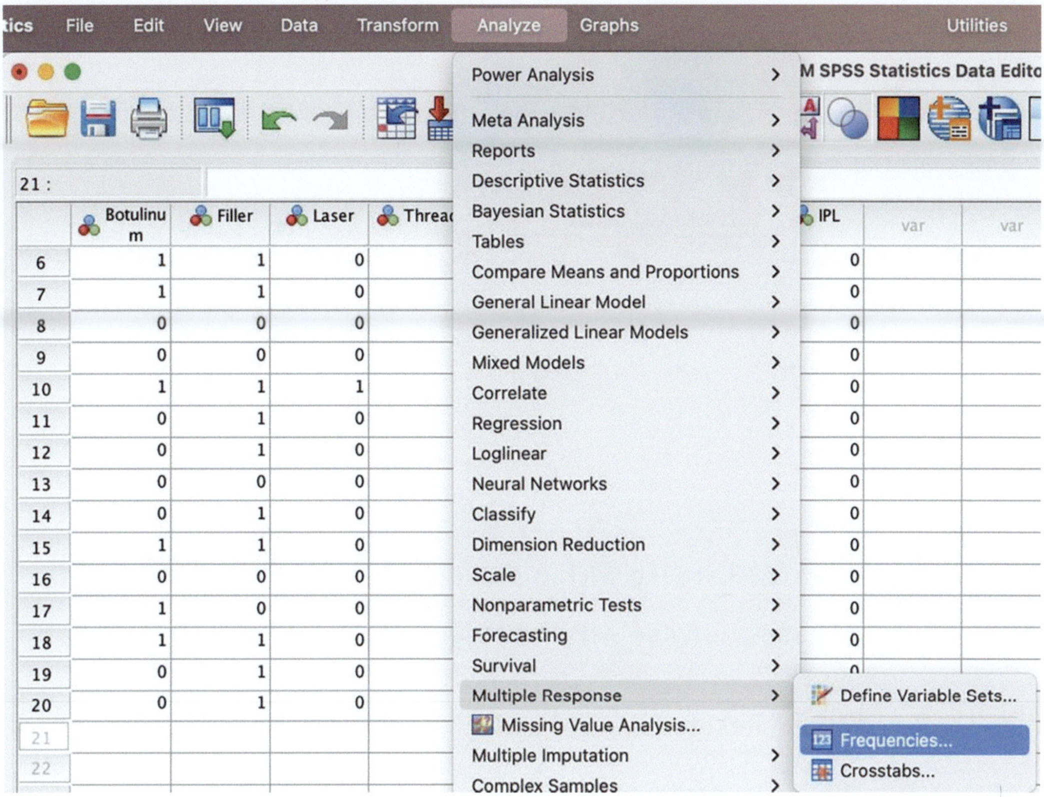

Fig. 11.22 Accessing the "Frequencies" option under Multiple Response in SPSS

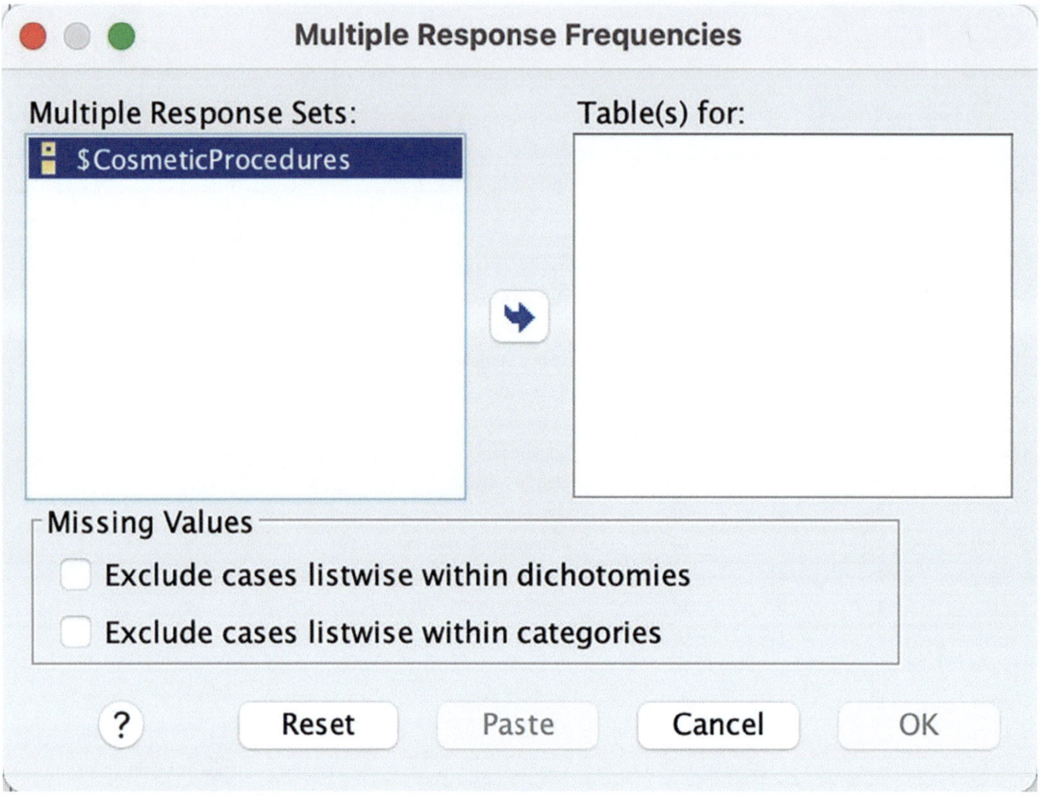

Fig. 11.23 “Frequencies” dialog box in SPSS for multiple response frequency analysis

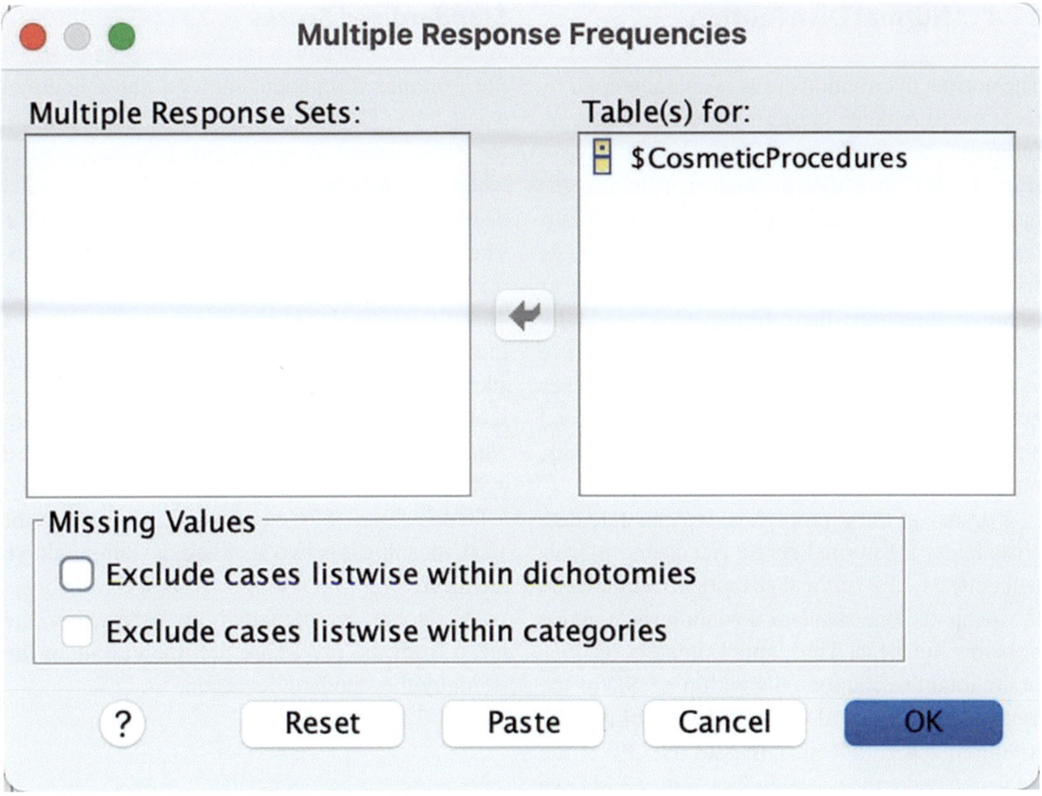

Fig. 11.24 Moving the $CosmeticProcedures variable to the "Table(s) for" box in SPSS for frequency analysis

Fig. 11.25 Output table generated from multiple response frequency analysis in SPSS

$CosmeticProcedures Frequencies

		Responses		Percent of Cases
		N	Percent	
Cosmetic Procedures Received[a]	Botulinum	9	23.1%	50.0%
	Filler	14	35.9%	77.8%
	Laser	2	5.1%	11.1%
	SkinBoost	2	5.1%	11.1%
	Microneedling	10	25.6%	55.6%
	ChemicalPeeling	2	5.1%	11.1%
Total		39	100.0%	216.7%

a. Dichotomy group tabulated at value 1.

11.4 Normal Distribution

The normal distribution curve is characterized by most measurements clustering around the mean, forming a symmetric, bell-shaped curve (Fig. 11.26). In a true normal distribution, the mean, median, and mode are identical. Both kurtosis and skewness are zero. As scores deviate further from the mean in either the positive or negative direction, their frequencies gradually decrease. Theoretically, the tails of the curve extend indefinitely; that is, the curve approaches but never actually touches the x-axis. The total area under the curve represents probability, meaning that the entire area equals 1.

Because of these properties, we can calculate areas under the normal curve. According to statisticians, 34.13% of the distribution lies between the mean and one standard deviation (SD) above or below the mean. Thus, approximately 68.26% of the total distribution falls within ±1 SD of the mean. Similarly, ±2 SD covers 95.44% of the distribution, and ±3 SD encompasses 99.73% of the total area under the curve. In fact, with ±3 SD, we can account for nearly the entire distribution. Using the characteristics of the normal distribution, we can interpret standard deviations. For example, if the mean $\underline{x} = 65$ and the standard deviation SD = 6.06, we can estimate that approximately 68% of the sample measurements fall between 58.94 and 71.06.

Standardized Scores

For example, if a patient shows a transepidermal water loss (TEWL) measurement of 58 g/m^2/h, the significance of this value becomes clearer when it is interpreted in relation to the normal distribution of TEWL values. If we know that the sample has a mean ($\bar{x}$) of 56 and a standard deviation (SD) of 10, we can see that a TEWL value of 46 falls within 1 SD below the mean. When a score is expressed using SD units, it is called a standardized score, or a *z-score*. In this case, a score of 46 corresponds to a *z*-score of −1.0, where the negative sign indicates that it is located one standard deviation below the mean. Similarly, a TEWL value of 76 corresponds to a z-score of +2.0, meaning it is two standard deviations above the mean.

A *z*-score is calculated by subtracting the mean from the raw score and then dividing the result by the standard deviation.

$$z = \frac{x - \underline{x}}{SD}$$

For instance, if the TEWL is 80, with $\bar{x} = 60$ and SD = 10,

$$z = \frac{80 - 60}{10}$$

Thus, a TEWL value of 80 is located two standard deviations above the mean.

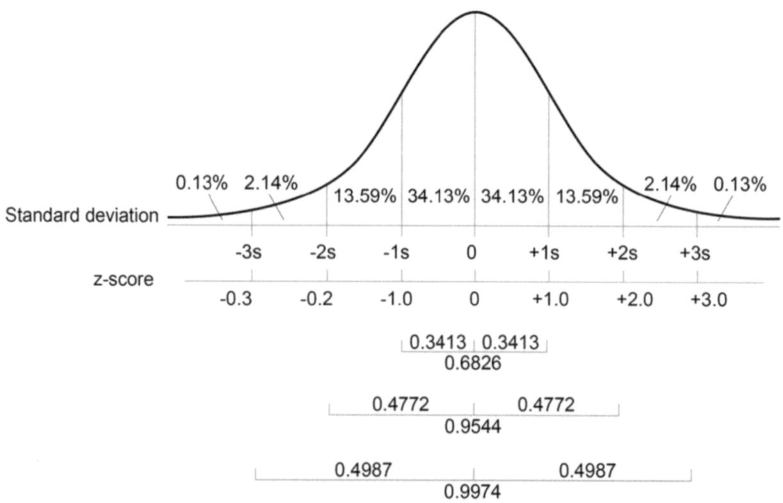

Fig. 11.26 Normal distribution curve

Standardized Normal Curve

A normal distribution can be represented using standardized scores. In a distribution of z-scores, the mean is always 0 and the standard deviation (SD) is always 1. As shown in the figure above, the area under the standardized normal curve between $z = 0$ and $z = +1.0$ is approximately 34%, which corresponds to the area between the mean ($z = 0$) and 1 SD. The total area within $z = \pm 2.0$ is 95.44% (±2 SD). Using this model, we can determine the proportional area under the curve between any two points within a normal distribution.

Suppose the TEWL value is given as $\bar{x} = 56$ g/m²/h with SD = 12. If we want to know what percentage of the sample has a TEWL greater than 34, we first calculate the z-score for a TEWL value of 34.

$$z = \frac{34 - 56}{12} = \frac{-22}{12} = -1.83$$

Thus, a TEWL of 34 falls approximately within 2 SD below the mean.

Refer to Fig. 11.27, where the shaded area represents all scores greater than 34, or equivalently, all scores greater than $z = -1.8$. To determine this area, we first calculate the area between 34 and 56, which corresponds to the area between $z = 0$ and $z = 1.8$. Since the area from the center to the right represents 50% of the curve, we proceed by referring to the standardized normal distribution table (Table 11.8).

This table is organized into three columns: the first column lists the z-scores, and the next two columns show the areas between 0 and z, and the areas beyond z, respectively. In this example, we are interested in the area from 0 to 1.8. Because the normal curve is symmetrical, the area from 0 to +1.8 is the same as that from 0 to –1.8.

From Table 11.8, for $z = 1.80$, the area between 0 and z is found to be 0.4641, or 46.41% of the curve.

Therefore, the total area corresponding to TEWL values above 34 is 50% + 46.41% = 96.41%.

As another example, suppose we want to find the area corresponding to TEWL values greater than 70.

The z-score for 72 is calculated as (70–56)/12 = 14/12 = 1.17. Referring again to Table 11.8, the area beyond $z = 1.2$ is 0.1151, or 11.51% of the curve (Fig. 11.28).

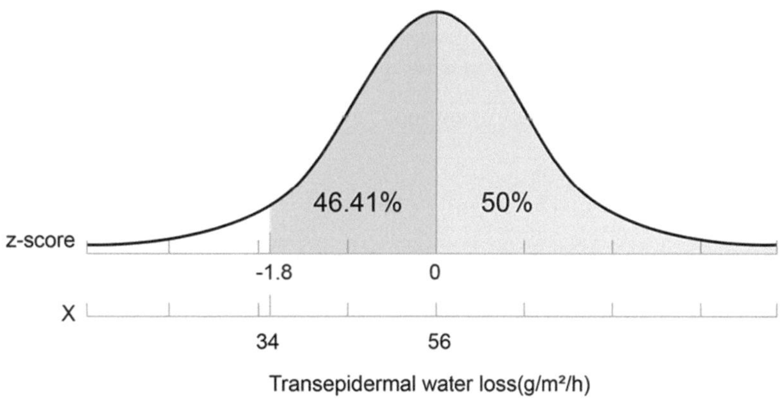

Fig. 11.27 *Z*-score for TEWL of 34 when the mean TEWL is 56 and the standard deviation is 12

Table 11.8 Areas under the standardized normal distribution curve

z	Area between 0 and z	Area above z	z	Area between 0 and z	Area above z	z	Area between 0 and z	Area above z
1.20	.3849	.1151	1.60	.4452	.0548	2.00	.4772	.0228
1.21	.3869	.1131	1.61	.4463	.0537	2.01	.4778	.0222
1.22	.3888	.1112	1.62	.4474	.0526	2.02	.4783	.0217
1.23	.3907	.1093	1.63	.4484	.0516	2.03	.4788	.0212
1.24	.3925	.1075	1.64	.4495	.0505	2.04	.4793	.0207
			1.645	.4500	.0500			
1.25	.3944	.1056	1.65	.4505	.0495	2.05	.4798	.0202
1.26	.3962	.1038	1.66	.4515	.0485	2.054	.4800	.0200
1.27	.3980	.1020	1.67	.4525	.0475	2.06	.4803	.0197
1.28	.3997	.1003	1.68	.4535	.0465	2.07	.4808	.0192
1.29	.4015	.0985	1.69	.4545	.0455	2.08	.4812	.0188
						2.09	.4817	.0183
1.30	.4032	.0968	1.70	.4554	.0446	2.10	.4821	.0179
1.31	.4049	.0951	1.71	.4564	.0436	2.11	.4826	.0174
1.32	.4066	.0934	1.72	.4573	.0427	2.12	.4830	.0170
1.33	.4082	.0918	1.73	.4582	.0418	2.13	.4834	.0166
1.34	.4099	.0901	1.74	.4591	.0409	2.14	.4838	.0162
1.35	.4115	.0885	1.75	.4559	.0401	2.15	.4842	.0158
1.36	.4131	.0869	1.751	.4600	.0400	2.16	.4846	.0154
1.37	.4147	.0853	1.76	.4608	.0392	2.17	.4850	.0150
1.38	.4162	.0838	1.77	.4606	.0384	2.18	.4854	.0146
1.39	.4177	.0823	1.78	.4625	.0375	2.19	.4857	.0143
			1.79	.4633	.0367			
1.40	.4192	.0808	1.80	.4641	.0359	2.20	.4861	.0139
1.41	.4207	.0793	1.81	.4649	.0351	2.21	.4864	.0136
1.42	.4222	.0778	1.82	.4656	.0344	2.22	.4868	.0132
1.43	.4236	.0764	1.83	.4664	.0336	2.23	.4871	.0129
1.44	.4251	.0749	1.84	.4671	.0329	2.24	.4875	.0125
1.45	.4265	.0735	1.85	.4678	.0322	2.25	.4878	.0122
1.46	.4279	.0721	1.86	04688	.0314	2.26	.4881	.0119
1.47	.4292	.0708	1.87	.4693	.0307	2.27	.4884	.0116
1.48	.4306	.0694	1.88	.4699	.0301	2.28	.4887	.01113
1.49	.4319	.0681	1.881	.4700	.0300	2.29	.4890	.0110

			1.89	.4706	.0294			
1.50	.4332	.0668	1.90	.4713	.0287	2.30	.4893	.0107
1.51	.4345	.0655	1.91	.4719	.0281	2.31	.4896	.0104
1.52	.4357	.0643	1.92	.4726	.0274	2.32	.4898	.0102
1.53	.4370	.0630	1.93	.4732	.0268	2.328	.4900	.0100
1.54	.4382	.0618	1.94	.4738	.0333	2.33	.4901	.0099
						2.34	.4904	.0096
1.55	.4394	.0606	1.95	.4744	.0256	2.35	.4906	.0094
1.56	.4406	.0594	1.96	.4750	.0250	2.36	.4909	.0091
1.57	.4418	.0582	1.97	.4756	.0244	2.37	.4911	.0089
1.58	.4429	.0571	1.98	.4761	.0239	2.38	.4913	.0087
1.59	.4441	.0559	1.99	.4767	.0233	2.39	.4915	.0084

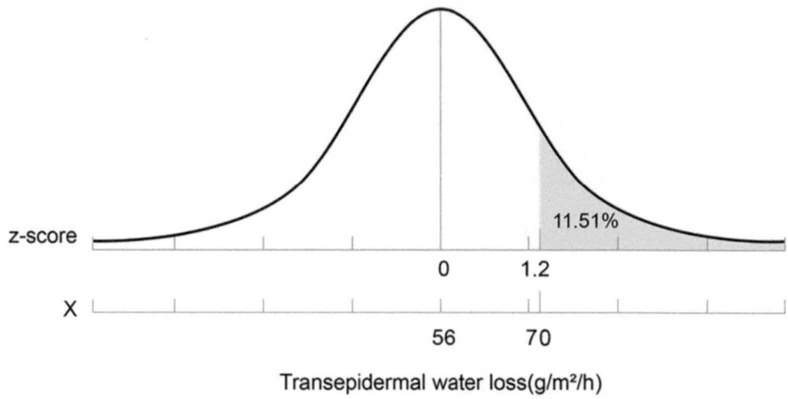

Fig. 11.28 *Z*-score for TEWL of 70 when the mean TEWL is 56 and the standard deviation is 12

Reference

Yancy JM. Ten rules for reading clinical research reports [Editorial]. *Am J Surg*. 1990;159(6):553–559

Basic Statistics (2) 12

12.1 Sampling and Sampling Distributions

1. *Why Do We Conduct Sampling?*

   In statistics, a population refers to the entire group that includes every individual we are interested in studying. In most cases, it is neither economically, temporally, nor logistically feasible to study every member of a population. Sometimes, it is even necessary to conceptualize hypothetical populations, such as "individuals who may receive treatment in the future," in which case it would be impossible to study the entire group directly. Therefore, researchers collect and analyze data from a sample that represents the population and make inferences about the entire population based on that sample.

   When data are collected through sampling from a population, the sample cannot perfectly represent the population. The discrepancy that arises from studying only a subset rather than the entire population is referred to as sampling error.

2. *Sampling for Representativeness*

   The most ideal method is simple random sampling. If a complete list of the population members (sampling frame) is created and individuals are selected randomly, each member will have an equal chance of being selected. However, for economic or time-related reasons, it is often difficult to obtain a complete list of the entire population. In such cases, researchers may choose a convenience sample, selecting subjects who are easily accessible. For example, when studying patients with rare conditions, a researcher might select a particular hospital and study some or all of the patients there. Sometimes, other sampling methods such as quota sampling or systematic sampling are used.

3. *Point Estimates and Interval Estimates*

   Estimation is concerned with parameters—values such as means or proportions—calculated from a population. Parameters are usually denoted by Greek letters: for example, the population mean is represented by μ, and the standard deviation by σ. Researchers estimate these parameters based on data obtained from samples.

   There are two main methods for estimating parameters: point estimation and interval estimation, both of which require an understanding of sampling distributions. Point estimation refers to the use of a single value calculated directly from sample data to estimate a population parameter. For example, estimating that the average life expectancy of women is 70 years or that the smoking rate among female college students is 30% are both examples of point estimates. However, using a single sample-derived value as an estimate for the true population parameter inevitably involves some error. Therefore, it is more

K.-H. Yi, *Statistical Research Methods for Dermatologists and Plastic Surgeons*,
https://doi.org/10.1007/978-981-95-5668-7_12

meaningful to provide a confidence interval (CI), which suggests a range within which the parameter is likely to fall, rather than relying solely on a point estimate.

For instance, suppose we measure the Melanin Index reduction after fractional laser treatment in individuals aged 30–39. If we randomly select 42 participants and find that the mean reduction is 15.0 units, with a standard deviation of 4.2 units, then the point estimate for the mean is 15.0. However, we cannot be fully confident about how closely this point estimate reflects the true population mean. Instead, it is preferable to present a confidence interval that indicates the plausible range where the true population mean is expected to lie.

Confidence intervals express the boundaries derived from the sample mean and the standard error (SE). The wider the confidence interval, the greater the likelihood that it contains the true parameter. Confidence levels are usually expressed as percentages, with 95% confidence intervals being the most commonly used.

For example, if the mean reduction is 15.0, the standard deviation is 4.2, and $n = 42$, then the standard error is calculated as $\mathrm{SE} = 4.2 / \sqrt{42} = 0.648$.

Thus, the 95% confidence interval (CI) is:

$$95\%\mathrm{CI} = \bar{x} \pm (1.96)\mathrm{SE}$$

$$95\%\mathrm{CI} = 15 \pm (1.96)(0.648) = 15 \pm 1.27$$

$$95\%\mathrm{CI} = 13.73 \le \mu \le 16.27$$

This means that the population mean for Melanin Index reduction after fractional laser treatment in individuals aged 30–39 is estimated to fall between 13.73 and 16.27, with approximately 95% confidence. For a 99% confidence interval, the calculation would be:

$$99\%\mathrm{CI} = \bar{x} \pm (2.58)\mathrm{SE}$$

$$99\%\mathrm{CI} = 15 \pm (2.58)(0.648) = 15 \pm 1.67$$

$$99\%\mathrm{CI} = 13.33 \le \mu \le 16.67$$

Thus, the population mean is estimated to lie between 13.33 and 16.67, with approximately 99% confidence.

Since single-sample estimates inherently involve error, presenting confidence intervals is significantly more meaningful. The interpretation of a 95% confidence interval is similar to stating that if we were to draw an infinite number of samples using the same method, approximately 95% of the resulting confidence intervals would contain the true population parameter. For example, suppose we conduct 100 sample surveys in the same manner and construct 100 confidence intervals. Among these, 95 of the confidence intervals would contain the population parameter.

4. *Sampling Distribution of the Mean*

When we repeatedly draw samples of the same size from a population, it is unlikely that the mean of each sample will exactly match the population mean (the parameter). If a researcher aims to estimate the population mean, they can repeatedly draw many samples from the population and calculate the mean for each sample. The distribution formed by all these sample means is called the sampling distribution of the mean. Theoretically, the mean of all the sample means will equal the population mean. Moreover, according to the Central Limit Theorem, as the sample size (n) increases, the distribution of the sample means will approximate a normal distribution regardless of the shape of the original population distribution.

The standard deviation of the sampling distribution of the mean is called the standard error of the mean (SEM). If the population standard deviation (σ) is known, SEM is calculated as $\mathrm{SEM} = \sigma / \sqrt{n}$. However, because the population standard deviation is rarely known in practice, the sample standard deviation (s) is typically used, and SEM is estimated as $\mathrm{SEM} = s / \sqrt{n}$, where s is the sample standard deviation and n is the sample size. Thus, as indicated by the formula, the larger the sample size, the smaller the SEM becomes.

In summary, if we were to draw all possible samples from a population and calculate the mean for each sample, the distribution of these sample means would ultimately approach a normal distribution. The mean of the sample means would equal the population mean, and the variance of the sample means would be equal to the population variance divided by the sample size. Taking the square root of this variance gives the standard error, which represents the standard deviation of the sample means.

5. *Interpretation of the Standard Error*

   A large standard error indicates that the estimate is less precise, whereas a small standard error suggests that the estimate is relatively accurate.

   If the sample size is large and the variability within the data is small, the standard error will decrease, allowing researchers to obtain a more accurate estimate of the population parameter.

6. *Should We Use Standard Deviation or Standard Error?*

   Although the standard deviation and the standard error may appear similar, they serve different purposes. The standard deviation reflects the variability within a set of data and is used to describe how widely data points are dispersed around the mean. In contrast, the standard error represents the precision of the sample mean as an estimate of the population mean.

12.2 Hypothesis Testing

A hypothesis is "a statement that predicts a relationship between two or more variables." When formulating a hypothesis, the following points must be observed:

First, the hypothesis must state a relationship between variables.
Second, it must be testable.
Third, it must be simple and clear.
Fourth, it should be stated in the present tense, as a hypothesis is a tentative conclusion. However, in cases where it predicts outcomes, it may also be expressed in the future tense.

Below are examples of research hypotheses adapted for studies in cosmetic dermatology and plastic surgery:

Example 1: In the general population, there is a correlation between skin elasticity and subjective satisfaction with facial appearance.
Example 2: In individuals with normal skin and those with photoaged skin, prior exposure to UV-protection education influences both immediate and voluntary sun-protection behaviors.
Example 3: In patients undergoing facial filler treatments, age impacts treatment satisfaction levels.
Example 4: The average improvement in melanin index among patients participating in a 6-week brightening skincare program will be significantly greater than that of patients who do not participate in the program.
Example 5: Patients with low self-esteem will report a higher level of dissatisfaction with cosmetic procedure outcomes than those with high self-esteem.
Example 6: Individuals with delayed wound healing times will achieve lower scores on scar assessment scales compared to peers with normal healing rates.
Example 7: Early application of skin hydration interventions will enhance recovery of skin barrier function following ablative laser procedures.
Example 8: Microneedling treatment will benefit skin texture improvement. Alternatively, microneedling treatment may have adverse effects on skin integrity.
Example 9: Patients using antioxidant serums in combination with sunscreen will show greater reduction in hyperpigmentation compared to those using sunscreen alone.
Example 10: Regular use of retinoid-based skincare products will be more effective in reducing fine wrinkles than vitamin C-based products.

12.3 Null Hypothesis and Alternative Hypothesis

In hypothesis testing, the researcher tests the null hypothesis (H_0). The null hypothesis assumes that there is no effect or no difference due to the treatment or intervention. In other words, it assumes that the difference in means between the respective populations is zero. For example, if the researcher's interest lies in comparing the prevalence of melasma between patients who have undergone chemical peeling and those who have not, the hypotheses could be stated as follows:

H_0: The prevalence of melasma is the same between patients who have received chemical peeling and those who have not.

Next, the researcher establishes the alternative hypothesis (H_1). The alternative hypothesis describes what would be true if the null hypothesis is not correct. It is directly related to the researcher's theory or research question. In the above example, the alternative hypothesis would be:

H_1: The prevalence of melasma differs between patients who have received chemical peeling and those who have not.

It should be noted that the alternative hypothesis stated above does not specify a direction. That is, it does not indicate whether melasma is more or less prevalent in the treated group. When no direction is specified, a two-tailed test is conducted. If the alternative hypothesis specifies the direction (e.g., the prevalence is lower in the treatment group), a one-tailed test is appropriate.

Generally, two-tailed tests are considered more conservative than one-tailed tests. For example, with a t-test at 10 degrees of freedom and a significance level of 0.05, the critical value for a two-tailed test is 2.228, while for a one-tailed test it is 1.812.

After collecting data, the researcher substitutes the observed data into the appropriate statistical formula to calculate the test statistic. The test statistic provides evidence against the null hypothesis; generally, the larger the absolute value of the test statistic, the stronger the evidence against H_0.

The researcher must determine how much evidence is necessary to reject the null hypothesis. A smaller p-value indicates stronger evidence against H_0. Traditionally, if the p-value is less than 0.05, there is sufficient evidence to reject the null hypothesis at the 5% level. This is because, if the null hypothesis is true, the probability of obtaining such a result would be less than 1 in 20. Therefore, when the p-value associated with the test statistic is less than 0.05, the researcher rejects the null hypothesis and concludes that the results are statistically significant at the 5% level.

In contrast, if the p-value is greater than 0.05, the conclusion is that there is not enough evidence to reject the null hypothesis. It is important to note that not rejecting H_0 does not mean H_0 is true. Rather, it means there is insufficient evidence to conclude that a difference exists. For example, if a p-value of 0.17 is obtained when comparing the mean melanin reduction between two skin treatment groups, it would be inappropriate to conclude "there is no difference." Instead, the correct interpretation would be: "There is not enough evidence to conclude a difference exists."

Choosing a 5% significance level is arbitrary. If rejecting the null hypothesis at the 5% level could lead to serious clinical implications—such as risks associated with a new cosmetic procedure—researchers may require stronger evidence, using a cutoff p-value of 0.01 or 0.001. This preset significance level (0.05, 0.01, etc.) is referred to as the significance level (α level) (Fig. 12.1).

When presenting results, simply stating "statistically significant at the 0.05 level" can be misleading. For instance, if the p-value is 0.049, the null hypothesis would be rejected; if it is 0.051, it would not. However, in reality, $p = 0.049$ and $p = 0.051$ are not substantially different. Because of this, it is now encouraged to report the exact p-value and allow readers to make their own judgments.

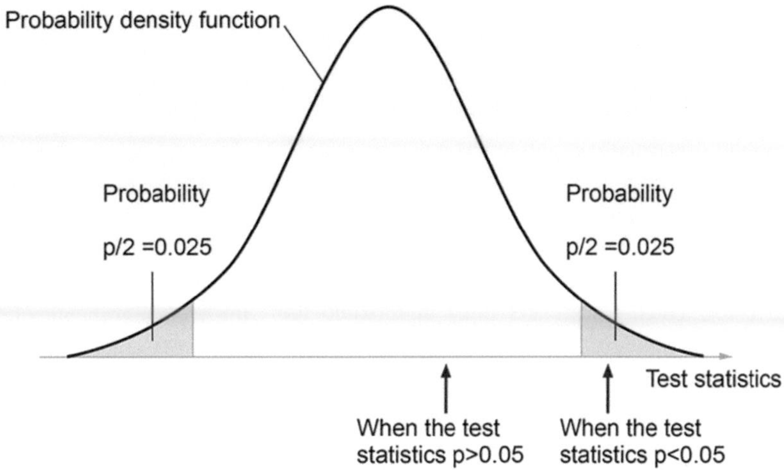

Fig. 12.1 Probability distribution for a two-tailed test at $p = 0.05$

Additionally, statistical significance and clinical significance do not always align. For example, even if a facial lifting procedure statistically improves skin elasticity by a small measurable degree, the improvement might be clinically meaningless if it falls within the margin of measurement error. In conclusion, hypothesis testing is a useful tool for interpreting results but should not be treated as the ultimate truth.

12.4 Errors in Hypothesis Testing

When testing the treatment effects between a treatment group and a control group using a two-tailed test, the null hypothesis (H_0) is stated as "there is no difference in treatment effect" or "the treatment effects are equal." The alternative hypothesis (H_1) states "the difference in treatment effect is not zero." The purpose of hypothesis testing is to determine whether there is sufficient evidence to reject the null hypothesis. The researcher has two choices: either to reject the null hypothesis or to fail to reject it.

Although researchers wish to reach correct conclusions about the null hypothesis, they must recognize that, because they rely on sample information rather than the entire population, there is always a risk of making incorrect decisions—either by rejecting or failing to reject the null hypothesis. The possible types of errors in hypothesis testing are summarized in Table 12.1.

Table 12.1 Outcomes of hypothesis testing

	Reject the null hypothesis	Fail to reject the null hypothesis
Null hypothesis is true	Type I error (α error)	Correct decision (no error)
Null hypothesis is false	Correct decision (power = $1 - \beta$)	Type II error (β error)

- *Type I error*: Rejecting the null hypothesis when it is actually true. This means concluding that a treatment effect exists when, in fact, it does not. The probability of committing a Type I error is denoted by α (alpha). α is also referred to as the significance level of the test. When the *p*-value from the test statistic is smaller than the significance level ($p < \alpha$), the null hypothesis is rejected. Researchers must decide on the α level before collecting data. Traditionally, $\alpha = 0.05$ is used, although more stringent criteria like $\alpha = 0.01$ are sometimes applied. The probability of making a Type I error does not exceed the predetermined α level. For example, if $\alpha = 0.05$, and the *p*-value is less than 0.05, the null hypothesis is rejected; if the *p*-value is greater than 0.05, the null hypothesis is not rejected, thereby avoiding a Type I error.
- *Type II error*: Failing to reject the null hypothesis when it is actually false. This means concluding that there is no treatment effect when, in fact, there is one. The probability of making

a Type II error is denoted by β (beta), and the complement $(1 - \beta)$ is called the *power* of the test. Statistical power refers to the probability of correctly rejecting a false null hypothesis, and it is usually expressed as a percentage.

Ideally, researchers aim for 100% power, but this is not realistically achievable because there is always a slight possibility of committing a Type II error. Thus, researchers must understand the statistical power of the method they intend to use during the study design phase. In clinical research, a power level of 70–80% is generally considered acceptable. If the power is as low as 40%, conducting a clinical trial would be considered a waste of time and resources.

Several factors affect statistical power: sample size (n), variability of observations (s^2), effect size (ES), and the significance level (α). Larger sample sizes increase statistical power, meaning it becomes easier to detect clinically meaningful effects with larger samples than with smaller ones. Lower variability among observations also increases power. Additionally, larger treatment effect sizes lead to higher power. Finally, the significance level affects power: when the significance level (α) is increased, the probability of a Type I error rises, but the probability of a Type II error (β) decreases, resulting in higher power $(1 - \beta)$. Thus, setting the significance level at 0.05 rather than a stricter 0.01 makes it more likely to achieve statistical significance before the experiment begins.

12.5 Statistical Power and Sample Size

In power analysis, factors such as significance level, sample size, sample variance, effect size, and statistical power are considered. Effect size refers to the magnitude of a difference or the strength of a relationship. When the number of participants is either very small or very large, statistical results can be distorted; effect size helps to correct for such distortions. For example, when the sample size is large, even a very small difference may become statistically significant. In such cases, reporting the effect size helps determine whether the result is truly meaningful. Effect sizes are also useful in meta-analyses, allowing comparisons across studies with different sample sizes.

The larger the observed effect difference, the more likely it is to be statistically significant at the same significance level. The effect size index refers to a standardized measure—such as t, F, or r—that is dimensionless and can be applied across different types of data. After a study is completed, information such as sample size, variance, means, and correlation coefficients becomes available, allowing researchers to calculate the statistical power. However, when such data are not available beforehand, the researcher must estimate the expected effect size. This estimation can be based on previous research findings or preliminary (pilot) studies that provide reasonable estimates for mean differences, correlations, or variances. If even preliminary data are unavailable, the researcher must rely on professional judgment to estimate what would constitute a clinically meaningful difference. For example, suppose two different treatment methods are being compared for improving post-inflammatory hyperpigmentation (PIH) following laser procedures. The researcher may determine that a reduction of at least 15 units in the melanin index between the two treatments would be considered clinically meaningful. In this case, a 15-unit difference would be used as the expected effect size. Similarly, in a correlational study, a researcher might judge that a correlation coefficient of $r = 0.6$ would represent a meaningful relationship. Such clinical judgments often serve as a guide for estimating the required sample size.

When no existing data are available for planning the sample size, researchers can use the conventional values suggested by Cohen. Cohen categorized effect sizes into small, medium, and large categories. These classifications are relative and should be considered in the context of the specific research setting.

In general, Cohen's d is commonly used to calculate effect size:

- 0.2 indicates a small effect
- 0.5 indicates a medium effect
- 0.8 indicates a large effect

There are five major types of methods for calculating effect size, each with its own formula:

1. Between two independent groups
2. Within two dependent groups (paired samples)
3. For correlation studies
4. For analysis of variance (ANOVA)
5. For meta-analysis

When comparing the effect size between two groups (e.g., experimental vs. control), Cohen's d is typically used. The formula is as follows:

$$d = \left(\bar{X}_1 - \bar{X}_2\right) / s$$

where $\bar{X}_1$ and $\bar{X}_2$ are the group means, and s is the standard deviation.

Let us illustrate how to calculate the statistical power and sample size in the case of an independent t-test assuming equal variances. Suppose we measure the improvement in skin brightness after a new skin rejuvenation procedure. The results are as follows: mean improvement score for Group 1 (treatment group) is $\bar{X}_1 = 10.11$, mean for Group 2 (control group) is $\bar{X}_2 = 5.45$, and the pooled variance (s_p^2) is 14.695. Assuming a directional hypothesis was set, the calculation would proceed as:

$$d = \left(\bar{X}_1 - \bar{X}_2\right) / s$$

$$s = \sqrt{s^2} = \sqrt{14.695} = 3.83,$$
$$d = \left(10.11 - 5.45\right) / 3.83 = 1.22$$

If $t = 2.718$ and the sample size for each group is $n = 10$, another way to calculate d is:

$$d = t\sqrt{\frac{n_1 + n_2}{n_1 n_2}} = 2.718\sqrt{\frac{10+10}{(10)(10)}}$$
$$= 2.718\sqrt{0.20} = 1.22$$

Based on this, to find the statistical power, we would refer to Cohen's power table. For $\alpha_1 = 0.05$ and $n = 10$ per group, the power for $d = 1.2$ would be approximately 83%. If we aim for a standard power of 80%, we would consult the second table, which indicates that each group would need about 9 participants (a total of 18 participants) to achieve sufficient power.

Power of the t-Test for α1 =0.05

	d										
n	0.10	0.20	0.30	0.40	0.50	0.60	0.70	0.80	1.00	1.20	1.40
8	07	10	13	19	25	31	38	46	61	74	85
9	07	11	15	20	27	34	41	50	66	79	88
10	08	11	16	22	29	36	45	53	70	83	91
11	08	12	17	23	31	39	48	57	74	86	94
12	08	12	18	25	33	41	51	60	77	89	96
13	08	13	18	26	34	44	54	63	80	91	97
14	08	13	19	27	36	46	57	66	83	93	98
15	08	13	20	28	38	48	59	69	85	94	98
16	09	14	21	30	40	51	62	72	87	95	99
17	09	14	22	31	42	53	64	74	89	96	99
18	09	15	22	32	43	55	66	76	90	97	99
19	09	15	23	33	45	57	68	78	92	98	
20	09	15	24	34	46	59	70	80	93	98	
30	10	19	31	46	61	74	85	92	99		
40	11	22	38	55	72	84	93	97			
50	12	26	44	63	80	91	97	99			
100	17	41	68	88	97						
200	26	64	91	99							

Sample Sizes Needed for the t-Test

	d										
Power	0.10	0.20	0.30	0.40	0.50	0.60	0.70	0.80	1.00	1.20	1.40
$\alpha_1 = .05$											
0.70	942	236	105	60	38	27	20	15	10	7	6
0.80	1237	310	138	78	50	35	26	20	13	9	7
0.90	1713	429	191	108	69	48	36	27	18	13	10

If, during the planning phase of the study, a two-tailed hypothesis test is to be conducted and a difference of approximately 5 kg is considered clinically meaningful, and if the standard deviation is assumed to be 8.0, then the effect size d would be calculated as $d = 5/8 = 0.625$. According to the second table, when alpha = 0.05 and d = 0.60, a sample size of 35 participants per group (a total of 70 participants) would be required to achieve 80% power.

The above example illustrates how to calculate statistical power and sample size for an independent t-test assuming equal variances. In actual studies, however, different formulas and tables must be used depending on the situation, such as for paired t-tests, when variances are unequal, analysis of variance (ANOVA), two-way ANOVA, correlation analysis, regression analysis, and chi-square tests.

To calculate the required sample size using a software program, you can use a tool called *G**Power. To download this program, you can search for "*G*Power" in the search bar at http://www.google.com or directly download it from http://www.psycho.uni-duesseldorf.de/abteilungen/aap/gpower3/ (Fig. 12.2).

To download the program, scroll down the website and select the appropriate version for your computer's operating system under the Download section. For users with Microsoft Windows, click on "Download *G**Power 3.1.9.7 for Windows" and follow the installation instructions (Fig. 12.3).

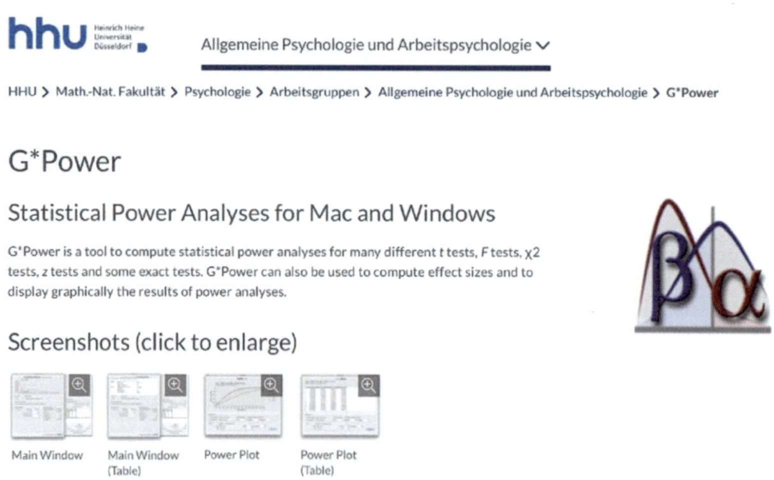

Fig. 12.2 Homepage of the *G**Power website, which provides access to the statistical software for sample size and power calculations

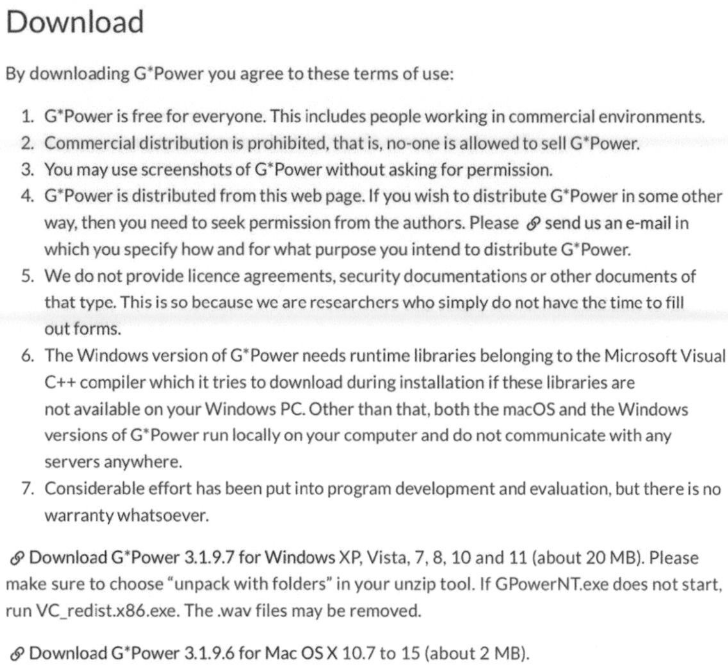

Download

By downloading G*Power you agree to these terms of use:

1. G*Power is free for everyone. This includes people working in commercial environments.
2. Commercial distribution is prohibited, that is, no-one is allowed to sell G*Power.
3. You may use screenshots of G*Power without asking for permission.
4. G*Power is distributed from this web page. If you wish to distribute G*Power in some other way, then you need to seek permission from the authors. Please send us an e-mail in which you specify how and for what purpose you intend to distribute G*Power.
5. We do not provide licence agreements, security documentations or other documents of that type. This is so because we are researchers who simply do not have the time to fill out forms.
6. The Windows version of G*Power needs runtime libraries belonging to the Microsoft Visual C++ compiler which it tries to download during installation if these libraries are not available on your Windows PC. Other than that, both the macOS and the Windows versions of G*Power run locally on your computer and do not communicate with any servers anywhere.
7. Considerable effort has been put into program development and evaluation, but there is no warranty whatsoever.

Download G*Power 3.1.9.7 for Windows XP, Vista, 7, 8, 10 and 11 (about 20 MB). Please make sure to choose "unpack with folders" in your unzip tool. If GPowerNT.exe does not start, run VC_redist.x86.exe. The .wav files may be removed.

Download G*Power 3.1.9.6 for Mac OS X 10.7 to 15 (about 2 MB).

Fig. 12.3 Instructions and links for downloading the *G**Power software from the official website

Let us now walk through the process of calculating statistical power for an independent t-test using the *G**Power program (Fig. 12.4). Suppose Group 1 consists of 20 participants with a mean of 10.1 and a standard deviation of 3.3, and Group 2 consists of 18 participants with a mean of 15.4 and a standard deviation of 5.5. We aim to determine the statistical power of this analysis.

	Group 1 ($n = 20$)	Group 2 ($n = 18$)
Mean	10.1	15.4
Standard deviation	3.3	5.5

From the main screen, click on Tests, select Means, and then choose Two independent groups (Fig. 12.5). In the middle of the screen, under Type of power analysis, click the downward arrow and select Post hoc: Compute achieved power—given α, sample size, and effect size (Fig. 12.6). Then click Determine, and in the newly opened window, select $n1 \neq n2$ (indicating unequal group sizes), enter 10.1 for Mean group 1, and enter 15.4 for Mean group 2 (Figs. 12.7 and 12.8). Since the group sizes differ ($n1 \neq n2$), a pooled standard deviation must be calculated using the following formula:

$$
\begin{aligned}
\text{SD pooled} &= \text{sqrt}\left(\left(n1-1\right)s1^2 + \left(n2-1\right)s2^2 / n1 + n2 - 2\right) \\
&= \text{sqrt}\left(\left(20-1\right)3.3^2 + \left(18-1\right)5.5^2 / 20 + 18 - 2\right) \\
&= \text{sqrt}\left(20.87\right) \\
&= \sqrt{20.87} = 4.57
\end{aligned}
$$

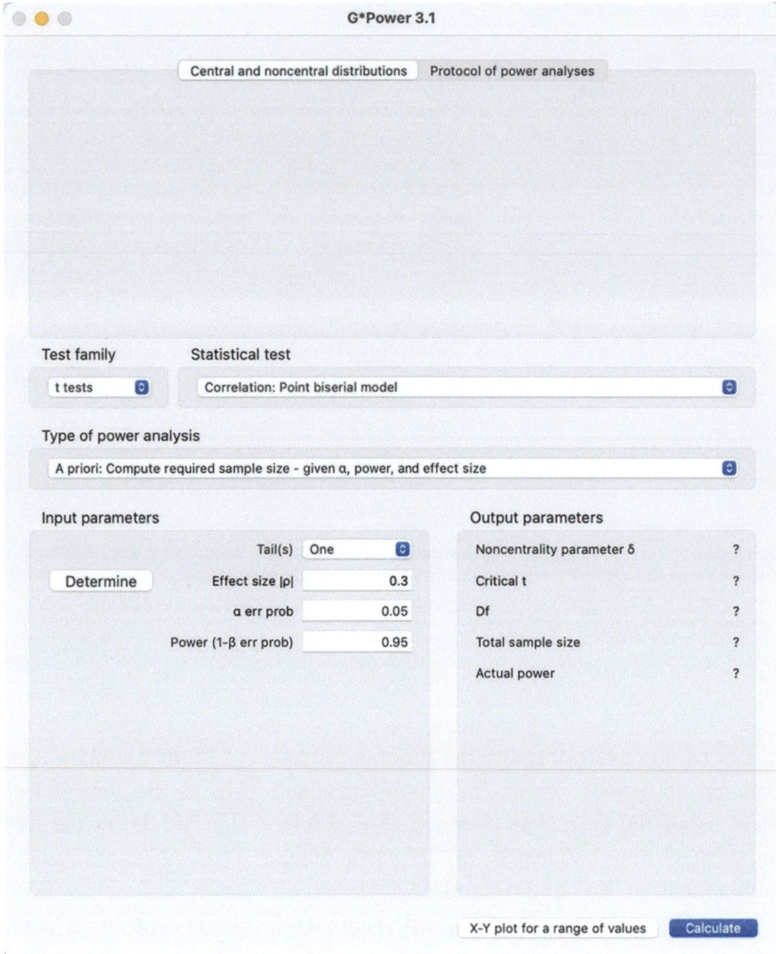

Fig. 12.4 Initial interface of the *G**Power 3.1 software

After calculating, input 4.57 into the SDσ within each group field. Click Calculate, then Calculate and transfer to the main window, and close the window. In the Input Parameters panel, set Tail(s) to Two, enter 20 for Sample size group 1, enter 18 for Sample size group 2, and click Calculate (Figs. 12.9 and 12.10).

The result displayed under Power ($1 - \beta$ err prob) is 0.93. A power of 0.93 is considered high and indicates that the test has a strong ability to detect a true effect (Fig. 12.11).

Let us now calculate the appropriate sample size for this experiment. From the initial screen in *G**Power, click on Tests, and then select Means: Difference between two independent means (two groups) (Fig. 12.12). Alternatively, instead of navigating through the menus, you may directly select Test family → t-tests and Statistical test → Means: Difference between two independent means (two groups). In the Type of power analysis field, choose A priori: Compute required sample size—given α, power, and effect size (Fig. 12.13). Then click Determine. In the pop-up window, select $n1 \neq n2$ (indicating unequal sample sizes). Enter the following values: Mean group 1: 10.1, Mean group 2: 15.4, and SDσ within each group: 4.57 (Fig. 12.14). Click Calculate, then Calculate and transfer to the main window, and close the window. Back in the main screen, set Tails to Two, enter 0.80 for Power ($1 - \beta$ err prob), and click Calculate (Fig. 12.15).

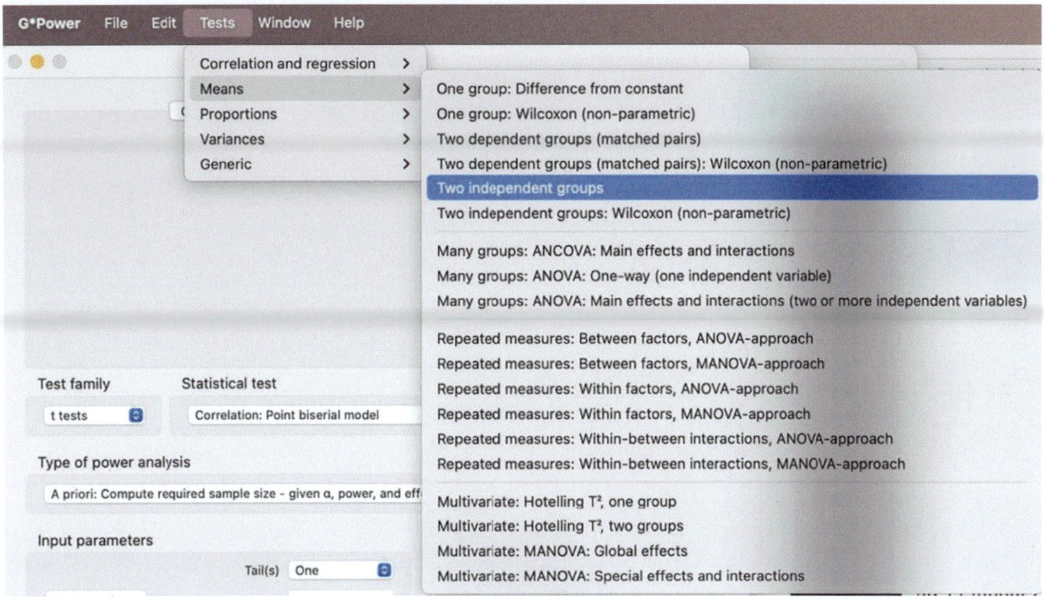

Fig. 12.5 Selecting "Two Independent Groups" under the "Means" test family in *G**Power

Fig. 12.6 Selecting "Post hoc: Compute achieved power – given *α*, sample size, and effect size" under Type of power analysis in *G**Power

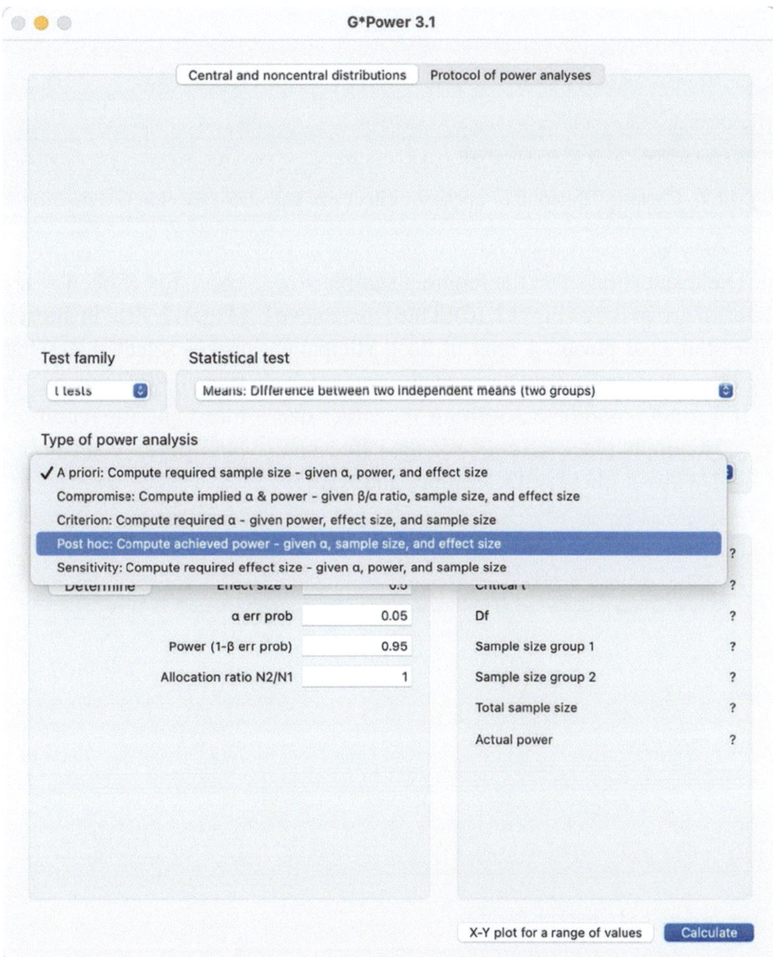

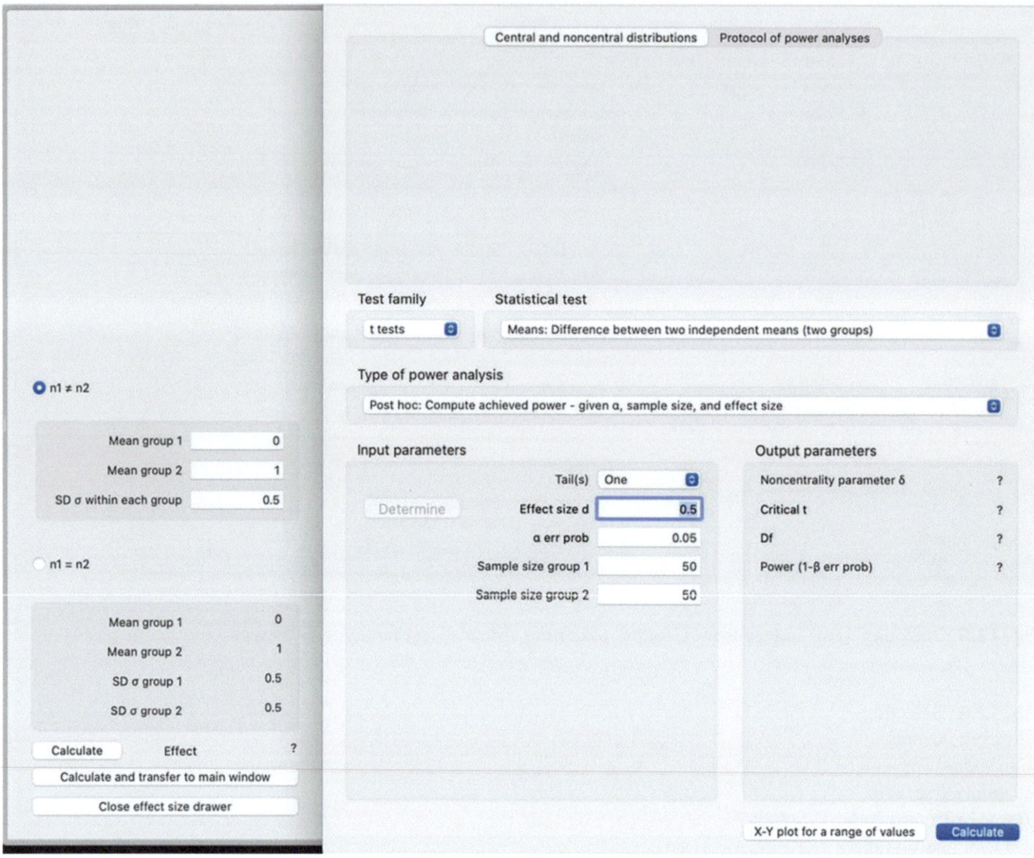

Fig. 12.7 Clicking "Determine" opens the effect size calculator panel in *G**Power

The result shows that the required sample size for each group is 13 (Fig. 12.16). Thus, to achieve 80% statistical power, a total of 26 participants (13 in each group) would be needed.

If it is not possible to determine the effect size directly, simply place the cursor in the Effect size d field without clicking Determine, and a reference for Cohen's *d* effect size will appear (Fig. 12.17). In most cases, the medium effect size is selected, and the Power ($1-\beta$ err prob) is set to 0.80. Then, by clicking Calculate at the bottom right, the required sample size for achieving 80% power can be obtained.

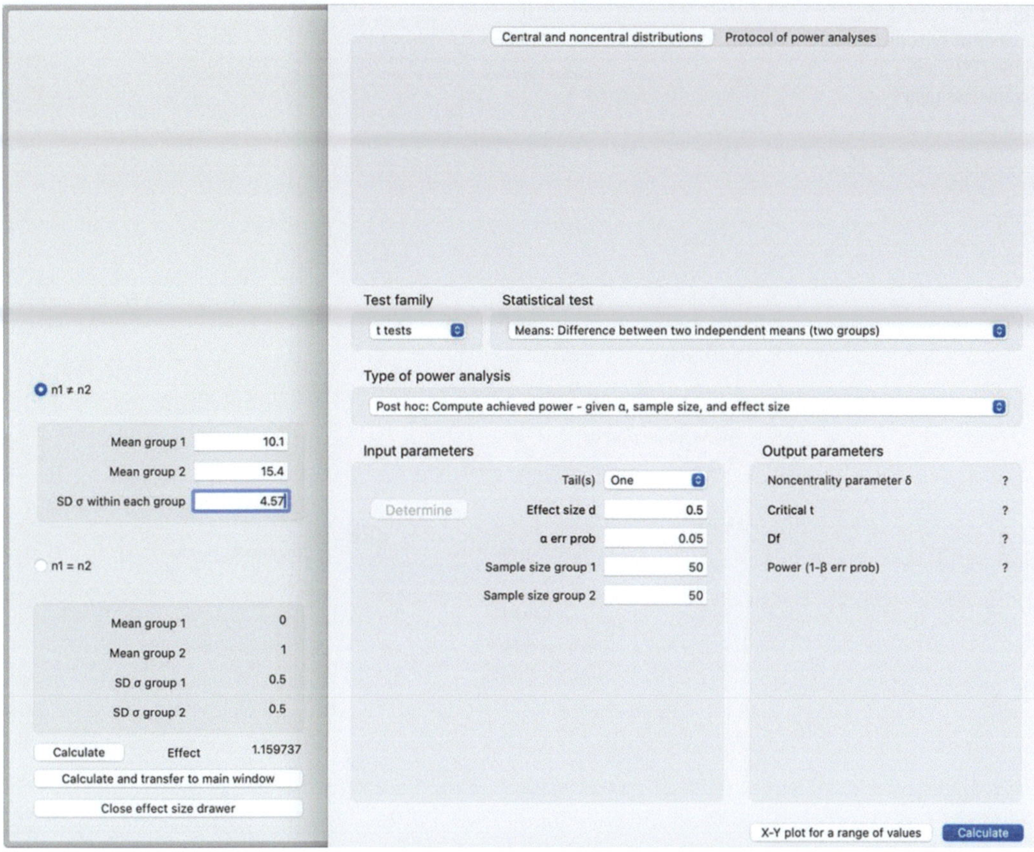

Fig. 12.8 Specifying unequal group sizes ($n1 \neq n2$) and entering group parameters in G*Power

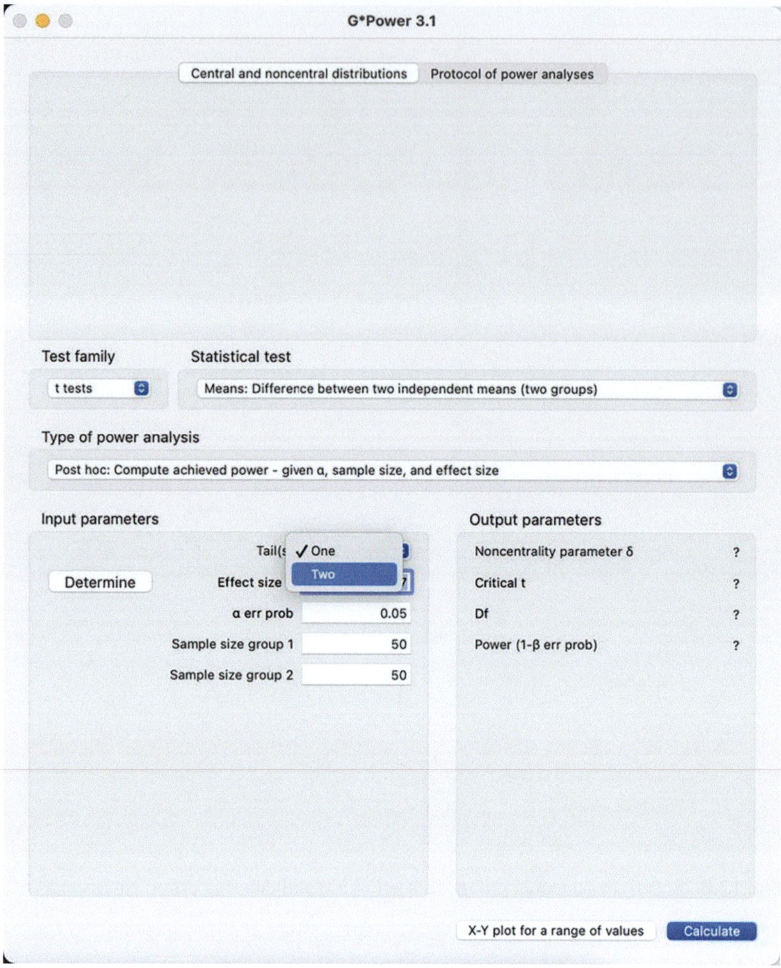

Fig. 12.9 Setting the number of tails to "Two" in the *G**Power Parameters panel

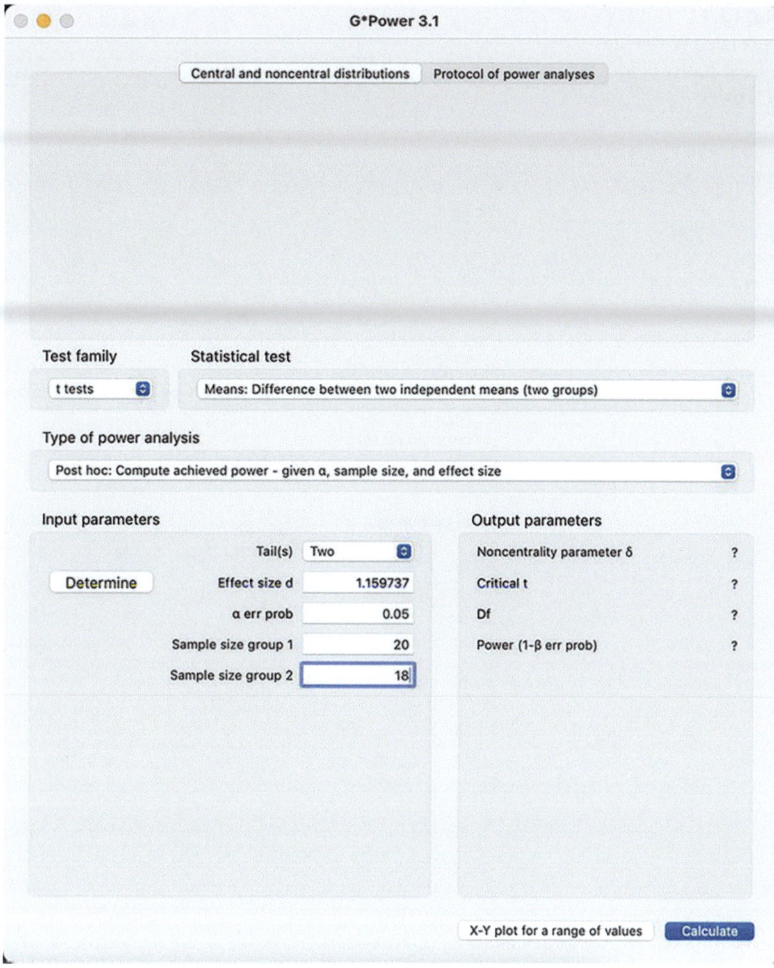

Fig. 12.10 Inputting sample sizes (Group 1: 20, Group 2: 18) and clicking "Calculate" in *G**Power

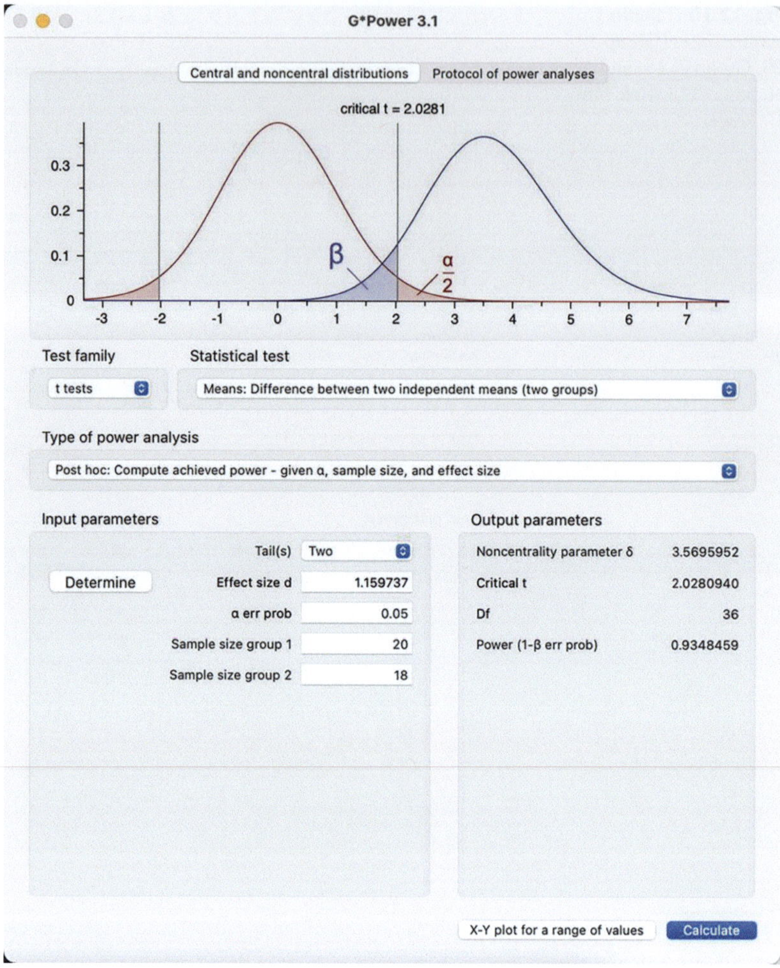

Fig. 12.11 Display of calculated power and related statistics in *G**Power

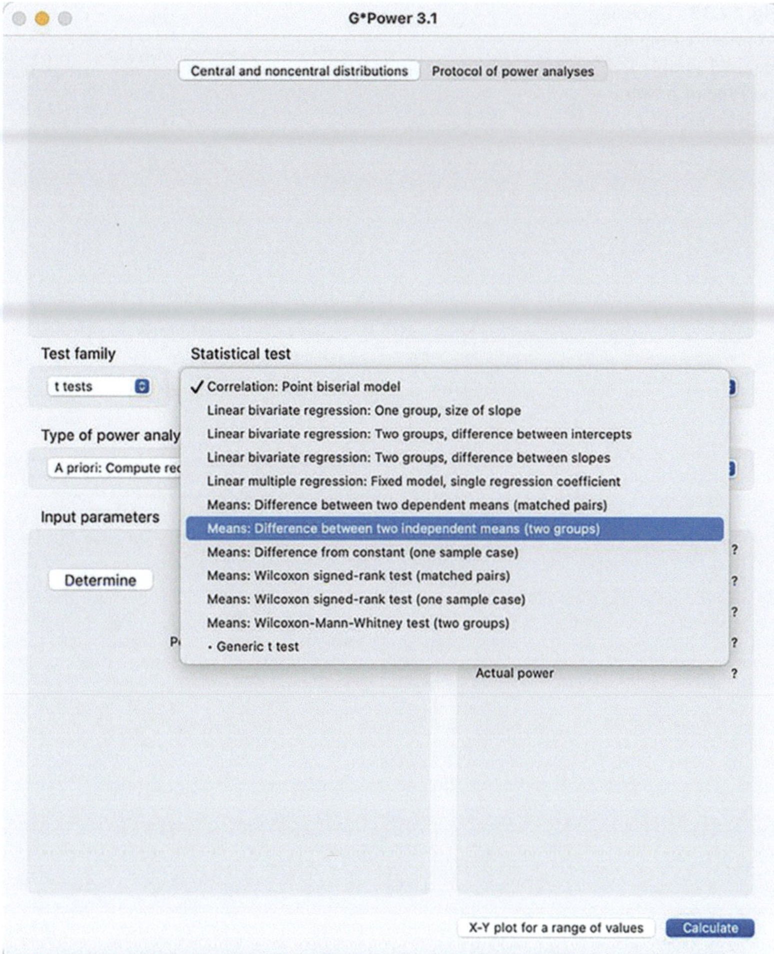

Fig. 12.12 Initial step for calculating sample size using two-group comparison in *G**Power

Fig. 12.13 Choosing "A priori: Compute required sample size" in the Type of power analysis menu

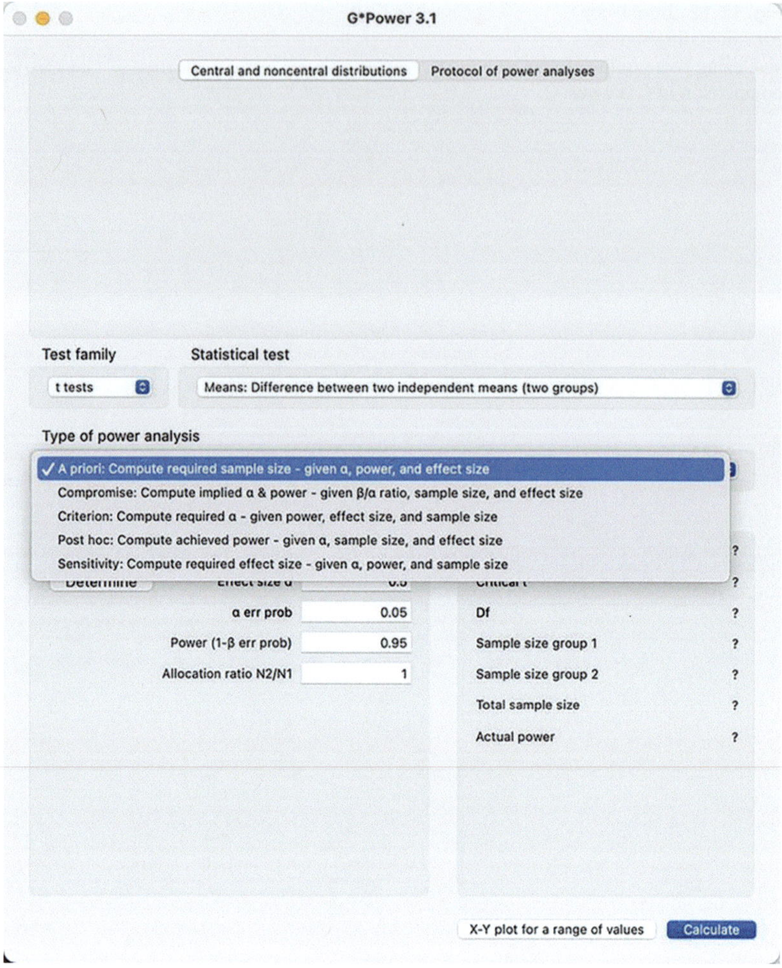

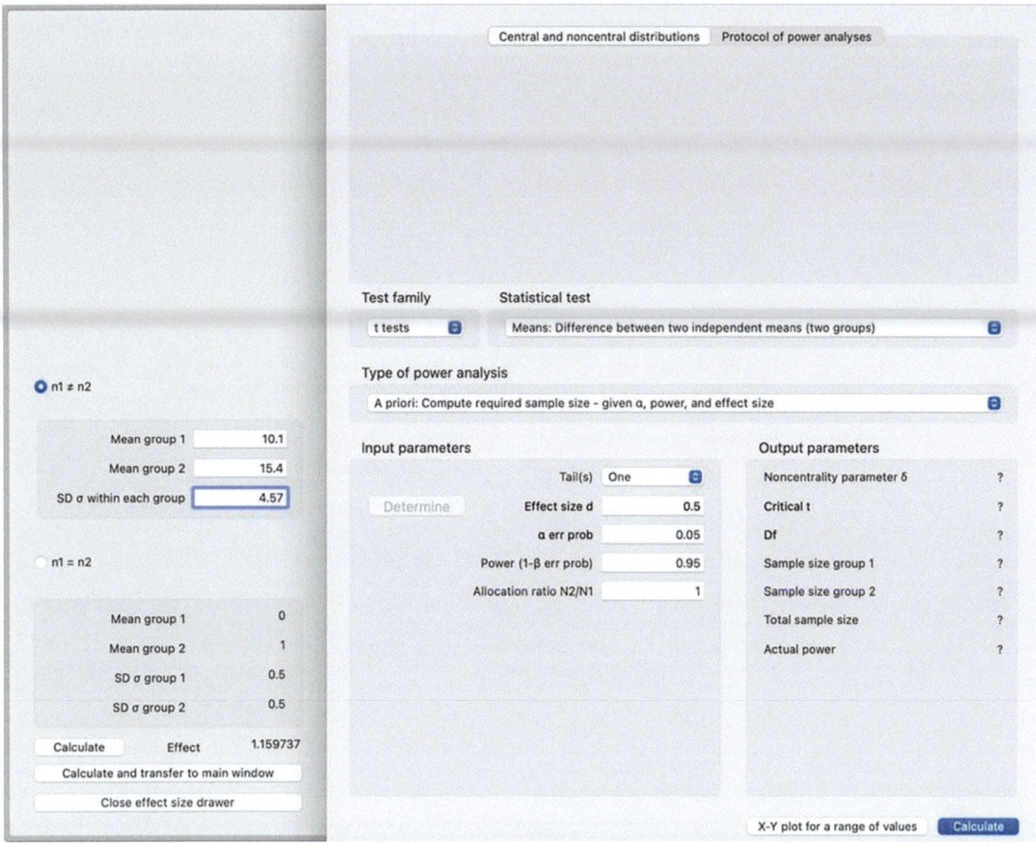

Fig. 12.14 Filling in example values for mean difference and pooled standard deviation

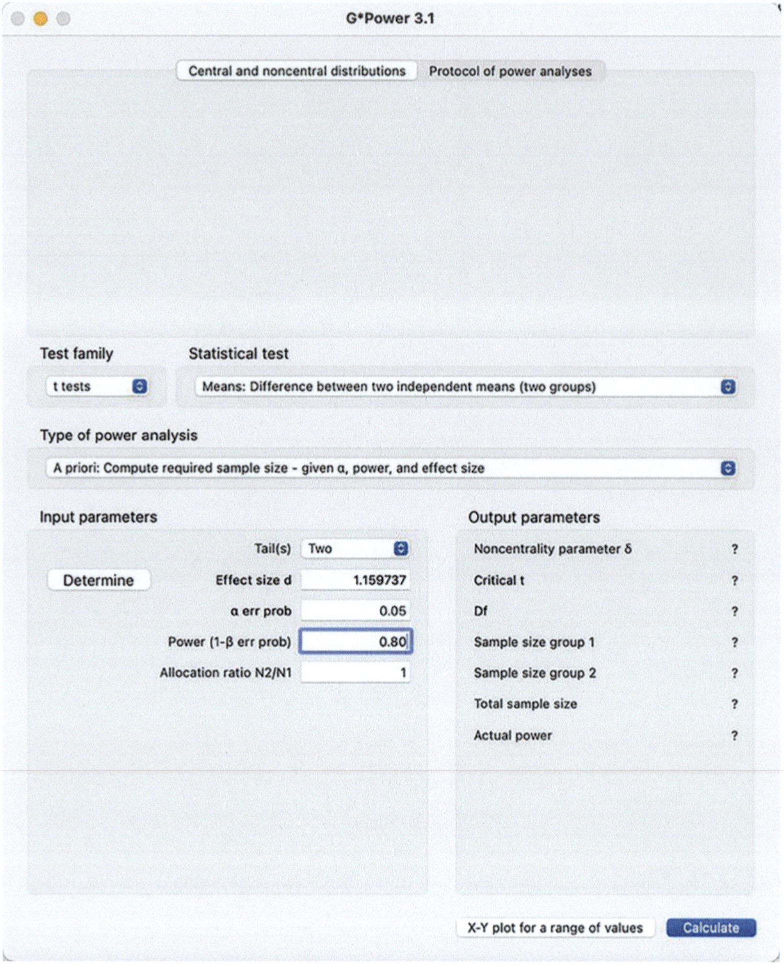

Fig. 12.15 Setting two-tailed test and desired power level in *G**Power main window

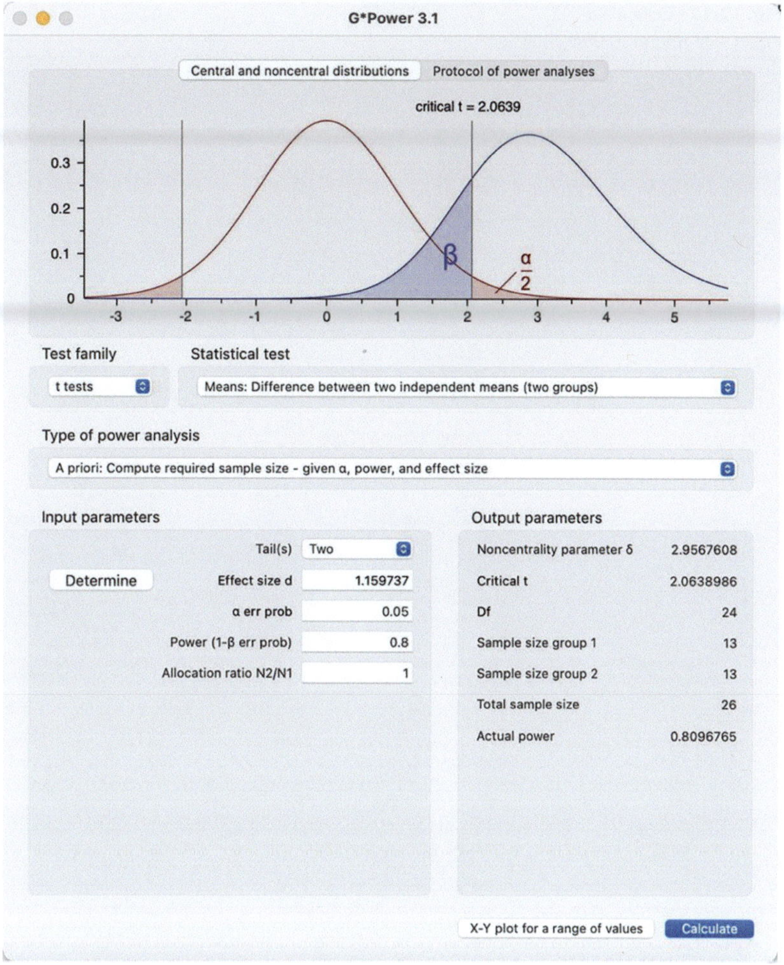

Fig. 12.16 Required sample size output from *G**Power for two independent means

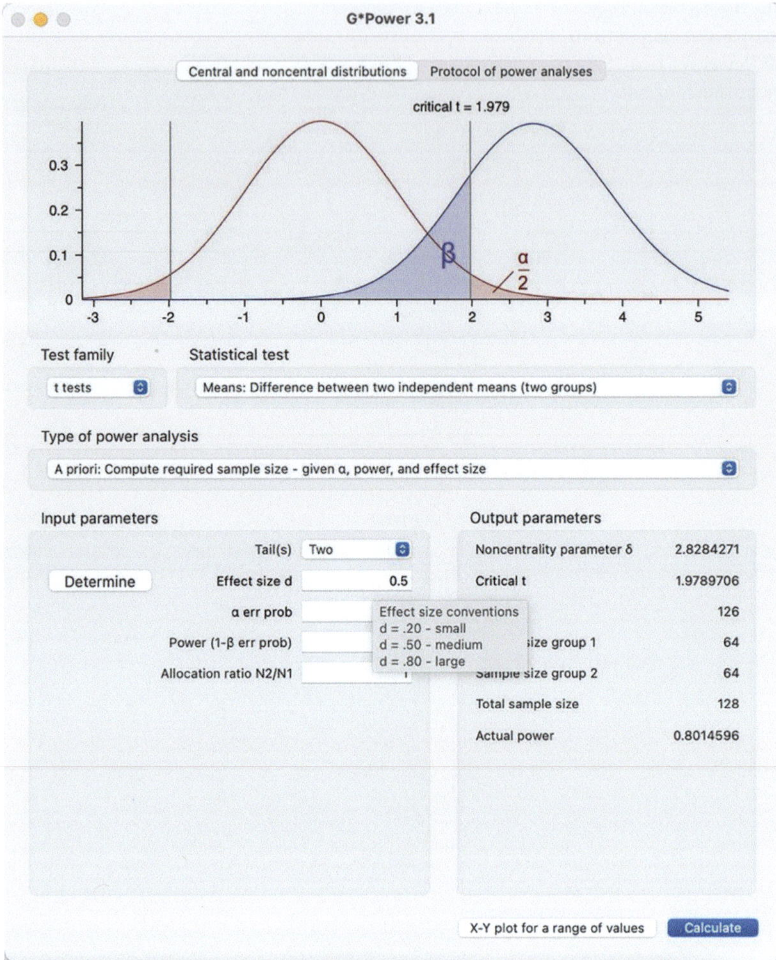

Fig. 12.17 Cohen's *d* effect size interpretation displayed in *G**Power interface

12.6 Procedures of Hypothesis Testing

Hypothesis testing refers to the process of deciding whether to accept or reject a given alternative hypothesis (H_1) based on sample data. This process generally follows the steps below:

First, establish the null hypothesis (H_0) and the alternative hypothesis (H_1). Then, collect data from the sample.

Second, determine the significance level α, which represents the probability of committing a Type I error—that is, rejecting the null hypothesis when it is actually true. The choice of α should be based on the potential consequences of making such an error. Common significance levels include $\alpha = 0.05$ or $\alpha = 0.01$.

Third, select an appropriate statistical method—either parametric or nonparametric—based on the characteristics of the data. If the data follow a normal distribution, parametric tests generally have greater statistical power than nonparametric ones.

Fourth, calculate the test statistic using the chosen statistical method, determine the corresponding *p*-value from the relevant probability distribution, and compare it to the significance level. If the *p*-value falls within the rejection region, reject the null hypothesis. If the *p*-value does not fall within the rejection region, do not reject the null hypothesis.

Fifth, interpret the p-value and the results. When reporting findings, it is preferable to express the conclusion in terms of the hypotheses being tested (e.g., "There is a significant difference between groups") rather than simply stating that a result is "statistically significant" or "not significant."

Null Hypothesis (H_0): There is no difference in language ability between men and women.
Alternative Hypothesis (H_1): There is a difference in language ability between men and women.
Critical Region: The range of values for the test statistic that leads to the rejection of the null hypothesis. The boundary value of the critical region is called the *critical value*.
Significance Probability (p-value):
When p-value < α: Reject the null hypothesis.
When p-value > α: Fail to reject (retain) the null hypothesis.
The larger the significance level α is set, the greater the probability of incorrectly rejecting the true null hypothesis. Conversely, setting a smaller α reduces the probability of such an error. Therefore, in studies where the results are expected to have major impacts on human life or welfare, it is advisable to select a smaller α to minimize the risk of wrongfully rejecting the null hypothesis.
One Sided Test (One Tailed Test): A test where the rejection region is located only on one side of the distribution.
Example: "The group receiving microneedling treatment will show greater improvement in skin elasticity compared to the control group."
Since the hypothesis specifies that the effect will be an increase (improvement), it is considered a *directional hypothesis*.
Two-Sided Test (Two-Tailed Test): A test where the rejection regions are located on both sides of the distribution.
If a computer output provides a p-value for a two-sided test, it must be divided by 2 to apply it for a one-sided test.
Type I Error (α-error): The probability of incorrectly rejecting a true null hypothesis.
Type II Error (β-error): The probability of failing to reject a false null hypothesis.
Statistical Power (Power of the Test): The probability of correctly rejecting the null hypothesis when it is false, denoted as $(1 - \beta)$. If the probability of a Type II error (β) is set at 0.2, the power is calculated as $(1 - \beta) = (1 - 0.2) = 0.8$.

Norton and Strube (2001)

12.7 Inferential Statistics

The following are methods classified under parametric statistical tests.

1. *t-Test*

A t-test is used when comparing the means of two populations. There are two main types of t-tests: the independent samples t-test and the paired samples t-test (also known as the dependent t-test). This test is sometimes referred to as the Student's t-test, a name originating from W. S. Gossett (1876–1937), who published the method under the pseudonym "Student" in 1908.

In a t-test, the dependent variable should be continuous, and the independent variable is typically a binary categorical (nominal) variable. It is generally assumed that the two populations follow a normal distribution and have equal variances, and that the two groups are independent. If the assumption of normality is violated, a nonparametric statistical method or data transformation (e.g., log transformation) may be applied. To assess the assumption of normality, one may examine skewness, kurtosis, or conduct goodness-of-fit tests such as the one-sample Kolmogorov–Smirnov test or the Shapiro–Wilk test. To evaluate whether the assumption of equal variances holds, statistical tests such as Bartlett's test, Hartley's test, or Levene's test can be used. Bartlett's and Hartley's tests are sensitive to violations of normality, making them less suitable when the assumption of normal distribution is not clearly met. In such cases, Levene's test is preferred because it is more robust even when the population distribution is non-normal. When the two groups are not independent or the experimental design involves paired observations, a paired t-test should be used instead of an independent samples t-test.

Thus far, we have described methods for comparing population means under the assumption of equal variances. However, if there is insufficient evidence to support the homogeneity of variance assumption, a test for equal variances should be conducted.

Table 12.2 Provides an example of how to report t-test results in a research publication

Group (*N*)	Mean	Standard deviation	*t*-value	Degrees of freedom	*p*-value
Experimental ($n = 29$)	37.55	10.02	3.40	56	0.001
Control ($n = 29$)	42.92	10.56			

1. *Steps of the t-Test*

First, establish the null hypothesis (H_0) and alternative hypothesis (H_1). For example, suppose a study is conducted on adult women with pronounced expression wrinkles caused by facial muscle tension. One group receives a biofeedback-based relaxation training, while the control group receives a placebo treatment. The primary outcome is the depth of facial wrinkles. The hypotheses can be stated as:

- H_0: $M_b \geq M_p$, where M_b is the mean wrinkle depth in the biofeedback group, and Mp is the mean wrinkle depth in the placebo group
- H_1: $M_b < M_p$

  In this case, the null hypothesis asserts that the wrinkle depth in the biofeedback group is the same as or greater than that in the placebo group, while the alternative hypothesis asserts that the wrinkle depth is smaller in the biofeedback group.

  Second, determine the appropriate statistical test. The choice of test depends on the type of variables, their distribution, the study design, and the research objective.

  Third, set the significance level (α).

  Fourth, calculate the test statistic. In the case of a t-test, this means computing the *t*-value.

  Fifth, consult the t-distribution table to find the critical *t*-value using the chosen significance level and degrees of freedom.

  Sixth, compare the computed *t*-value with the critical *t*-value from the table. Based on this comparison, determine whether to reject or fail to reject the null hypothesis (Table 12.2).

2. *Example of Independent t-test Using SPSS*

Launch SPSS and enter the data as shown in Fig. 12.18. The following dataset is a hypothetical example that represents skin elasticity improvement scores after two types of facial treatments. Group 1 received a standard microneedling procedure, while Group 2 received microneedling combined with radiofrequency.

After launching the program, a blank data entry screen appears (Fig. 12.19). Variable names are not yet specified.

Click on the Variable View tab at the bottom of the screen, and the following window will appear (Fig. 12.20).

Enter Score and Group into the first two rows under the "Name" column. Other attributes such as "Type" and "Width" are auto-filled (Fig. 12.21).

To include a description for the grouping variable, click the cell where "Values" intersects with the "Group" variable. Then, the following window will appear (Fig. 12.22).

A value label window will appear (Fig. 12.23).

Click "+" and enter 1 as the value and "Microneedling only" as the label (Fig. 12.24).

Then enter 2 as the value and "Microneedling + RF" as the label (Fig. 12.25). Then click "OK."

Now the data entry screen will show variables named Score and Group (Fig. 12.26).

Enter the corresponding data (Fig. 12.27).

Once data entry is complete, click Analyze → Compare Means → Independent-Samples T Test (Fig. 12.28).

In the dialog box that appears (Fig. 12.29), select Score (the dependent variable) and move it to the "Test Variable(s)" box using the top middle arrow (Fig. 12.30). Then select Group (the independent variable) and move it to the "Grouping Variable" box using the lower arrow.

Click "Define Groups," and enter 1 for Group 1 and 2 for Group 2 (Fig. 12.31). Click "Continue."

When the following window appears, click OK (Fig. 12.32).

The SPSS output window will display the results of the independent t-test (Fig. 12.33). The first table shows that each group had 8 partici-

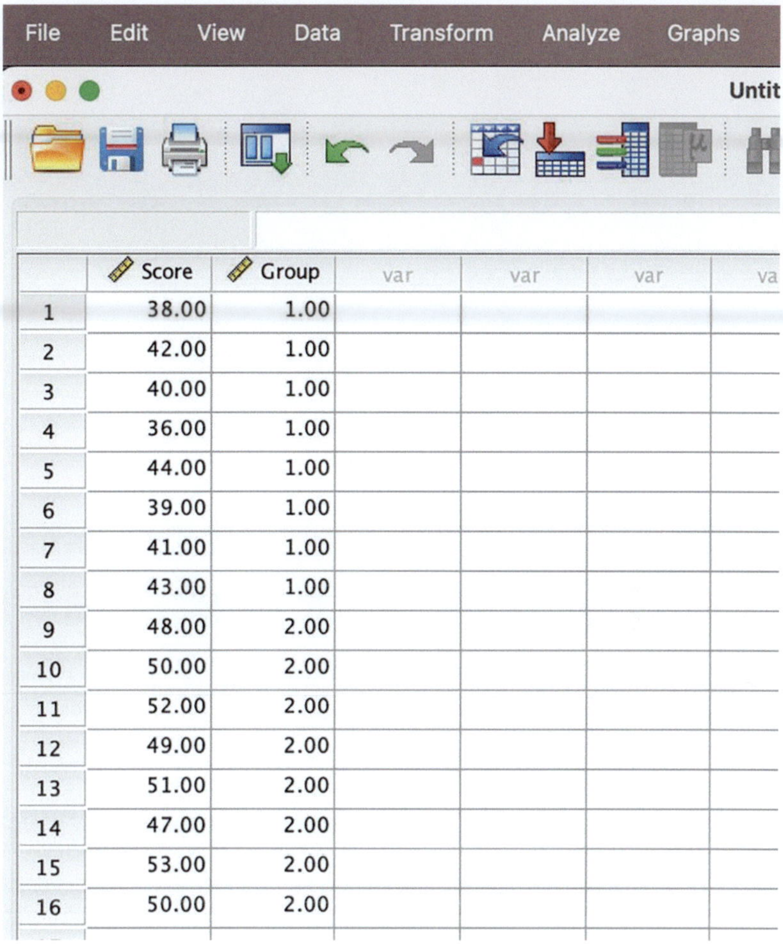

Fig. 12.18 SPSS data entry for skin elasticity scores

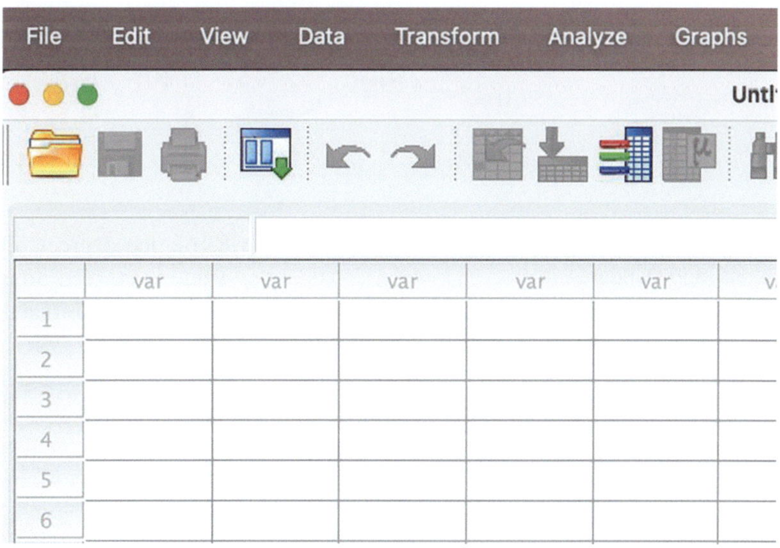

Fig. 12.19 Initial screen after launching SPSS

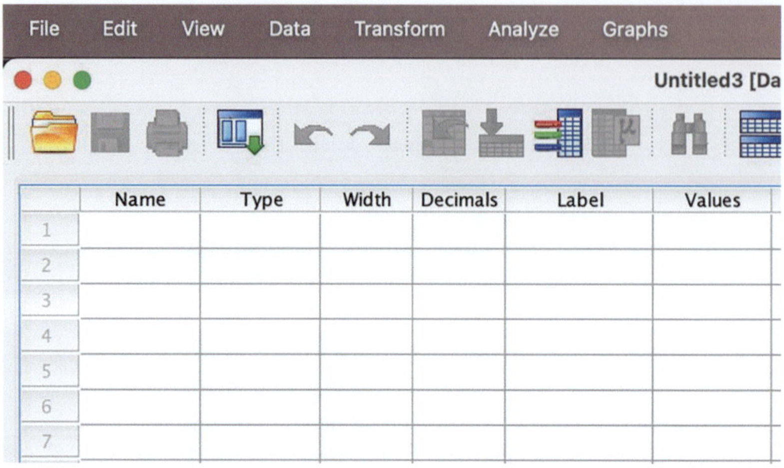

Fig. 12.20 Variable view tab in SPSS

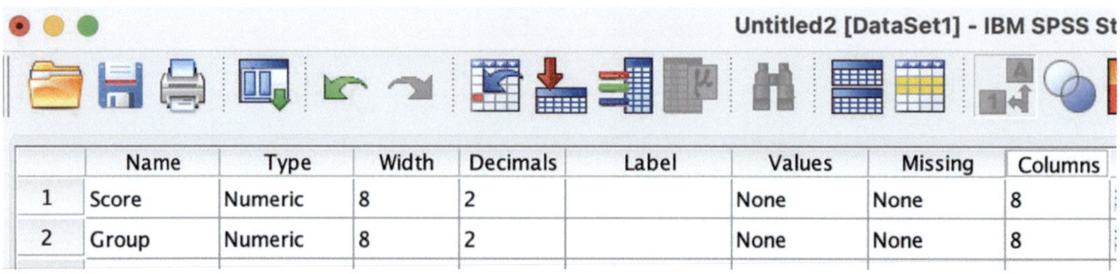

Fig. 12.21 Example of data entry in variable view

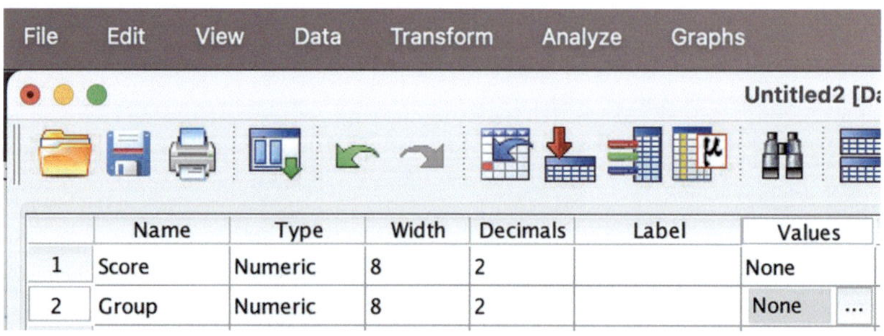

Fig. 12.22 Assigning value labels to the grouping variable in SPSS

pants, along with the group means, standard deviations, and standard errors.

The Levene's test for equality of variances yields a p-value of 0.353, which is greater than the 0.05 significance level (Fig. 12.34). Therefore, equal variances can be assumed. The t-value is −8.162, the degrees of freedom are 14, and the p-value is <0.001. Since the p-value is less than 0.05, we conclude that the skin elasticity improvement in Group 2 (Microneedling + RF) is significantly greater than that in Group 1 (Microneedling only).

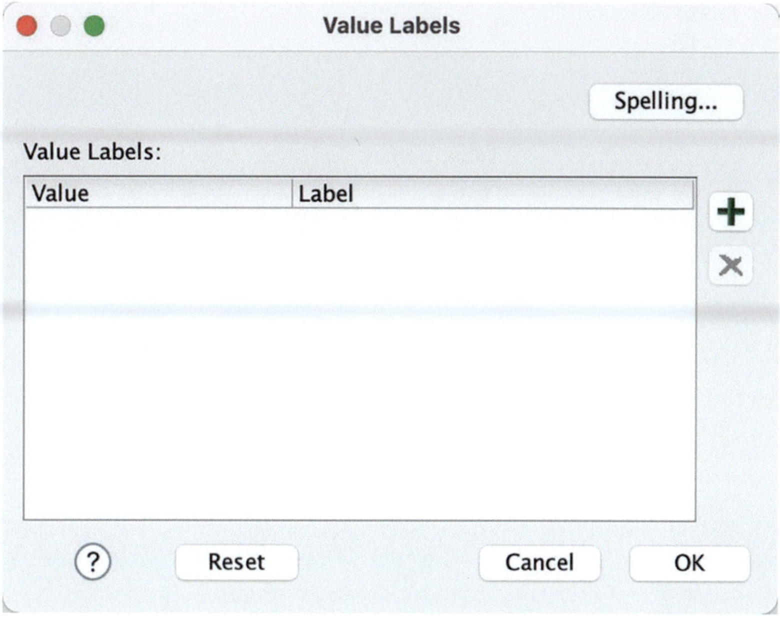

Fig. 12.23 Value Labels Dialog Box in SPSS

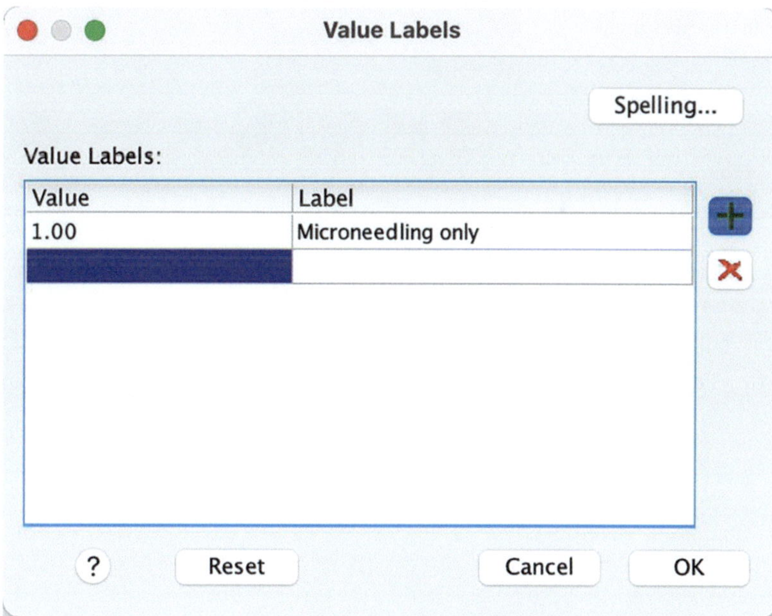

Fig. 12.24 Value label entry example

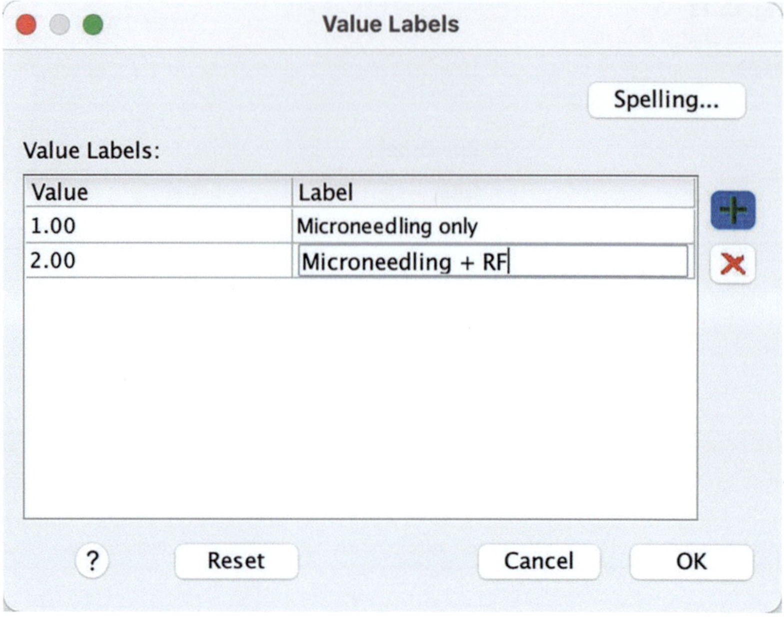
Value Labels
Spelling...
Value Labels:
Value
Label
1.00
Microneedling only
2.00
Microneedling + RF
?
Reset
Cancel
OK

Fig. 12.25 Value label entry example

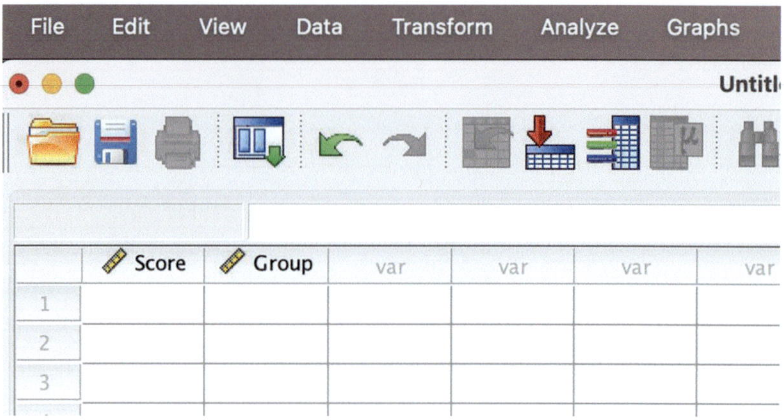

Fig. 12.26 Data view with score and group variables

Fig. 12.27 Entered dataset in SPSS

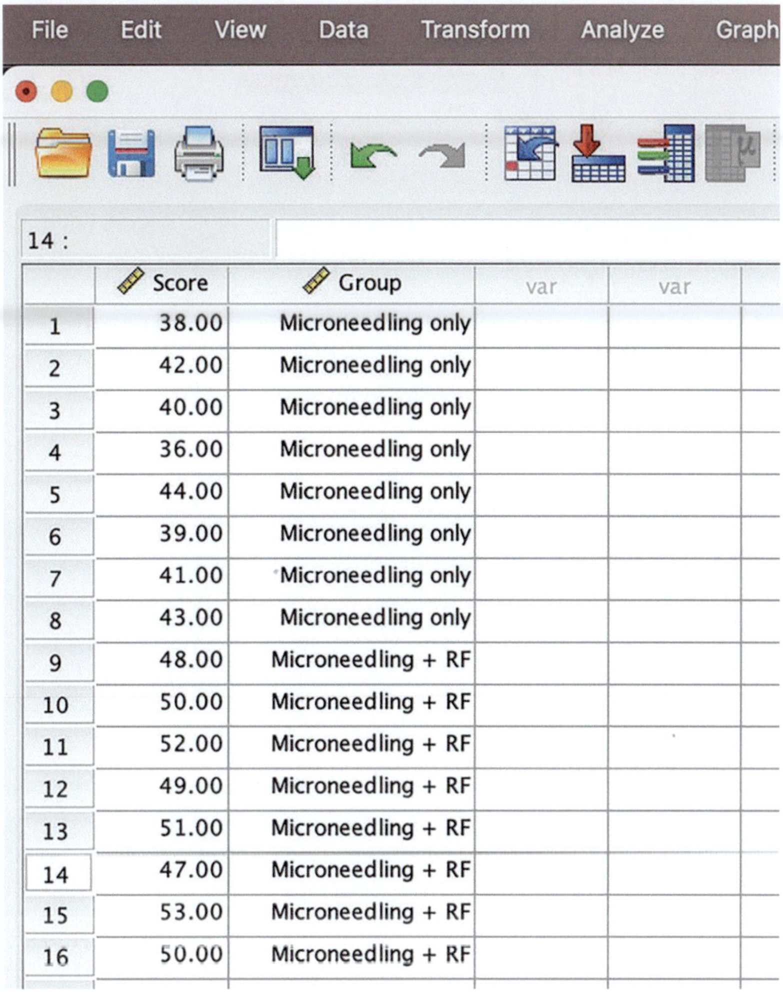

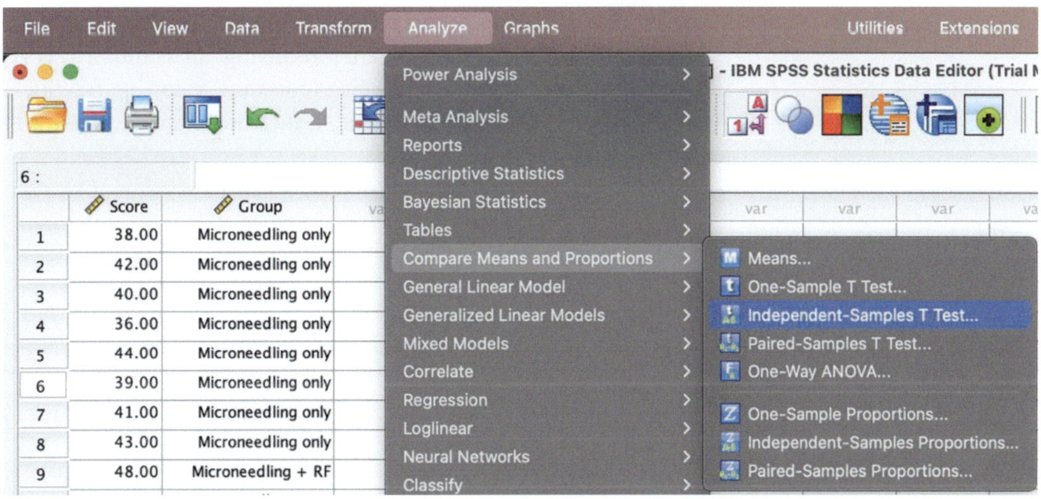

Fig. 12.28 Menu path for conducting independent-samples T test

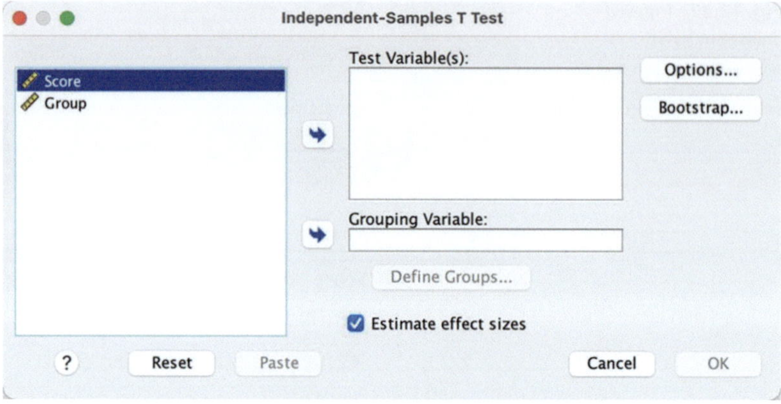

Fig. 12.29 Independent-samples T test dialog box in SPSS

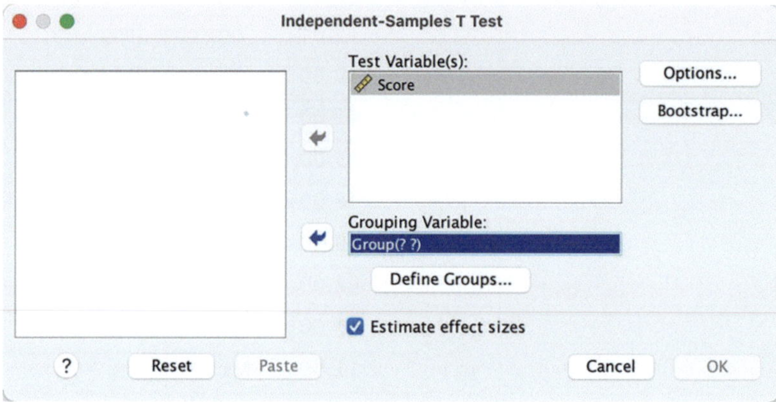

Fig. 12.30 Specifying test and grouping variables in SPSS T test dialog

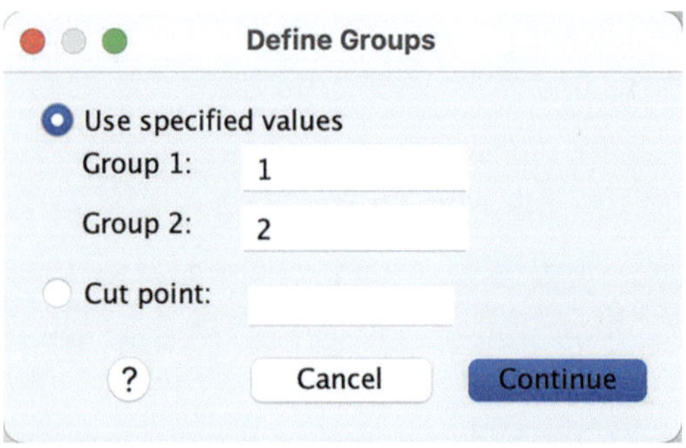

Fig. 12.31 Defining groups for independent-samples T test

2. *Example of Paired t-Test Using SPSS*

Start SPSS and enter the following data. The following example compares transepidermal water loss (TEWL) in the same ten participants before and after receiving an additional post-treatment cooling procedure following fractional laser resurfacing. Data were entered as shown in Fig. 12.35.

From the menu, go to *Analyze → Compare Means → Paired-Samples T Test* (Fig. 12.36).

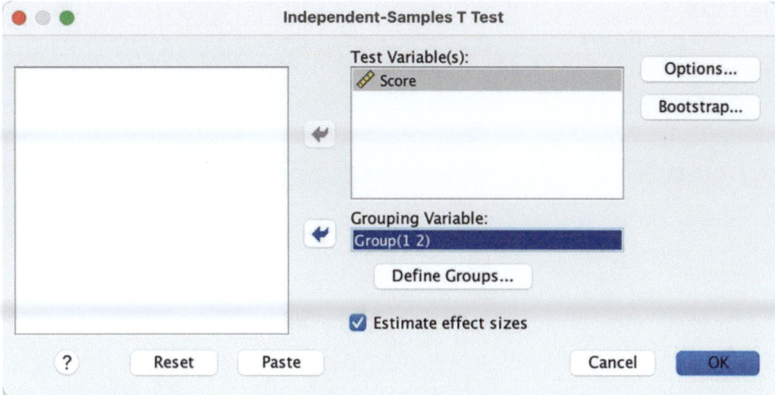

Fig. 12.32 Groups defined and ready for analysis

Fig. 12.33 SPSS output window displaying independent-samples T test results

Group Statistics

	Group	N	Mean	Std. Deviation	Std. Error Mean
Score	Microneedling only	8	40.3750	2.66927	.94373
	Microneedling + RF	8	50.0000	2.00000	.70711

Independent Samples Test

		Levene's Test for Equality of Variances		t-test for Equality of Means							
						Significance				95% Confidence Interval of the Difference	
		F	Sig.	t	df	One-Sided p	Two-Sided p	Mean Difference	Std. Error Difference	Lower	Upper
Score	Equal variances assumed	.921	.353	-8.162	14	<.001	<.001	-9.62500	1.17925	-12.15423	-7.09577
	Equal variances not assumed			-8.162	12.976	<.001	<.001	-9.62500	1.17925	-12.17309	-7.07691

Fig. 12.34 SPSS output window displaying independent-samples T test results

Click on the variables “nocooling” and “cooling” in the left window, then click the middle arrow to move them to the paired variables window (Figs. 12.37 and 12.38).

Click *OK*.

The result table will appear as shown in Fig. 12.39. In the first table, the mean TEWL without cooling treatment is shown as 21.42 g/m^2/h, and after cooling treatment, it is 21.27 g/m^2/h. The standard deviation and standard error for each condition are also presented. The second table shows the correlation between the two sets of scores, with $r = 0.99$ and the significance level $p < 0.001$. In the third table, the t-value is 1.964 with 9 degrees of freedom, and the p-value is 0.081 (Fig. 12.40). Since the p-value is greater than the significance level of 0.05, we conclude that there is no statistically significant difference in TEWL between the two treatments.

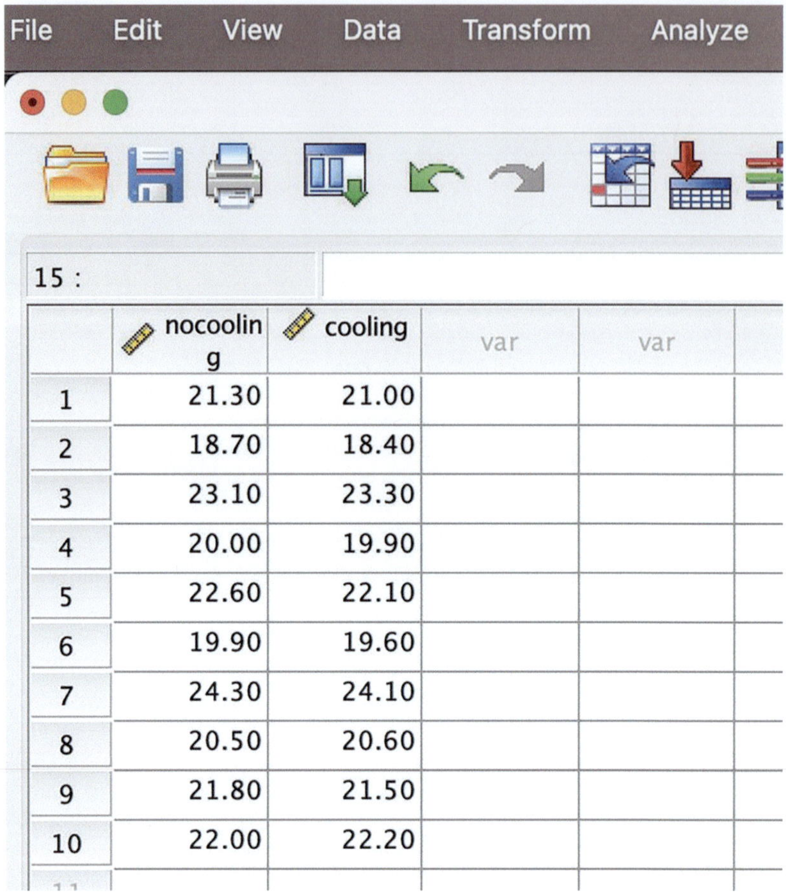

Fig. 12.35 Example dataset for paired t-test entered in SPSS

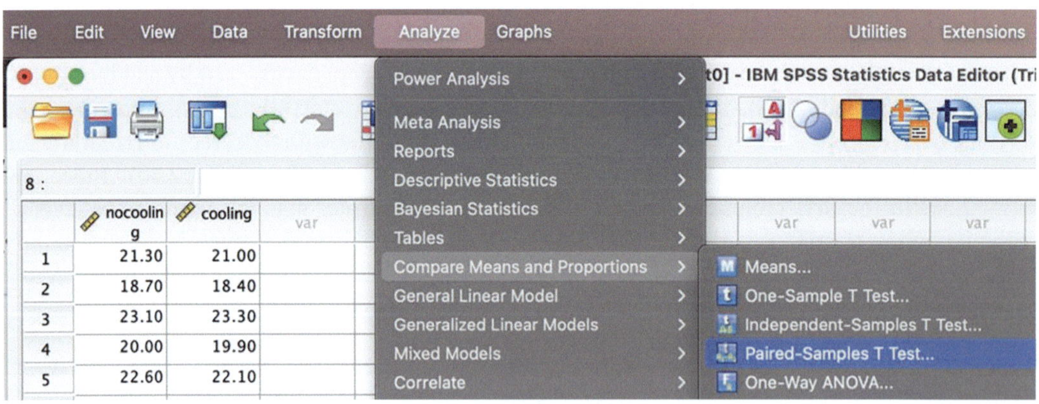

Fig. 12.36 Navigation path to perform a paired-samples t-test in SPSS

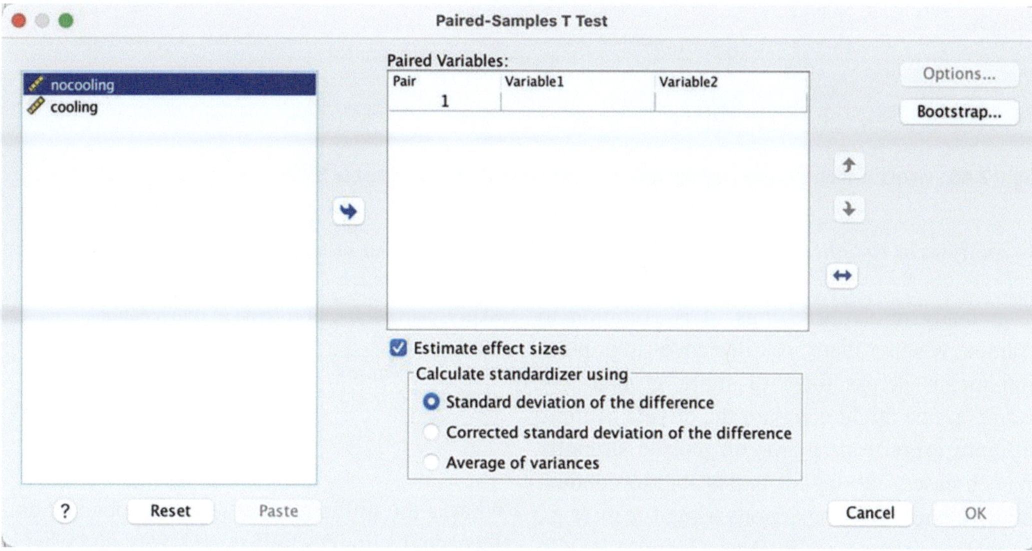

Fig. 12.37 Paired-samples T test dialog window in SPSS

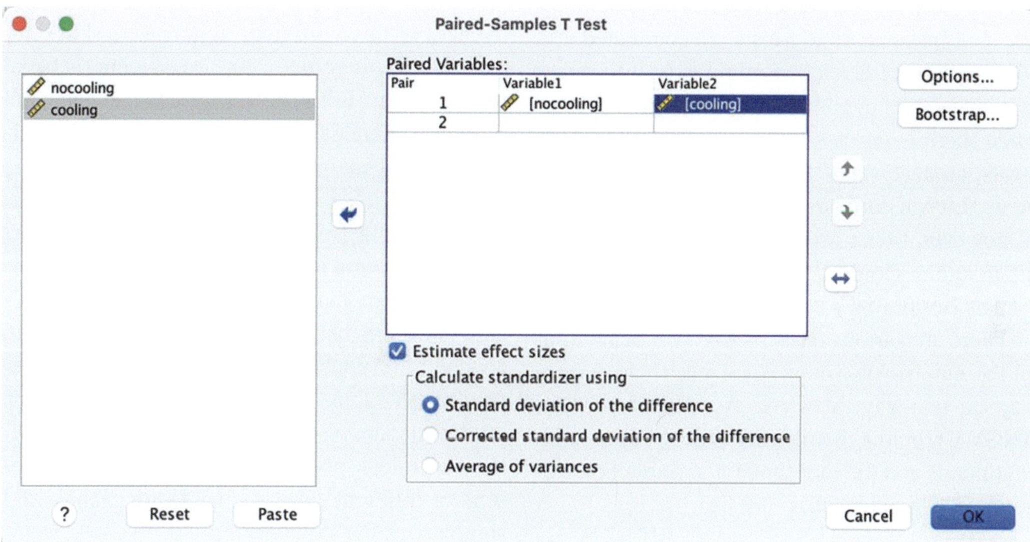

Fig. 12.38 Assigning paired variables for the paired-samples T test in SPSS

Fig. 12.39 Output window displaying the results of the paired-samples T test in SPSS

Paired Samples Statistics

		Mean	N	Std. Deviation	Std. Error Mean
Pair 1	nocooling	21.4200	10	1.68576	.53308
	cooling	21.2700	10	1.73721	.54935

Paired Samples Correlations

		N	Correlation	Significance One-Sided p	Significance Two-Sided p
Pair 1	nocooling & cooling	10	.990	<.001	<.001

Paired Samples Test

		Paired Differences					t	df	Significance	
					95% Confidence Interval of the Difference					
		Mean	Std. Deviation	Std. Error Mean	Lower	Upper			One-Sided p	Two-Sided p
Pair 1	nocooling – cooling	.15000	.24152	.07638	−.02278	.32278	1.964	9	.041	.081

Fig. 12.40 Output window displaying the results of the paired-samples T test in SPSS

3. *Analysis of Variance (ANOVA)*

In many research settings, it is common to examine whether there are differences in population means across three or more groups. For example, one might compare the effects of three different exercise programs on muscle strength. In such cases, although it is possible to conduct multiple pairwise comparisons using t-tests (e.g., comparing group A vs. B, B vs. C, and A vs. C), performing multiple t-tests increases the likelihood of committing a Type I error—incorrectly rejecting the null hypothesis when it is actually true. For instance, if 20 t-tests are conducted at a 5% significance level, one might expect to reject at least one null hypothesis by chance alone, even when there is no true difference. To avoid such errors, an analysis of variance (ANOVA) should be used when comparing more than two groups. If, however, t-tests are used instead of ANOVA, the *p*-values should be adjusted using a method such as Bonferroni's correction.

There are various types of ANOVA depending on the number of factors involved, such as one-way or two-way ANOVA. As with the t-test, ANOVA requires that the dependent variable be continuous and the independent variable be categorical (nominal level).

1. *One-Way Analysis of Variance (One-Way ANOVA)*

One-way ANOVA is a statistical method used to determine whether the mean scores of a dependent variable differ significantly across groups that are defined by a single factor or independent variable. To understand ANOVA, it is important to first clarify several key terms: What is variance? What constitutes independent groups?

Table 12.3 An example of skin treatment factor and levels

Skin Treatment Factor *A* (type of rejuvenation procedure)		
Level A_1 (chemical peeling) ($n_1 = 10$)	Level A_2 (fractional laser) ($n_2 = 10$)	Level A_3 (IPL) ($n_3 = 10$)

What is the difference between independent and dependent variables? What are levels, and what is a factor?

Consider the following example: Suppose a researcher is interested in comparing the effectiveness of three different noninvasive skin rejuvenation programs in reducing facial pigmentation. Let's assume the three treatment types are chemical peeling, fractional laser therapy, and intense pulsed light (IPL) therapy. The outcome variable is defined as the melanin index measured via spectrophotometry, with lower scores indicating reduced pigmentation.

In this case, the dependent variable is the melanin index—a measurable trait that is expected to change in response to an intervention. The independent variable, or factor, is the type of skin treatment administered. Each treatment modality—chemical peeling, laser, and IPL—represents a different level of the factor. Table 12.3 summarizes the study design.

The term independent groups refers to a type of research design in which the groups are separate from one another. However, the participants are considered homogeneous, and each belongs to only one of the levels that constitute the factor. Ideally, this means that participants are randomly selected from a population with no prior exposure (e.g., to treatment or exercise) and are then randomly assigned to one of several groups. Being assigned to only one group implies that each participant is exposed to only one level of the factor. Furthermore, it also means that the dependent variable is measured only once for each participant.

In our example, each subject undergoes only one of the three rejuvenation treatments. After completing the respective treatments, all participants have their melanin index measured, and the effectiveness of the three interventions is evaluated using ANOVA.

In contrast, repeated-measures designs involve measuring the dependent variable more than once—either before and after exposure to an intervention level, or after exposure to multiple levels of the independent variable over time. Although repeated-measures designs are more economical in terms of sample size, they risk carryover effects—that is, the effect of one level of the independent variable may persist and influence the response to another level, leading to biased results. Because repeated-measures ANOVA involves additional complexities, this section will focus only on between-group ANOVA, where each group is independent.

Importantly, ANOVA is not designed to tell us which group means are higher or lower. Rather, it examines whether the variability between group means is significantly greater than the variability within groups. Therefore, to fully understand ANOVA, we must first understand the concept of variance.

2. *Variance*

What is variance? Simply put, variance refers to the variations or differences in scores observed among subjects. Regardless of what is being measured, it is rare for all individuals to have the same score. People are inherently different—height, weight, IQ, and muscular strength all vary from person to person. Variance is a numerical value that quantifies the degree of variability observed among individuals when a dependent variable is measured. Of course, there are many reasons why these differences in numerical values occur; there are various sources of variation. In analysis of variance (ANOVA), the goal is to isolate one specific source of variation—the variation produced by the independent variable—from among all possible causes of variability in the dependent variable. Once this is achieved, the researcher can determine whether the independent variable makes a significant contribution to the variability of the dependent variable, thus affecting the differences in group means.

Let us illustrate this concept using Table 12.4. Suppose 30 participants are randomly assigned to three different skin rejuvenation treatment groups: chemical peeling, fractional laser therapy, and intense pulsed light (IPL) therapy, with 10 individuals per group. Each participant undergoes a post-treatment assessment of skin brightness score, denoted by X_{ij} and each group has a mean score $\overline{X}_j$, and k represents the number of groups. To calculate the variance, we first subtract the group mean from each individual score in the group ($X_{ij} - \overline{X}_j$). Then, we square each difference and sum them to obtain the sum of squares (SS).

$$\sum_{i=1}^{k}\left(X_{ij} - \overline{X}_j\right)^2$$

Dividing this total by the number of scores minus one yields the group variance $\left(s_j^2\right)$. Taking the square root of the variance gives the standard deviation (s_j) for that group. While the group mean and group variance are themselves useful descriptive statistics, they are even more important for understanding the theoretical basis of analysis of variance (ANOVA).

$$\text{SSB} = n\sum_{j=1}^{k}\left(\overline{X}_j - \overline{X}\right)^2 = 10\left(130.10 - 133.37\right)^2 + 10\left(135.50 - 133.37\right)^2 + 10\left(134.50 - 133.37\right)^2$$

$$= 10\left(10.69 + 4.54 + 1.28\right) = 165.10$$

$$df_{\text{B}} = k - 1 = 3 - 1 = 2$$

$$\text{MSB} = \text{SSB} / df_{\text{B}} = 165.10 / 2 = 82.55$$

Table 12.4 An example of ANOVA

	Chemical peeling group			Fractional laser therapy group			Intense pulsed light therapy group		
	X_{j1}	$(X_{j1}-\bar{X}_1)$	$(X_{j1}-\bar{X}_1)^2$	X_{j2}	$(X_{j2}-\bar{X}_2)$	$(X_{j2}-\bar{X}_2)^2$	X_{j3}	$(X_{j3}-\bar{X}_3)$	$(X_{j3}-\bar{X}_3)^2$
	130	−0.10	0.01	135	−0.50	0.25	131	−3.50	12.25
	129	−1.10	1.21	136	0.50	0.25	135	0.50	0.25
	133	2.90	8.41	132	−3.50	12.25	134	−0.50	0.25
	132	1.90	3.61	134	−1.50	2.25	137	2.50	6.25
	130	−0.10	0.01	135	−0.50	0.25	135	0.50	0.25
	132	1.90	3.61	139	3.50	12.25	137	2.50	6.25
	127	−3.10	9.61	135	−0.50	0.25	133	−1.50	2.25
	128	−2.10	4.41	134	−1.50	2.25	136	1.50	2.25
	129	−1.10	1.21	137	1.50	2.25	133	−1.50	2.25
	131	0.90	0.81	138	2.50	6.25	134	0.50	0.25
Sum	$\sum_{i=1}^{n}$ 1301	0	32.90	1355	0	38.5	1345	0	32.5
Mean	X_j 130.1			135.5			134.5		
Variance	s_j^2 3.66			4.28			3.61		
Total Mean	$\bar{X}..$ 133.37								

$$\mathrm{SSW} = \sum_{j=1}^{k}\sum_{j=1}^{k}\left(X_{ij} - \bar{X}_j\right)^2 = \left(130.00 - 130.10\right)^2 + \left(129.00 - 130.10\right)^2 + \cdots + \left(134.00 - 134.5\right)^2 = 103.90$$

$$df_{\mathrm{W}} = k\left(n-1\right) = 3\left(9\right) = 27$$

$$\mathrm{MSW} = \mathrm{SSW} \,/\, df_{\mathrm{W}} = 103.90 \,/\, 27 = 3.85$$

$$F = \mathrm{MSB} \,/\, \mathrm{MSW} = 82.55 \,/\, 3.82 = 21.44$$

3. *Partitioning of Variance*

In analysis of variance (ANOVA), the goal is to isolate the effect of the independent variable from all the other sources of variation observed in the dependent variable. In other words, the total variation in the dependent variable is divided into two components: the between-groups component and the within-groups component. What does the within-groups component represent? It reflects the normal and random fluctuations in the dependent variable that would occur even in the absence of any intervention by the independent variable. That is, it represents the amount of variability we would expect if the independent variable had no effect at all.

It is important to remember that within each group, all participants are exposed to the same level of the independent variable. Thus, theoretically, the independent variable has no influence on variability within the group because every participant is equally affected. Adding a constant to all scores within a group does not affect the variance. How then is the within-groups component calculated? We estimate it by calculating the variance within each group. Due to random fluctuations, the variances within groups are not identical.

To obtain a better estimate, we sum the sum of squares (SS) from each group, resulting in the within-groups sum of squares (SSW). Next, we sum the degrees of freedom from each group, which is the number of participants in each group minus one, yielding the within-groups degrees of freedom (df_{w}). Dividing SSW by df_{w} gives us the within-groups mean square (MSW). This MSW is also referred to as the error mean square, residual mean square, or error variance. Conceptually, it represents the variability expected in participant outcomes when the independent variable has no effect.

But what if the independent variable does have an effect? How can we detect its influence? As we discussed earlier, within a group, the effect of the independent variable would uniformly shift all scores by a certain amount, affecting the group mean without necessarily increasing within-group variance. Therefore, we examine the variability between the group means to assess the impact of the independent variable.

The between-groups component is calculated similarly to how we calculate variance within a group. Between-groups variance measures how much each group mean deviates from the overall mean $\bar{X}$ across all participants. In essence, it evaluates how different the group means are from one another relative to the grand mean. Here is a simplified outline of how the between-groups component is calculated: Like the within-groups component, it involves calculating a sum of squares (SSB), a mean square (MSB), and degrees of freedom. The between-groups degrees of freedom are equal to the number of groups minus one.

4. *F Ratio*

The final step in the analysis of variance (ANOVA) is to calculate the *F* ratio. In this ratio, the mean square between groups (MSB) is placed in the numerator, and the mean square within groups (MSW) is placed in the denominator. As the *F* ratio indicates, ANOVA involves comparing the between-groups variance to the within-groups variance. Under the null hypothesis, it is assumed that all group means are equal. In this case, the variance among the means and the variance within the groups are both considered estimates of the total variance. The effect of the independent variable refers to the variability among the group means, not to the variability among scores within each group. Therefore, if the variance between the group means is substantially larger than the variance within the groups, the F value will be relatively large. When the null hypothesis—stating that all group means are equal—is true, the F ratio should be close to 1.0. The larger the F value, the more likely it is that the differences in scores among the three skin treatment groups are not due to chance or normal random fluctuations. In the example presented in this chapter, the F ratio is 21.44.

5. *Interpretation of Results*

What does an F ratio of 21.44 mean? It answers the question: *Are the differences among the group means likely to have occurred by chance?* To answer this, the calculated F value (21.44) must be compared to the theoretical F distribution under the null hypothesis. By referring to the F distribution table in the appendix, and finding the critical value corresponding to the appropriate significance level (α) and degrees of freedom, we can determine whether the observed F is statistically significant.

In this example, the degrees of freedom (df) are 2 and 27, and the significance level (α) is set at 0.05. The critical value from the F table is 3.35. Since the calculated F value (21.44) is greater than the critical value, we conclude that there is a statistically significant difference among the group means. In other words, the effects observed among the three facial rejuvenation treatment groups are not the same. Put differently, the three treatment methods do not yield the same effects on skin improvement. We can interpret this to mean that if the same experiment were repeated 100 times, we would expect to see such a large difference among group means less than 5 times purely by chance. However, ANOVA does not tell us which treatment method was the most or least effective. For such specific information, a post-hoc test must be conducted.

6. *Post-Hoc Comparison After ANOVA*

A post-hoc test is conducted to determine which specific group means differ from each other after a statistically significant F ratio has been found in ANOVA. Commonly used post-hoc tests include Tukey's HSD, Newman–Keuls, Bonferroni, Scheffé, and Duncan's multiple range test. The choice of method depends on whether pairwise or nonpairwise comparisons are to be made, and on the degree of Type I error protection desired. In the present example, the Newman–Keuls procedure was applied. The results showed that Group 1 (chemical peeling group) differed significantly from Group 2 (fractional laser therapy group) and Group 3 (intense pulsed light therapy group). However, there was no significant difference between Group 2 and Group 3. This can be interpreted to mean that fractional laser therapy and IPL therapy have comparable effects in improving skin appearance, whereas chemical peeling is less effective than either fractional laser therapy or IPL therapy.

7. *Assumptions of ANOVA*

There are three commonly stated assumptions for analysis of variance (ANOVA). First, the dependent variable must be normally distributed within each group (normality). Second, the variances of the dependent variable across groups must be equal (homogeneity of variance). Even if this assumption is moderately violated, it may be compensated by applying data transformations or by increasing the sample size. Third, the cases included in the analysis must be independent of one another (independence). When repeated measures are taken from the same participants, this assumption is violated. Applying standard ANOVA to such data can lead to serious errors. In such cases, an alternative method such as repeated-measures ANOVA should be used.

In SPSS, when conducting a one-way ANOVA, homogeneity of variance can be tested by selecting the option for "Test of Homogeneity of Variance" under the statistics settings. If the assumption of homogeneity is not met, Tamhane's

T2, Dunnett's T3, Games–Howell, or Dunnett's C can be used for post hoc multiple comparisons. Among these, Games–Howell is most commonly used.

Logically, ANOVA is an extension of the two-tailed t-test, and even when comparing only two groups, either an F-test (ANOVA) or a t-test may be used. The advantage of ANOVA over the t-test is that it can be used for three or more group comparisons. Like the t-test, ANOVA is only applicable to data measured on an interval or ratio scale. Technically, it may also be applied to ordinal scales if the intervals are assumed to be equal, although this remains a topic of debate among experts.

8. *What Should Be Included in the Results Section of an ANOVA Report*

What should be included in the results section following an analysis of variance (ANOVA)? First, in the introduction, the research hypothesis should be clearly stated. In the methods section, the report should describe the following: characteristics of the sample, sampling methods, randomization procedures, number of participants in each group, operational definition of the dependent variable, description of the factor (independent variable), levels of the factor, significance level (α), and the post-hoc test method used. In the results section, the report should present group means, variances (or standard deviations), sums of squares (between-groups and within-groups), mean squares, the F-value, degrees of freedom, and post-hoc comparison results. A results table can be formatted as shown in Table 12.5.

9. *Variance*

Variance is generally classified into two categories: systematic variance and error variance. Systematic variance refers to variations in measurement values that occur in a consistent direction due to known or unknown factors. These influencing factors may be artificial or natural in origin. For example, when a well-balanced die is rolled repeatedly, each number from 1 to 6 is expected to appear with equal frequency. However, if a poorly manufactured die is rolled repeatedly, a particular number may appear more frequently than others. This outcome reflects the influence of a systematic factor—specifically, a bias in weight distribution that causes the die to favor a certain side. Systematic variance can be further subdivided into between-group variance, and variance caused by bias.

1. Between-groups variance

   A concept closely related to between-groups variance is experimental variance. Experimental variance refers to the variation that occurs between groups as a result of an experiment. Manipulation (i.e., the experimental intervention) is essentially an act intended to increase between-groups variance. The larger the experimental variance, the more likely it is that the manipulation (independent variable) had an effect on the outcome.

2. Bias (also considered as error)

   Bias refers to the difference from the true value or the process by which such a difference arises. Bias can occur throughout all phases of a study—including participant selection, data collection, and data analysis—and is typically caused by a flawed or inadequate system or method. Bias is generally categorized into three types such as selection bias, measurement bias (or information bias), and confounding.

   Selection bias occurs during the subject recruitment process. For example, it arises when the study sample does not accurately

Table 12.5 Results of ANOVA

Source of variation	Degrees of freedom	Sum of squares	Mean square	F-value	p-value
Between groups	2	165.07	82.53	21.44	<0.05
Within groups	27	103.90	3.85		
Total	29	268.97			

represent the target population. Measurement bias (or information bias) occurs during the data collection process and often results from a lack of standardized measurement criteria. Examples include instrumental bias (due to measuring equipment) and interviewer bias. Although not originally a statistical term, confounding refers to bias introduced during the data analysis phase. It occurs when multiple factors, not just the variable of interest, influence the outcome. For instance, blood pressure is affected not only by salt intake but also by sex, age, ethnicity, socioeconomic status, and more. Therefore, to isolate the effect of salt intake on blood pressure, the variance caused by other factors must be controlled. Only the remaining variance—after removing the influence of these confounding variables—can be considered as the true effect of salt intake.

3. Error Variance (or Random Variance)

   Error variance refers to the portion of variability in measurement values that arises randomly and probabilistically due to chance.

10. *Problems When Using t-Tests Instead of ANOVA*

Suppose we want to test whether there are differences among the population means of six groups. If we decide to apply t-tests to compare the means of each pair of groups, the number of possible pairwise comparisons is $6 \text{C} 2 = 6 \times (6 - 1)/2 = 15$. This means we would need to conduct 15 separate t-tests. However, deriving a conclusion based on this method would be problematic. When performing multiple comparisons like this, the risk of making a Type I error (incorrectly rejecting a true null hypothesis) significantly increases. For instance, if the significance level is set at $\alpha = 0.05$, then the probability of not rejecting the null hypothesis for any one test is $1 - \alpha = 0.95$. Assuming the tests are independent (even though in reality they are not), the probability of not rejecting the null hypothesis across all 15 tests would be $(0.95)^{15} = 0.46$. Thus, the probability of rejecting at least one null hypothesis among the 15 comparisons is 0.54. This is much higher than the originally intended significance level of 0.05. Therefore, repeatedly applying t-tests leads to a situation where the effective significance level is substantially inflated, making the results statistically unreliable.

Let's consider another example. Suppose we are comparing three groups at $\alpha = 0.05$. The number of pairwise comparisons is $k(k - 1)/2 = 3(3-1)/2 = 3$. The familywise error rate (α_{FW}) becomes $\alpha_{FW} = 1 - (1 - 0.05)^3 = 1 - (0.95)^3 = 0.143$. This means that if the researcher finds significant differences in all three comparisons, there's at least a 14.3% chance that one of those results occurred by random chance—far above the conventional 5% Type I error threshold. As the number of comparisons increases, so does the probability of obtaining at least one false positive:

- To compare 4 means (6 comparisons available): $\alpha_{FW} = 1 - (1 - 0.05)^6 = 0.26$
- To compare 5 means (10 comparisons available): $\alpha_{FW} = 1 - (1 - 0.05)^{10} = 0.40$
  (Interpretation: 4 of 10 results may be false positives)
- To compare 6 means (15 comparisons available): $\alpha_{FW} = 1 - (1 - 0.05)^{15} = 0.54$

To prevent such inflation of Type I error, the Bonferroni method is used, where the significance level is adjusted by dividing α by the number of comparisons (e.g., $\alpha' = 0.05 / 6$), or by multiplying each *p*-value by the number of comparisons.

Since Bonferroni is often criticized for being overly conservative and lowering statistical power, a Modified Bonferroni test is sometimes applied to maintain the familywise error rate at 0.05 while improving power.

Suppose we conducted 15 pairwise comparisons on the same dataset and obtained the following *p*-values:

$p = 0.20$
$p = 0.30$
$p = 0.0035$
$p = 0.57$

$p = 0.16$
$p = 0.09$
$p = 0.002$
$p = 0.10$
$p = 0.10$
$p = 0.36$
$p = 0.04$
$p = 0.58$
$p = 0.04$
$p = 0.16$
$p = 0.40$

Among these, there are four p-values less than 0.05, which would traditionally be considered statistically significant. However, when the same hypothesis is tested 15 times, the risk of committing a Type I error increases—that is, we might incorrectly conclude that a difference or association exists in the population when it does not. Even if the significance level was set at $\alpha = 0.05$, the effective familywise error rate becomes $0.05 \times 15 = 0.75$.

To address this problem, Bonferroni proposed a correction method in which the significance level is adjusted by dividing it by the number of comparisons: $0.05/15 = 0.003$. Under this correction, only one 7th p-value in the list—$p = 0.002$—is less than 0.003 and thus considered statistically significant. However, a trade-off of using Bonferroni correction is a reduction in statistical power, meaning that even if a real difference or association exists, we are more likely to fail to detect it.

To overcome this limitation, a modified Bonferroni method was proposed, one of which is the Holm procedure. This method increases statistical power while still controlling the familywise error rate.

The Holm method follows these steps:

1. Rank the p-values from smallest to largest.
2. Compute the adjusted significance level for each p-value by dividing 0.05 by (number of comparisons − rank + 1).
3. Starting from the smallest p-value, compare each one to its corresponding adjusted significance level.
4. Continue until a p-value is greater than its adjusted α level; stop at that point. All remaining p-values are considered not significant. For example, if the third smallest p-value is 0.04 and the corresponding adjusted α is 0.0038, then because $0.04 > 0.0038$, all p-values ranked below it are not significant. When significance and nonsignificance are mixed and the cutoff is unclear, the rule is to determine the point where the first nonsignificant result appears (when scanning from top to bottom), and consider all lower-ranked results as nonsignificant.

Another approach is the Hochberg procedure, which is similar in calculation to the Holm method but proceeds in reverse. In this method, p-values are reviewed from bottom to top. The moment a p-value is found that is less than its corresponding adjusted significance level, all p-values above it are considered significant (Table 12.6).

11. *Selection of an Appropriate Multiple Comparison Method*

Analysis of variance (ANOVA) is a statistical method used to compare the means of three or more groups. The initial hypothesis typically tests whether all group means are equal, or whether at least one group differs from the others. When ANOVA yields a statistically significant result, the researcher must further investigate which specific group means differ.

However, ANOVA alone cannot identify which groups are significantly different from each other. Performing multiple t-tests for each pairwise comparison inflates the familywise error rate, thereby increasing the likelihood of Type I error. To address this issue, researchers must perform either a priori contrasts, post hoc contrasts, or multiple comparison procedures.

Once a significant effect among treatments has been established through ANOVA, the next step involves conducting pairwise comparisons between treatment groups to determine where the differences lie. This process is known as multiple

Table 12.6 An example of the Holm method

Rank	*P*-value	Adjusted significance level	Decision
1	0.002	0.05/(15 – 1 + 1) = 0.0033	Significant
2	0.0035	0.05/(15 – 2 + 1) = 0.0036	Significant
3	0.04	0.05/(15 – 3 + 1) = 0.0038	Not Significant
4	0.04	0.05/(15 – 4 + 1) = 0.0042	Not Significant
5	0.09	0.05/(15 – 5 + 1) = 0.0045	Not Significant
6	0.10	0.05/(15 – 6 + 1) = 0.0050	Not Significant
7	0.10	0.05/(15 – 7 + 1) = 0.0056	Not Significant
8	0.20	0.05/(15 – 8 + 1) = 0.0063	Not Significant
9	0.16	0.05/(15 – 9 + 1) = 0.0071	Not Significant
10	0.16	0.05/(15 – 10 + 1) = 0.0083	Not Significant
11	0.30	0.05/(15 – 11 + 1) = 0.0100	Not Significant
12	0.40	0.05/(15 – 12 + 1) = 0.0125	Not Significant
13	0.36	0.05/(15 – 13 + 1) = 0.0167	Not Significant
14	0.57	0.05/(15 – 14 + 1) = 0.0250	Not Significant
15	0.58	0.05/(15 – 15 + 1) = 0.0500	Not Significant

Table 12.7 Methods for multiple comparisons

Method	Timing of comparison	Comparison groups	Sample size
Fisher's Least-Significant-Difference (LSD) method	Post hoc	All pairwise comparisons[a]	Different sample sizes
Duncan's Multiple-Range Procedure	Post hoc	All pairwise comparisons	Equal sample sizes
Newman–Keuls (NK) or Student–Newman–Keuls (SNK) Procedure	Post hoc	All pairwise comparisons	Equal sample sizes
Tukey's Honestly Significant Difference (HSD) Procedure	Post hoc	All pairwise comparisons	Equal sample sizes
Scheffé Method	Post hoc	All combinations	Different sample sizes
Bonferroni Test	Post hoc	All combinations	Different sample sizes
Dunnett's Test	A priori[b]	Comparisons with a control group	Different sample sizes

[a]All pairwise comparisons mean that when there are k groups, there are kC2 possible comparisons. All combinations refer to comparisons of all possible linear combinations. Comparisons with a control group refer to comparing the control group with each of the other $k - 1$ groups. For example, 7C3 = (7 × 6 × 5)/3! = 35: choosing 3 out of 7 groups. 10C4 = (10 × 9 × 8 × 7)/4! = 210: choosing 4 out of 10 groups

[b]A priori contrasts refer to cases where comparisons between groups are planned before analyzing the data, whereas post hoc comparisons are made after finding significant results from ANOVA

comparison testing. Common multiple comparison methods include Least Significant Difference (LSD) Test, Tukey's Honestly Significant Difference (HSD) Test, Scheffé's Test, and Fisher's Protected Least Significant Difference Test.

A summary of these methods is shown in Table 12.7.

There is no definitive standard for determining which multiple comparison method is "superior." Researchers often select methods based on their preference or based on the default options available in statistical software packages. The appropriateness of a particular method should be determined in consideration of the study's design and objective. However, two key considerations must be taken into account: whether the comparisons are planned (a priori) or unplanned (post hoc), and whether the researcher is more concerned about Type I error or Type II error.

If the study involves one control group and multiple treatment groups, it may not be necessary to compare all possible group combinations. Instead, comparisons may be focused on the difference between the control group and each treatment group. In such cases, Dunnett's multiple comparison test is an appropriate choice.

12. *Points to Consider in ANOVA*

If the result of the F-test in ANOVA is not significant, the analysis of the data is essentially concluded. However, if the F-test result is significant, additional post hoc analyses can be performed to gather the necessary information, specifically to determine which means differ significantly from each other. The process of comparing individual means after finding a significant overall F-test result is called a post hoc comparison (posterior comparison or post-hoc comparison).

If the researcher has prior information regarding the effects of the treatments or is not interested in an overall comparison, it is not necessary to conduct an overall F-test. Instead, an experimental design focused on comparing the specific treatment effects of interest should be used, and the data should be analyzed accordingly. The process of comparing the means of planned experimental groups instead of performing an overall F-test is referred to as an a priori comparison (planned comparison).

Both a priori and post hoc comparisons are collectively referred to as multiple comparison tests. Multiple comparison analysis is applicable only to fixed-effect models and mixed-effect models. In particular, it is meaningful when applied to treatment groups that represent fixed factors.

13. *Test of Homogeneity of Variance*

To determine whether the assumption of normality in ANOVA is met, researchers may use a normal probability paper or apply the one-sample Kolmogorov–Smirnov test. To test for homogeneity of variance, commonly used methods include Bartlett's test, Hartley's test, and Levene's test.

- Terminology:
  - *Within-group variation* = *Unexplained variation* = *Residual variation* = *Variation due to error*
  - *Among-group variation* = *Variation due to the factor* = *Variation explained by the factor*

In this context, the term factor may also be referred to as a treatment.

14. *Hypothesis Testing Procedure in ANOVA*

Step 1: Formulate the statistical hypotheses.
Null hypothesis H_0: $\mu_1 = \mu_2 = \mu_3$
Alternative hypothesis H_1: Not all population means are equal.

Step 2: Select the test statistic.
Since ANOVA relies on the F-distribution, the F-value is used as the test statistic.

Step 3: Determine the level of significance.
$\alpha = 0.01$

Step 4: Calculate the test statistic.

$$F = \frac{\text{Between} - \text{group variance}}{\text{Within} - \text{group variance}} = \frac{\frac{\text{SSB}}{K-1}}{\frac{\text{SSW}}{N-K}}$$

$$= \frac{\text{MSB}}{\text{MSW or error}}$$

Step 5: Make a decision.
If the *p-value* $< \alpha \rightarrow$ Reject the null hypothesis $\rightarrow$ Conduct post-hoc comparisons
If the *p-value* $\geq \alpha \rightarrow$ Fail to reject the null hypothesis

As various terms are often used interchangeably in ANOVA, the terminology is summarized in Table 12.8.

Table 12.8 Abbreviations and synonyms used in ANOVA

Term	Abbreviation	Meaning
Sum of Squares	SS	Variation
Between	SSB	Between-group variation
Within	SSW	Within-group variation
TOTAL	SST	Total variation = Between + Within
Mean Square	MS	Variance
Between	MSB	Between-group or systematic variance
Within	MSW	Within-group or error variance
Factor	A	Independent variable
Level	a	Subcategory of independent variable
Subjects	Ss	
Degrees of freedom	df	Number of elements free to vary
n		Number of subjects in a group
N		Total number of subjects in the study
k		Number of groups in the study (levels of Factor A for one-way ANOVA)
Group mean	X_j	Average of scores in a group
Grand mean	X	Average of all scores in the study
Group variance	S_j^2	$\left(\sum_{j=1}^{n}(X_{ij}-X_j)^2(n-1)\right)$
Group standard deviation		Square root of variance
Sigma	Σ	Instructions to sum scores
		$\sum_{j=1}^{n} X_{ij}$ within a group
		$\sum_{j=1}^{k} X_{ij}$ across groups

15. *Special Models in Analysis of Variance*

In the example presented in Table 12.4, 30 participants were randomly assigned to three different skin treatment protocols—chemical peeling, fractional laser therapy, and IPL therapy—with 10 individuals allocated to each group. That is, each participant was exposed to only one of the three treatment types. However, this design requires a relatively large number of subjects. A commonly used alternative in analysis of variance is the repeated-measures design, in which all three skin treatments are applied to the same 10 subjects in a randomized order. This repeated-measures approach is advantageous in that it requires fewer participants and controls for inter-subject variability. However, several assumptions must be satisfied. Specifically, the administration of one treatment should not influence the effects of the subsequent treatments, and the order of treatments must not result in carry-over effects, such as learning effects or lasting physiological responses that confound the next measurement.

A repeated-measures ANOVA model offers certain advantages over traditional between-subjects ANOVA. Since the same individuals are exposed to all treatment levels, the influence of external or individual differences is reduced, and the required sample size is smaller.

In ANOVA, a fixed-effects model refers to a scenario where the experimenter is only interested in the specific treatments used in the study. For example, if a significant difference in skin elasticity improvement is found among the three skin treatment methods—chemical peeling, fractional laser, and IPL therapy—the generalization of the result is limited to those three interventions.

In contrast, a random-effects model assumes that the levels of the independent variable (e.g., types of therapists or clinics) are randomly selected from a larger population, and the goal is to generalize the findings to the broader group beyond those included in the study. For instance, a study assessing the efficacy of various skincare programs delivered by different dermatologists might be considered a random-effects model if the intent is to generalize beyond those specific providers.

In one-way ANOVA, there is no computational difference between fixed and random models. However, in two-way or higher-order ANOVAs, the models differ in how the error term is defined and interpreted, particularly in the calculation and interpretation of the F-statistic. When an ANOVA includes both fixed and random factors, it is called a mixed-effects model.

12.8 Example of Analysis of Variance (ANOVA) Using SPSS

This dataset is a hypothetical example measuring changes in dermal temperature following four different cosmetic procedures: chemical peeling, radiofrequency treatment, IPL therapy, and fractional laser therapy. In SPSS, enter the data as follows (Fig. 12.41). In the treatment method variable, 1 represents chemical peeling, 2 represents radiofrequency treatment, 3 represents IPL therapy, and 4 represents fractional laser therapy.

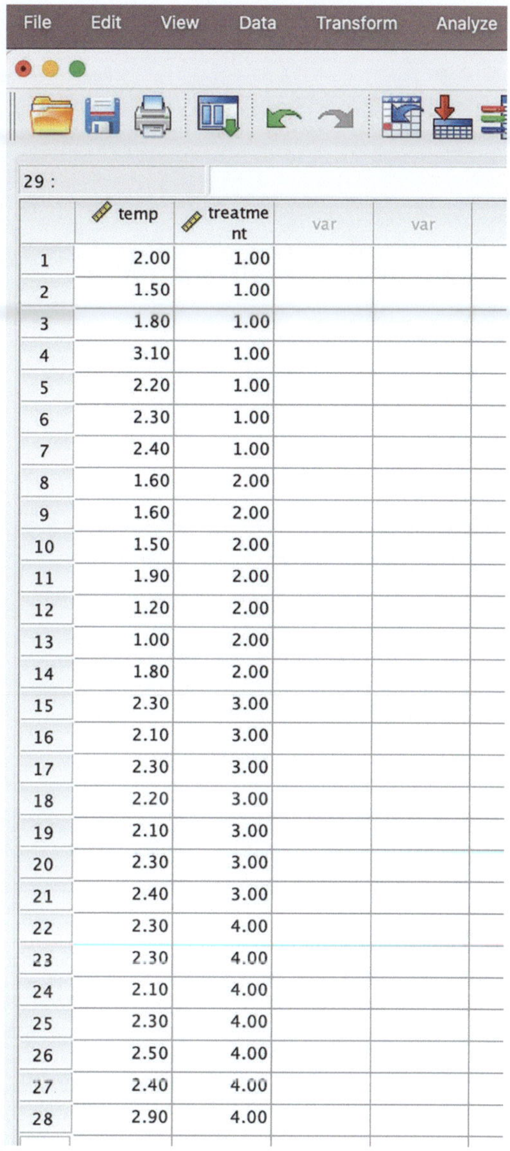

	temp	treatment	var	var
1	2.00	1.00		
2	1.50	1.00		
3	1.80	1.00		
4	3.10	1.00		
5	2.20	1.00		
6	2.30	1.00		
7	2.40	1.00		
8	1.60	2.00		
9	1.60	2.00		
10	1.50	2.00		
11	1.90	2.00		
12	1.20	2.00		
13	1.00	2.00		
14	1.80	2.00		
15	2.30	3.00		
16	2.10	3.00		
17	2.30	3.00		
18	2.20	3.00		
19	2.10	3.00		
20	2.30	3.00		
21	2.40	3.00		
22	2.30	4.00		
23	2.30	4.00		
24	2.10	4.00		
25	2.30	4.00		
26	2.50	4.00		
27	2.40	4.00		
28	2.90	4.00		

Fig. 12.41 Example dataset for conducting a one-way ANOVA using SPSS

After completing data entry, go to Analyze → Compare Means → One-Way ANOVA (Fig. 12.42).

The dialog box will appear. Select the dependent variable (e.g., temp) from the list on the left, and click the top-center arrow to move it into the Dependent List field on the right. Likewise, click on the independent variable (treatment), and use the bottom center arrow to move it into the Factor field. Then click OK (Fig. 12.43).

The resulting ANOVA table will appear (Fig. 12.44). The table shows that $p < 0.001$, indicating a statistically significant difference in dermal temperature changes among the four treatment groups. Although we do not yet know which groups differ from each other, the p-value being less than 0.05 suggests that a significant difference exists somewhere.

Since the p-value is less than 0.05, click on the Post Hoc button in the dialog box to determine where the differences lie (Fig. 12.45).

The following screen will appear (Fig. 12.46). And then choose the Scheffé method from the available options. Click Continue, then OK.

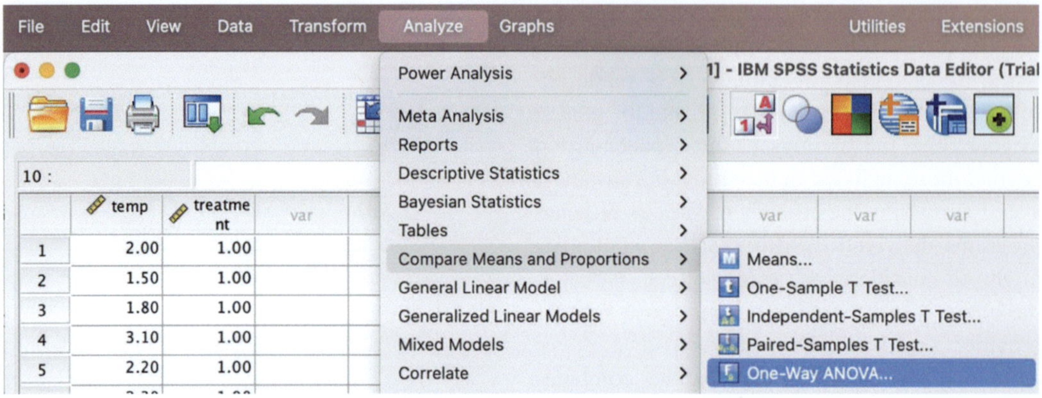

Fig. 12.42 Navigating to one-way ANOVA via Analyze → Compare Means in SPSS

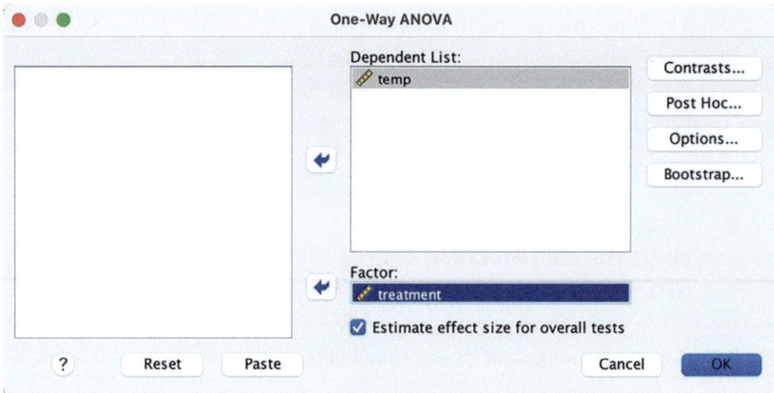

Fig. 12.43 One-way ANOVA dialog box in SPSS

ANOVA

temp

	Sum of Squares	df	Mean Square	F	Sig.
Between Groups	3.220	3	1.073	9.854	<.001
Within Groups	2.614	24	.109		
Total	5.834	27			

Fig. 12.44 SPSS output window displaying results of the one-way ANOVA

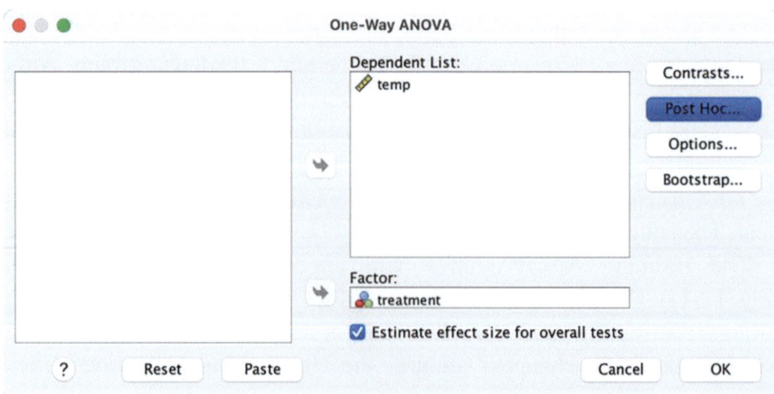

Fig. 12.45 Clicking the "Post Hoc…" button in the one-way ANOVA dialog

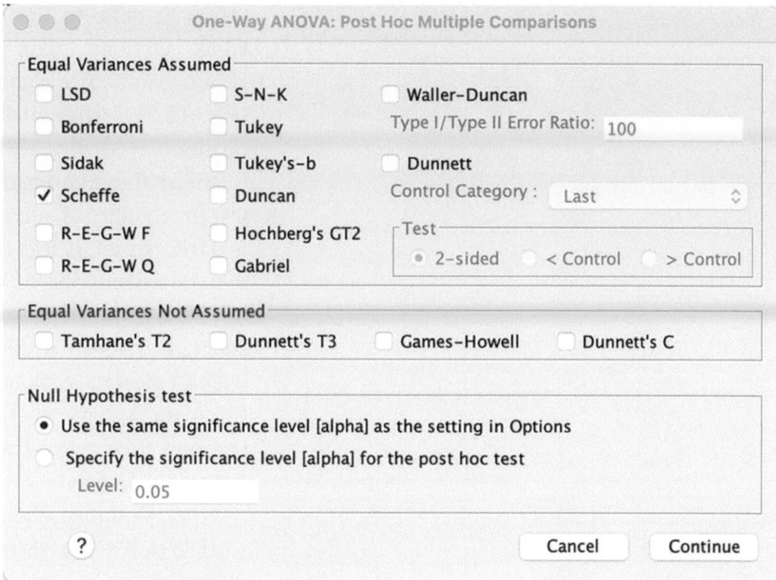

Fig. 12.46 Available options for post hoc multiple comparisons in SPSS's one-way ANOVA dialog box

Multiple Comparisons

Dependent Variable: temp
Scheffe

(I) treatment	(J) treatment	Mean Difference (I-J)	Std. Error	Sig.	95% Confidence Interval Lower Bound	95% Confidence Interval Upper Bound
chemical peeling	radiofrequency	.67143*	.17642	.009	.1414	1.2014
	IPL	-.05714	.17642	.991	-.5872	.4729
	fractional laser	-.21429	.17642	.691	-.7443	.3157
radiofrequency	chemical peeling	-.67143*	.17642	.009	-1.2014	-.1414
	IPL	-.72857*	.17642	.004	-1.2586	-.1986
	fractional laser	-.88571*	.17642	<.001	-1.4157	-.3557
IPL	chemical peeling	.05714	.17642	.991	-.4729	.5872
	radiofrequency	.72857*	.17642	.004	.1986	1.2586
	fractional laser	-.15714	.17642	.850	-.6872	.3729
fractional laser	chemical peeling	.21429	.17642	.691	-.3157	.7443
	radiofrequency	.88571*	.17642	<.001	.3557	1.4157
	IPL	.15714	.17642	.850	-.3729	.6872

*. The mean difference is significant at the 0.05 level.

Fig. 12.47 Post hoc multiple comparison results table from SPSS one-way ANOVA output

The output table will show the results of multiple comparisons (Fig. 12.47). According to the Scheffé test, radiofrequency treatment shows statistically significant differences in temperature changes compared to chemical peeling, IPL therapy, and fractional laser therapy at the 0.05 level.

Now, suppose we want to analyze a dataset that violates the assumption of homogeneity of variances. Enter the data accordingly and proceed as before (Figs. 12.48 and 12.49).

In the dialog box, move the dependent variable (e.g., score) to the Dependent List and the

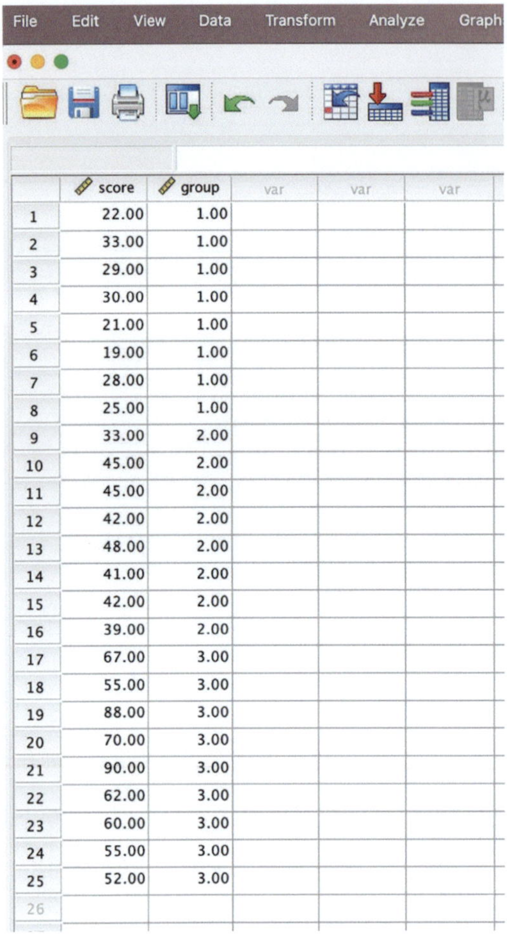

	score	group	var	var	var
1	22.00	1.00			
2	33.00	1.00			
3	29.00	1.00			
4	30.00	1.00			
5	21.00	1.00			
6	19.00	1.00			
7	28.00	1.00			
8	25.00	1.00			
9	33.00	2.00			
10	45.00	2.00			
11	45.00	2.00			
12	42.00	2.00			
13	48.00	2.00			
14	41.00	2.00			
15	42.00	2.00			
16	39.00	2.00			
17	67.00	3.00			
18	55.00	3.00			
19	88.00	3.00			
20	70.00	3.00			
21	90.00	3.00			
22	62.00	3.00			
23	60.00	3.00			
24	55.00	3.00			
25	52.00	3.00			
26					

Fig. 12.48 Example dataset for the following analysis in SPSS

group variable to the Factor field (Fig. 12.50). Click Options, then check Descriptive and Homogeneity of variance test, and click Continue (Fig. 12.51). After clicking OK, you will see the results.

Since the significance level of the Levene's test for equality of variances "based on the mean" is 0.012, which is less than 0.05, it is determined that the assumption of homogeneity of variances has been violated (Fig. 12.52). In this case, the standard ANOVA results are no longer valid. Go back to the data view and navigate to Analyze → Compare Means → One-Way ANOVA. Click Options, then select Brown–Forsythe and Welch tests (Fig. 12.53).

Click Continue, then OK.

If Welch's test shows a p-value of 0.000, it indicates that at least one group differs significantly from the others (Fig. 12.54). To determine where these differences occur, proceed with a post hoc test. If the results of Brown–Forsythe and Welch differ, interpret the results based on Welch, as it generally has greater statistical power (Fig. 12.55). However, when sample sizes are equal across groups, some researchers may prefer Brown–Forsythe.

Click Post Hoc, and under Equal variances not assumed, choose Games–Howell, then click Continue, then OK (Fig. 12.56).

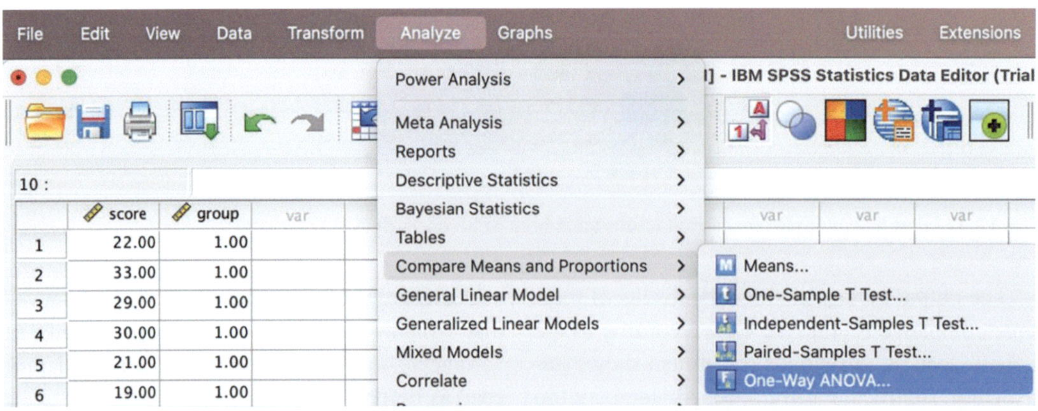

Fig. 12.49 Navigation path for one-way ANOVA in SPSS

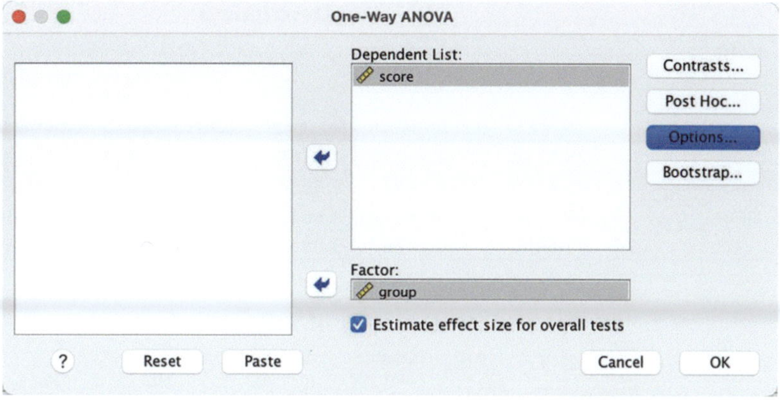

Fig. 12.50 One-way ANOVA dialog box in SPSS

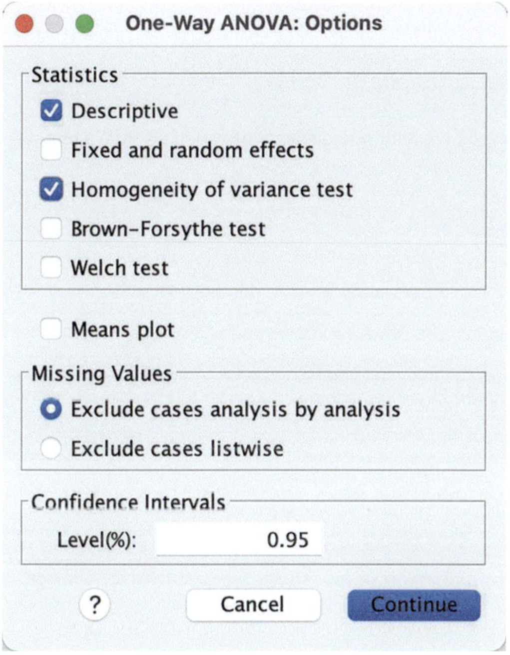

Fig. 12.51 Options dialog box in SPSS one-way ANOVA, used to specify descriptive statistics, homogeneity tests, and other display preferences

The post hoc results will indicate significant differences between the following group pairs: Group 1 and Group 2, Group 1 and Group 3, and Group 2 and Group 3 (Fig. 12.57).

Descriptives

score

	N	Mean	Std. Deviation	Std. Error	95% Confidence Interval for Mean		Minimum	Maximum
					Lower Bound	Upper Bound		
1.00	8	25.8750	4.91172	1.73656	21.7687	29.9813	19.00	33.00
2.00	8	41.8750	4.54933	1.60843	38.0717	45.6783	33.00	48.00
3.00	9	66.5556	13.98312	4.66104	55.8072	77.3039	52.00	90.00
Total	25	45.6400	19.42267	3.88453	37.6227	53.6573	19.00	90.00

Tests of Homogeneity of Variances

		Levene Statistic	df1	df2	Sig.
score	Based on Mean	5.498	2	22	.012
	Based on Median	3.243	2	22	.058
	Based on Median and with adjusted df	3.243	2	10.110	.082
	Based on trimmed mean	5.312	2	22	.013

Fig. 12.52 SPSS output showing descriptive statistics and Levene's test for homogeneity of variances from a one-way ANOVA analysis

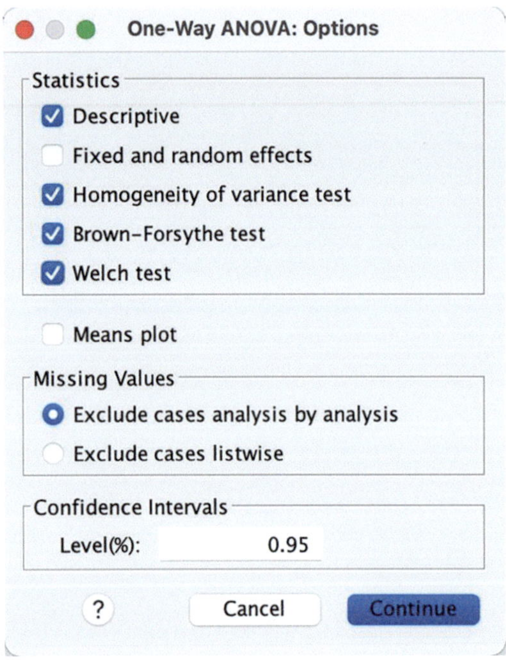

Fig. 12.53 Selection of additional options in the one-way ANOVA options dialog box in SPSS

Fig. 12.54 Output window displaying the results of the one-way ANOVA in SPSS

ANOVA

score

	Sum of Squares	df	Mean Square	F	Sig.
Between Groups	7175.788	2	3587.894	42.031	<.001
Within Groups	1877.972	22	85.362		
Total	9053.760	24			

Fig. 12.55 SPSS output displaying the robust tests of equality of means

Robust Tests of Equality of Means

score

	Statistic[a]	df1	df2	Sig.
Welch	43.033	2	13.957	<.001
Brown-Forsythe	46.112	2	11.964	<.001

a. Asymptotically F distributed.

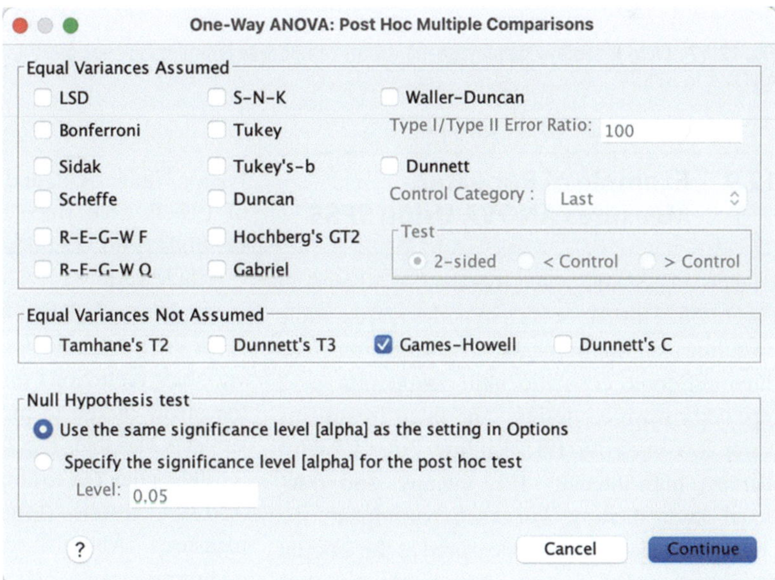

Fig. 12.56 Selection of alternative post hoc test options in the SPSS post hoc dialog box

Post Hoc Tests

Multiple Comparisons

Dependent Variable: score
Games–Howell

(I) group	(J) group	Mean Difference (I–J)	Std. Error	Sig.	95% Confidence Interval Lower Bound	95% Confidence Interval Upper Bound
1.00	2.00	-16.00000*	2.36700	<.001	-22.1992	-9.8008
	3.00	-40.68056*	4.97403	<.001	-54.2825	-27.0786
2.00	1.00	16.00000*	2.36700	<.001	9.8008	22.1992
	3.00	-24.68056*	4.93076	.001	-38.2290	-11.1321
3.00	1.00	40.68056*	4.97403	<.001	27.0786	54.2825
	2.00	24.68056*	4.93076	.001	11.1321	38.2290

*. The mean difference is significant at the 0.05 level.

Fig. 12.57 Output window displaying the results of multiple comparison tests (post hoc analysis) following one-way ANOVA in SPSS

12.9 Example of Repeated-Measures ANOVA Using SPSS

Launch SPSS and enter the data as shown in Fig. 12.58. This dataset is a hypothetical example involving six participants who each received three different cosmetic skin treatments in a repeated-measures design. The three treatments were: low-intensity IPL (Intense Pulsed Light) therapy, high-intensity IPL therapy, and fractional laser therapy. For each participant, the change in melanin index (measured as the amount of reduction before and after treatment) was recorded as an indicator of pigmentation improvement.

After entering the data, go to Analyze → General Linear Model → Repeated Measures (Fig. 12.59).

When the following window appears, enter a name that is easy to understand such as txtype (short for treatment type) in the Within-Subject Factor Name field, and enter "3" in the Number of Levels field since there are three treatment methods (Figs. 12.60 and 12.61).

Click Add.

And then click Define (Fig. 12.62).

In the next window, use your mouse to select variables reduction1 through reduction3, and use the arrow button to move them into the within-subjects variables box (Fig. 12.63).

Then click *OK* to obtain the repeated-measures ANOVA results (Fig. 12.64). The repeated-measures ANOVA output includes several assumption tests, and it is advisable to consult with a statistical expert when interpreting the results. Generally, if the assumption of sphericity is met, univariate tests are used; if not, multivariate tests are applied.

Figure 12.65 shows the results when repeated measures are used. It begins with the test for the assumption of sphericity. Just as Levene's test is used to assess the equality of variances in an

Fig. 12.58 Example dataset used for repeated-measures ANOVA analysis in SPSS

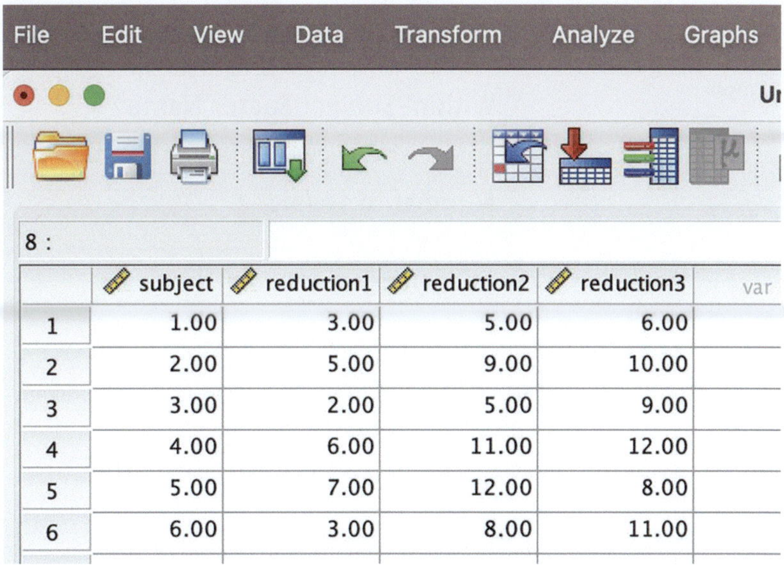

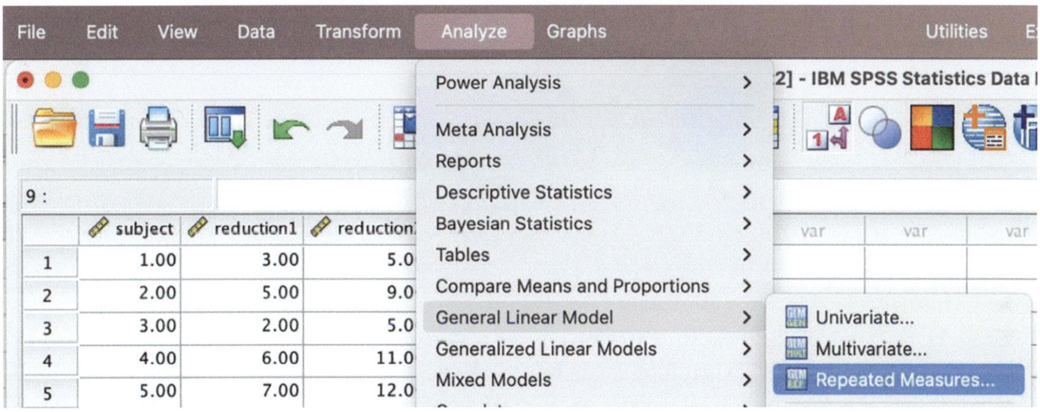

Fig. 12.59 Navigation path for conducting repeated-measures ANOVA in SPSS

independent t-test, Mauchly's test is used in repeated-measures ANOVA to check for sphericity. If the Mauchly statistic is not significant ($p > 0.05$), sphericity is assumed. If the assumption of sphericity is met—specifically, when Mauchly's test statistic is not significant ($p > 0.05$ or $p > 0.01$)—the results under the Sphericity Assumed condition can be used. However, if the assumption of sphericity is violated—i.e., when Mauchly's test statistic is significant ($p < 0.05$ or $p < 0.01$)—there are two options for interpreting the results: one is to refer to the multivariate test table, and the other is to use the epsilon (ε) value to adjust the degrees of freedom and interpret the results accordingly (e.g., using the Greenhouse–Geisser correction). If the epsilon is less than 0.75, use the Greenhouse–Geisser correction; if greater than 0.75, use the Huynh–Feldt correction. In the Mauchly's test of sphericity table below, the p-value is 0.253, which is greater than

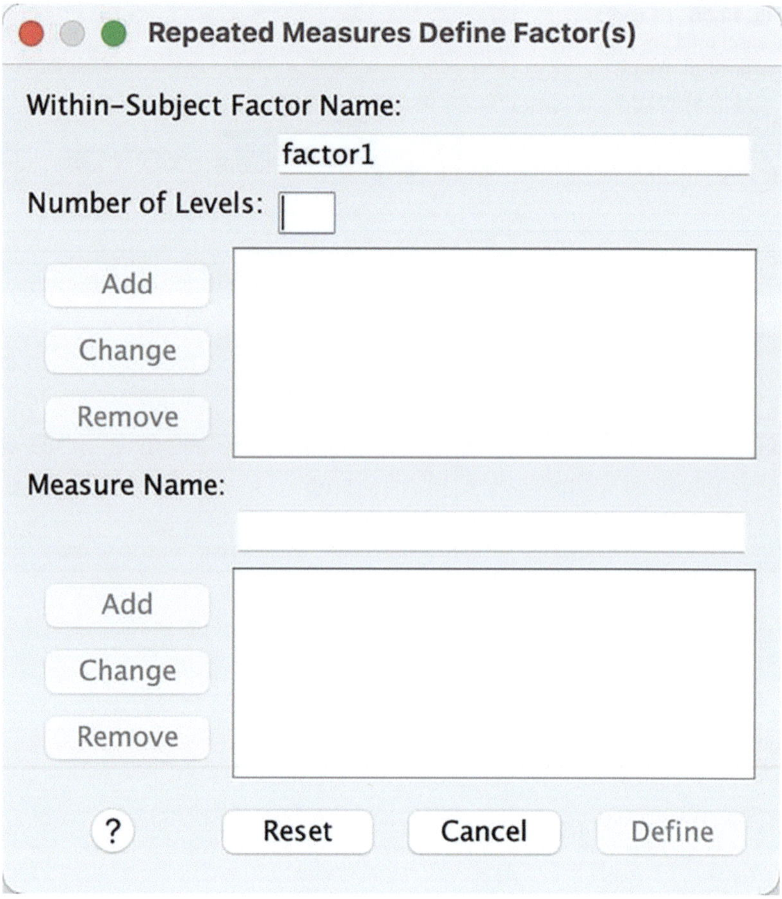

Fig. 12.60 "Repeated Measures Define Factors" dialog window in SPSS

the significance level of 0.05. Therefore, it can be concluded that the assumption of sphericity is satisfied, and the results under the Sphericity Assumed condition should be referred to. In general, the multivariate test can be used regardless of whether the assumption of sphericity is met. However, it should be noted that when the epsilon value is large, multivariate tests may have lower statistical power compared to univariate repeated-measures ANOVA with adjusted degrees of freedom (e.g., Greenhouse-Geisser). If the assumption of sphericity is not satisfied, one can use a multivariate test, adjust the degrees of freedom in univariate repeated-measures analysis, or apply a nonparametric test such as the Friedman test.

Even if the assumption of sphericity is not satisfied according to Mauchly's test, if the deviation of the epsilon values from 1 is small, the adjusted values from the test of within-subjects effects can be used (Fig. 12.66). If the epsilon value is close to 0, the results of the multivariate test should be reported. An epsilon value of 1 indicates perfect sphericity. If the epsilon value is less than 0.75, the Greenhouse–Geisser values should be referred to in the test of within-subjects effects table. If the epsilon value is 0.75 or greater, the Huynh–Feldt values should be used as the corrected values. In this example, the Greenhouse–Geisser epsilon is 0.668, which is less than 0.75, so the Greenhouse–Geisser row in the test of within-subjects effects table should be

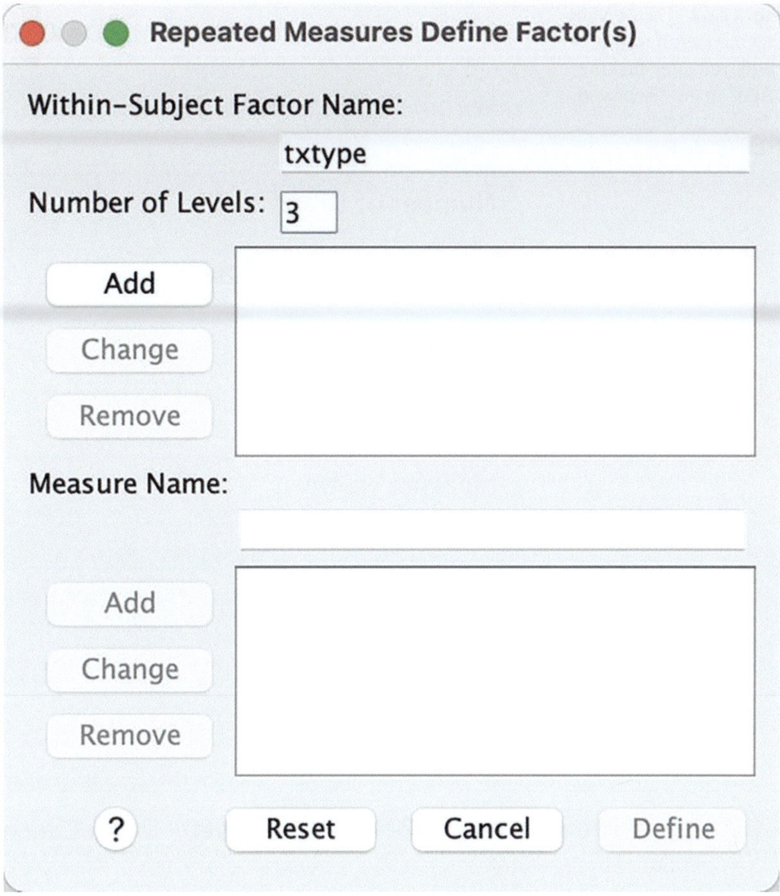

Fig. 12.61 Entering the factor name and number of levels in the "Repeated Measures Define Factors" dialog

consulted. The result shows a *p*-value of 0.004, and since $p < 0.005$, the null hypothesis is rejected. This indicates that there is a statistically significant difference among the three treatment methods. To determine specifically which treatment methods differ from one another, a post hoc analysis should be conducted.

All four multivariate tests in the output yield the same result because only one dependent variable was used. In general, Wilks' Lambda is reported. In this table, Wilks' Lambda = 0.063 and $p = 0.004$, indicating statistically significant differences among the three treatments. However, it is still unclear which specific treatment methods differ significantly from one another.

The degrees of freedom in the sphericity-assumed row are $F(2,10)$, while the Greenhouse–Geisser degrees of freedom are $F(1.336, 6.678)$, calculated by multiplying the original degrees of freedom by the epsilon value (0.668).

The within-subjects contrasts section evaluates which polynomial regression model fits the data best (Fig. 12.67). In the output, both linear and quadratic trends are shown. The linear term has a significant *p*-value ($p = 0.005$), while the quadratic term does not ($p = 0.083$), suggesting that the data follows a linear trend.

Between-subject effects are not interpreted in this repeated-measures ANOVA because there was no between-subject factor included in the design (Fig. 12.68).

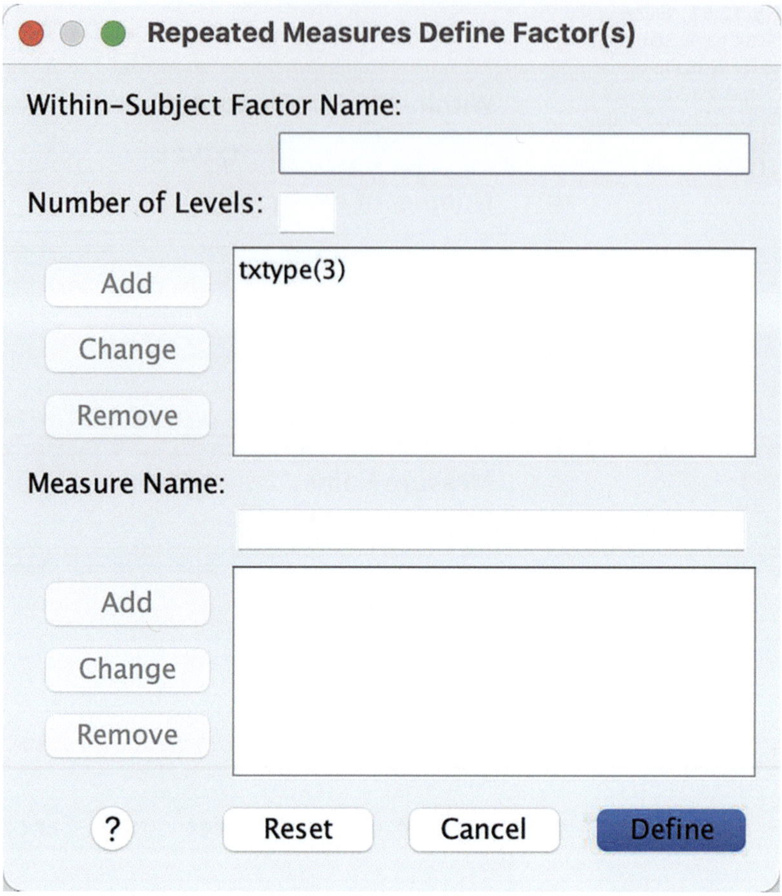

Fig. 12.62 Factor name and number of levels displayed after clicking "Add" in the "Repeated Measures Define Factors" dialog

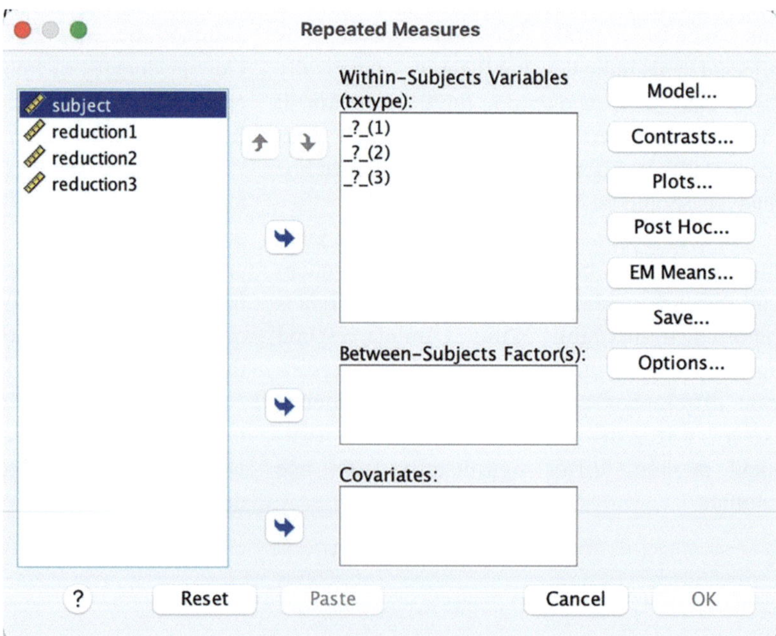

Fig. 12.63 Setting within-subjects variables in the repeated measures

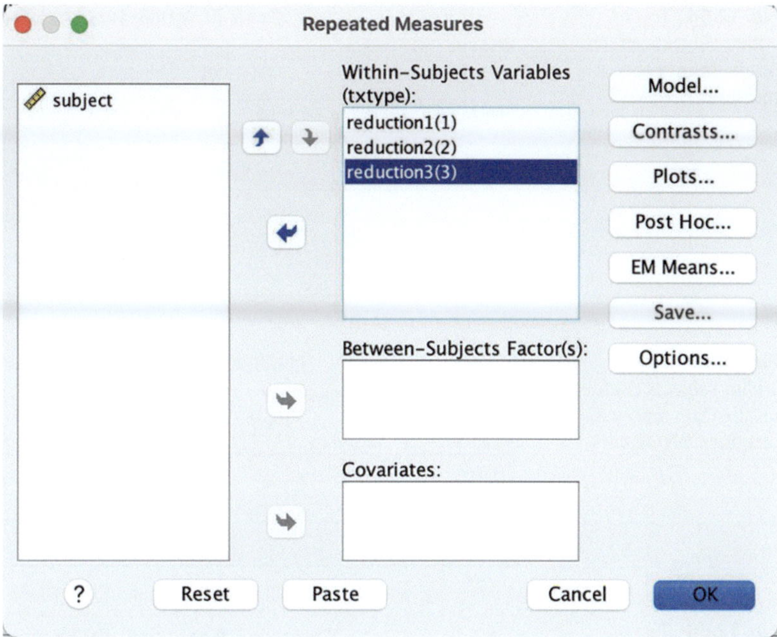

Fig. 12.64 All relevant variables assigned to the within-subjects variables

Multivariate Tests[a]

Effect		Value	F	Hypothesis df	Error df	Sig.
txtype	Pillai's Trace	.937	29.731[b]	2.000	4.000	.004
	Wilks' Lambda	.063	29.731[b]	2.000	4.000	.004
	Hotelling's Trace	14.866	29.731[b]	2.000	4.000	.004
	Roy's Largest Root	14.866	29.731[b]	2.000	4.000	.004

a. Design: Intercept
Within Subjects Design: txtype

b. Exact statistic

Mauchly's Test of Sphericity[a]

Measure: MEASURE_1

					Epsilon[b]		
Within Subjects Effect	Mauchly's W	Approx. Chi-Square	df	Sig.	Greenhouse-Geisser	Huynh-Feldt	Lower-bound
txtype	.503	2.753	2	.253	.668	.821	.500

Tests the null hypothesis that the error covariance matrix of the orthonormalized transformed dependent variables is proportional to an identity matrix.

a. Design: Intercept
Within Subjects Design: txtype

b. May be used to adjust the degrees of freedom for the averaged tests of significance. Corrected tests are displayed in the Tests of Within-Subjects Effects table.

Fig. 12.65 Mauchly's test of sphericity results from repeated-measures ANOVA

Fig. 12.66 Test of within-subjects effects results from repeated-measures ANOVA

Tests of Within-Subjects Effects

Measure: MEASURE_1

Source		Type III Sum of Squares	df	Mean Square	F	Sig.
txtype	Sphericity Assumed	84.000	2	42.000	15.750	<.001
	Greenhouse-Geisser	84.000	1.336	62.895	15.750	.004
	Huynh-Feldt	84.000	1.641	51.188	15.750	.002
	Lower-bound	84.000	1.000	84.000	15.750	.011
Error(txtype)	Sphericity Assumed	26.667	10	2.667		
	Greenhouse-Geisser	26.667	6.678	3.993		
	Huynh-Feldt	26.667	8.205	3.250		
	Lower-bound	26.667	5.000	5.333		

Fig. 12.67 Test of within-subjects contrasts results from repeated-measures ANOVA

Tests of Within-Subjects Contrasts

Measure: MEASURE_1

Source	txtype	Type III Sum of Squares	df	Mean Square	F	Sig.
txtype	Linear	75.000	1	75.000	22.059	.005
	Quadratic	9.000	1	9.000	4.655	.083
Error(txtype)	Linear	17.000	5	3.400		
	Quadratic	9.667	5	1.933		

Fig. 12.68 Test of between-subjects effects results from repeated-measures ANOVA

Tests of Between-Subjects Effects

Measure: MEASURE_1

Transformed Variable: Average

Source	Type III Sum of Squares	df	Mean Square	F	Sig.
Intercept	968.000	1	968.000	81.573	<.001
Error	59.333	5	11.867		

If the goal is not to compare all three treatment methods with one another, but rather to examine whether there is a difference between the first or last level and the remaining levels, a contrast test can be performed. Before running a contrast test, setting up plots in advance is helpful, as the output will include graphs that visually display the changes in mean values across levels.

Click on Plots in the dialog box shown in Fig. 12.69.

Click on txtype and move it to the horizontal axis field (Figs. 12.70 and 12.71).

Click Add (Fig. 12.72).

Then click Continue (Fig. 12.73).

In repeated-measures ANOVA, post hoc analysis options do not appear by default. If you wish to compare specific treatment levels, click on EM Means (Fig. 12.74).

Move the txtype variable to Display Means for: by clicking the right arrow button, then click Continue (Fig. 12.75).

Click on Contrasts on the right side of the screen (Fig. 12.76).

A polynomial contrast is typically selected when there is a meaningful order among the three conditions (e.g., low, medium, high). However, since there is no inherent order among the treatment methods in this example, click the ▼ icon next to Polynomial and select Simple instead (Fig. 12.77).

Since the reference category for comparison is the first level, select First. Click Continue. The output table will display the following results (Fig. 12.78):

There is a statistically significant difference between Level 1 and Level 2 at the $\alpha = 0.05$ significance level. A significant difference is also found between Level 1 and Level 3 at the same significance level. The accompanying graph illustrates the differences between the levels (Fig. 12.79).

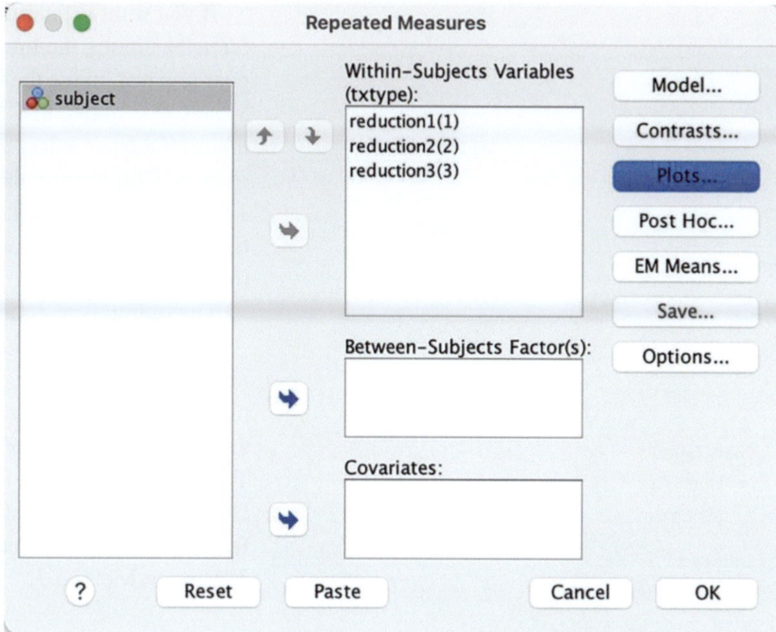

Fig. 12.69 Accessing the "Plots" option in the repeated-measures ANOVA dialog box

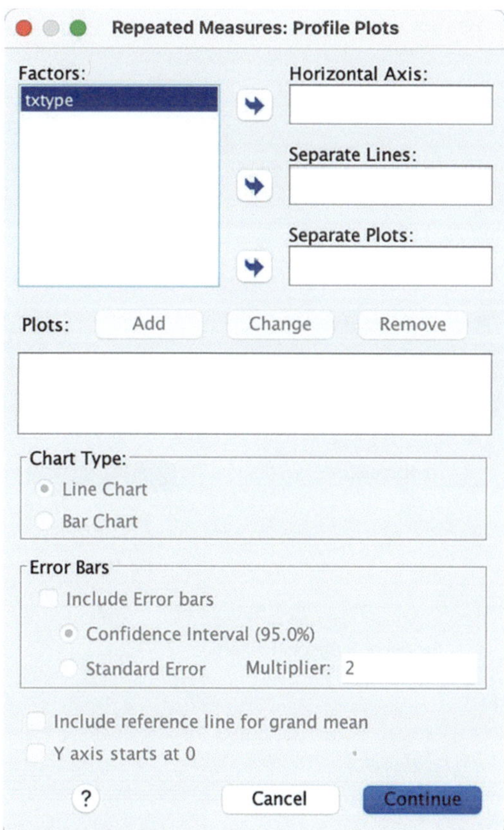

Fig. 12.70 The "Profile Plots" dialog box displayed after selecting the Plots option in repeated-measures ANOVA

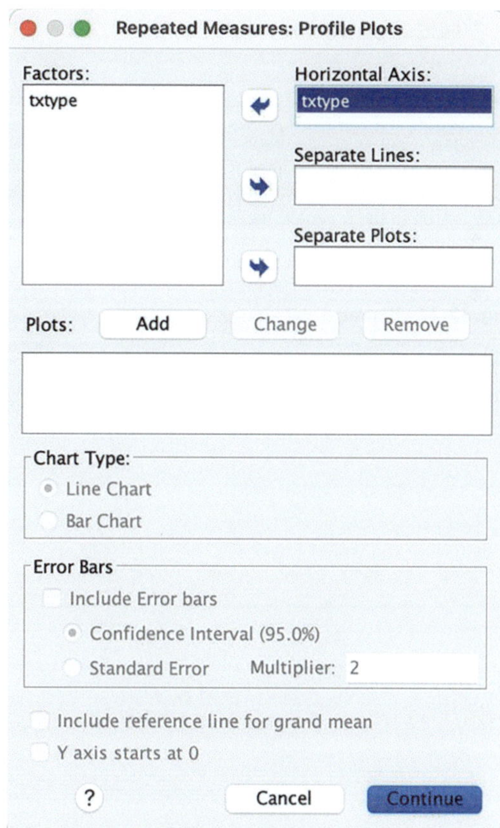

Fig. 12.71 Assigning a variable to the horizontal axis in the profile plots dialog

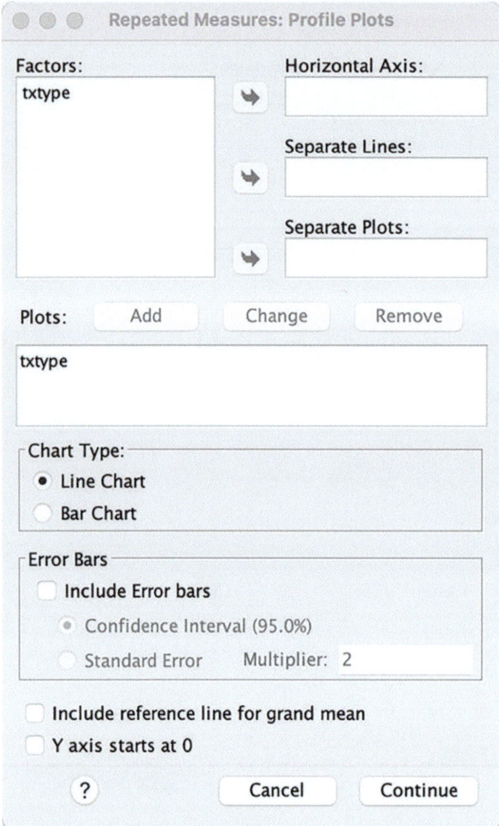

Fig. 12.72 Profile plot variable added after clicking the Add button in the repeated-measures ANOVA dialog

If you want to determine whether there are differences among the three treatment types using a post-hoc test, move the variable txtype to Display Means for: under EM Means → click Compare main effects → select either LSD or Bonferroni → click Continue → then click OK (Figs. 12.80, 12.81, and 12.82). To also display descriptive statistics, go to Options and check Descriptive statistics (Fig. 12.83).

The output is as follows (Fig. 12.84).

The results in Fig. 12.85 indicate that, at a significance level of 0.05, there is a statistically significant difference between Treatment Method 1 and Treatment Method 2, as well as between Treatment Method 1 and Treatment Method 3. However, there is no statistically significant difference between Treatment Method 2 and Treatment Method 3.

Fig. 12.73 Repeated Measures dialog window after configuring plots and clicking the Continue button

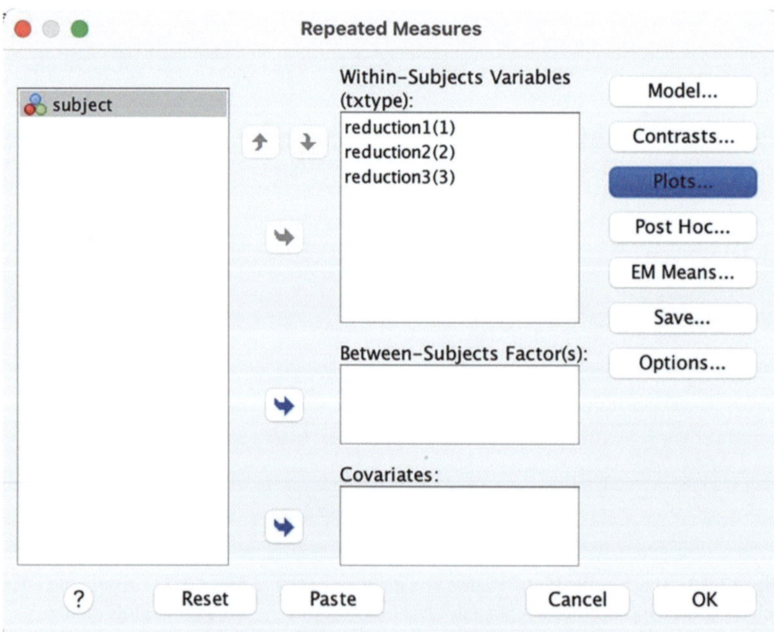

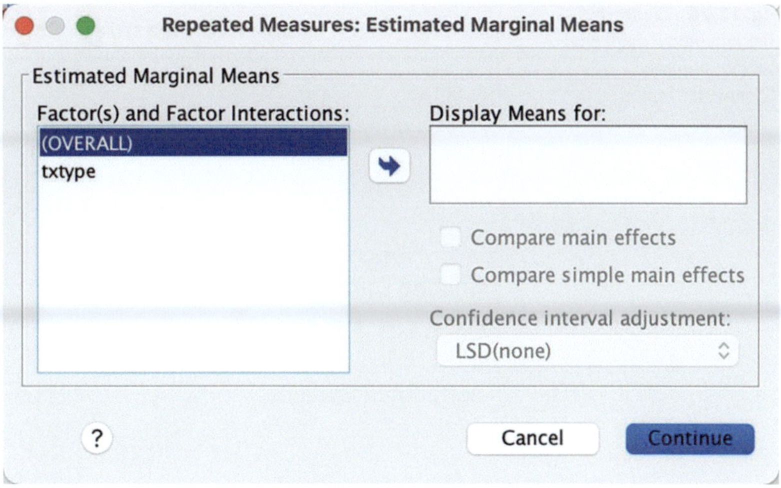

Fig. 12.74 Estimated marginal means (EM Means) dialog window accessed during repeated-measures ANOVA

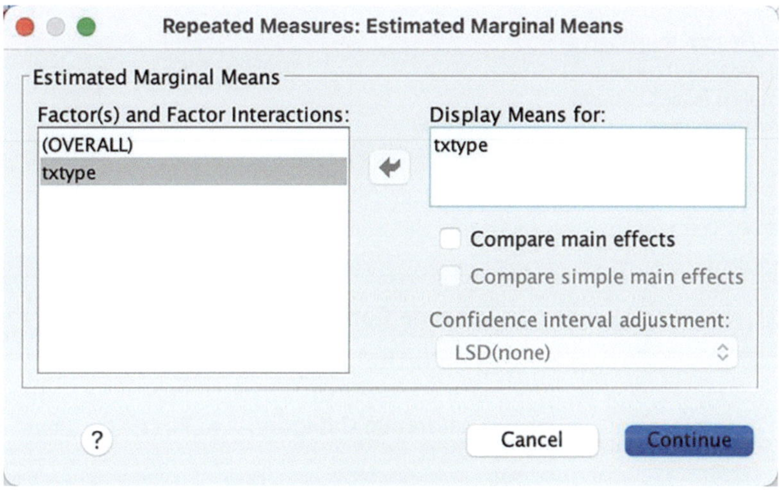

Fig. 12.75 Variable entered into the "Display Means for" box in the Estimated Marginal Means dialog

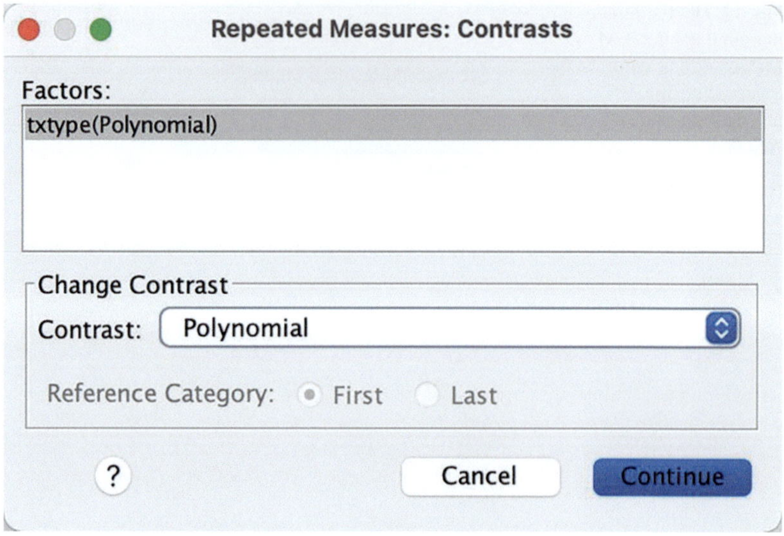

Fig. 12.76 Contrasts dialog window displayed after clicking the "Contrasts" button

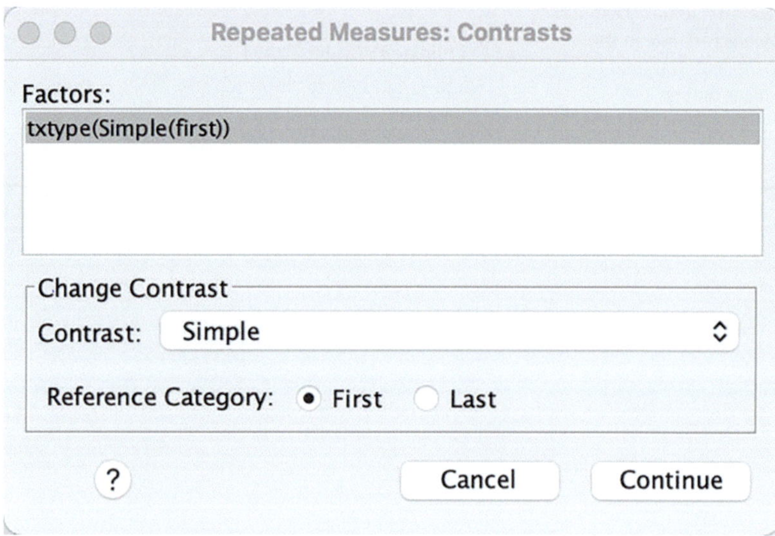

Fig. 12.77 Selection of the "Simple" contrast method in the Contrasts dialog window

Tests of Within-Subjects Contrasts

Measure: MEASURE_1

Source	txtype	Type III Sum of Squares	df	Mean Square	F	Sig.
txtype	Level 2 vs. Level 1	96.000	1	96.000	60.000	<.001
	Level 3 vs. Level 1	150.000	1	150.000	22.059	.005
Error(txtype)	Level 2 vs. Level 1	8.000	5	1.600		
	Level 3 vs. Level 1	34.000	5	6.800		

Fig. 12.78 Output window displaying the results of tests of within-subjects contrasts

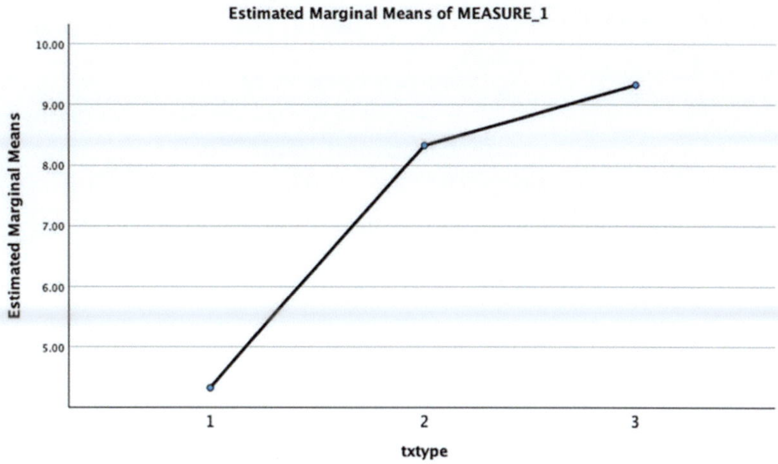

Fig. 12.79 Output window displaying the results of tests of within-subjects contrasts

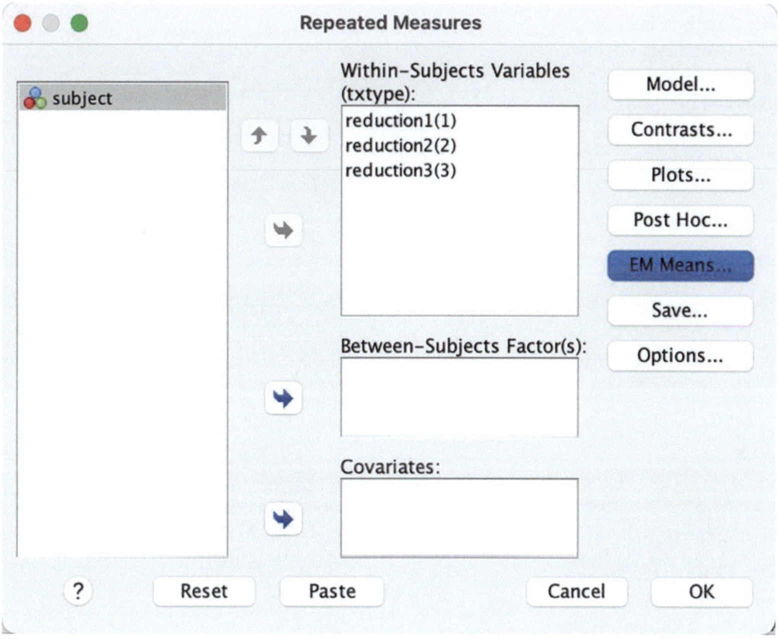

Fig. 12.80 Returning to the repeated measures dialog for post hoc multiple comparisons setup

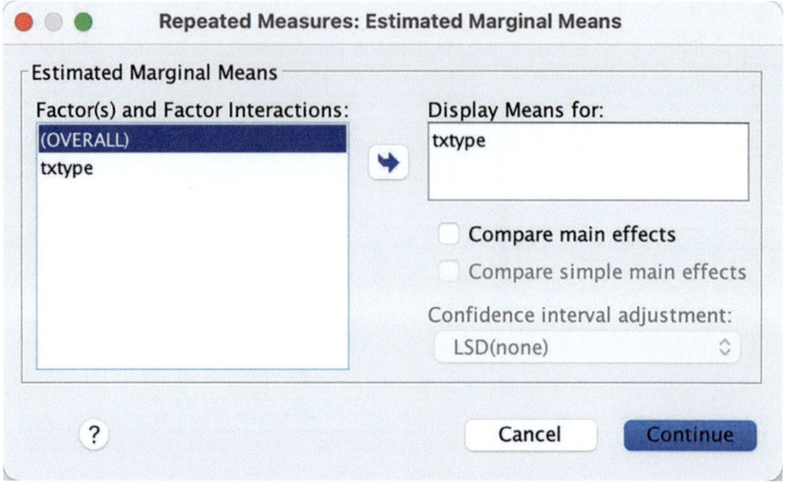

Fig. 12.81 Estimated marginal means (EM Means) dialog window in repeated-measures ANOVA

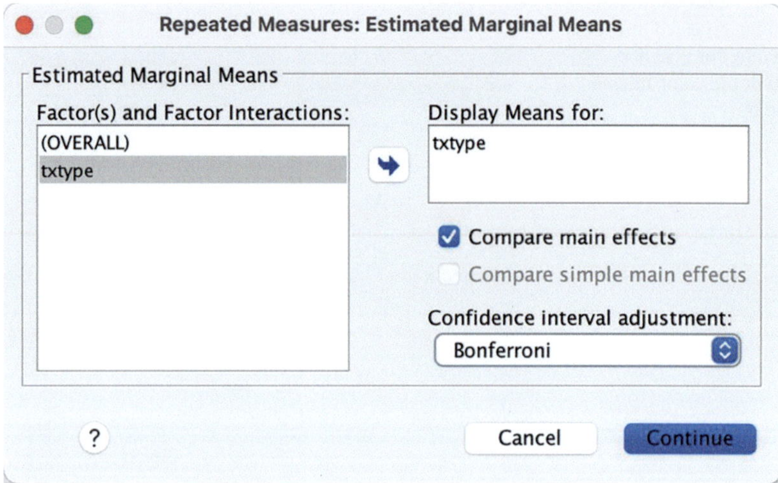

Fig. 12.82 Clicking "Compare main effects" in the estimated marginal means dialog

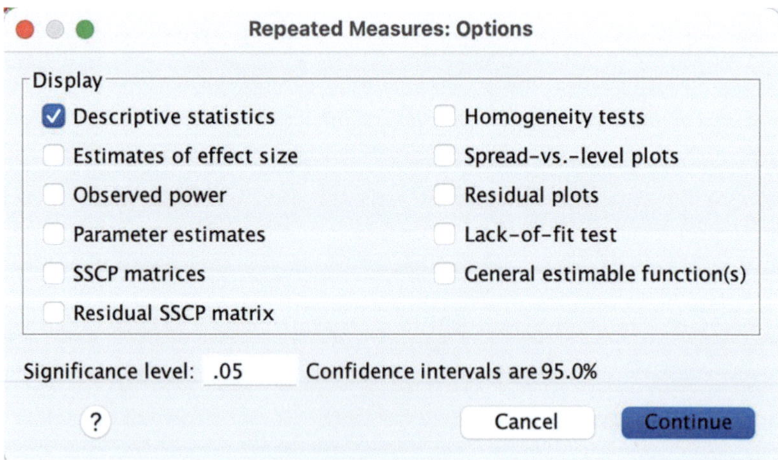

Fig. 12.83 Dialog window displayed after clicking "Options" in the repeated-measures ANOVA setup

Estimates

Measure: MEASURE_1

txtype	Mean	Std. Error	95% Confidence Interval	
			Lower Bound	Upper Bound
1	4.333	.803	2.270	6.397
2	8.333	1.202	5.244	11.423
3	9.333	.882	7.066	11.600

Fig. 12.84 Post hoc multiple comparisons output from repeated-measures ANOVA in SPSS

Pairwise Comparisons

Measure: MEASURE_1

(I) txtype	(J) txtype	Mean Difference (I-J)	Std. Error	Sig.[b]	95% Confidence Interval for Difference[b]	
					Lower Bound	Upper Bound
1	2	-4.000*	.516	.002	-5.825	-2.175
	3	-5.000*	1.065	.016	-8.762	-1.238
2	1	4.000*	.516	.002	2.175	5.825
	3	-1.000	1.125	1.000	-4.978	2.978
3	1	5.000*	1.065	.016	1.238	8.762
	2	1.000	1.125	1.000	-2.978	4.978

Based on estimated marginal means

*. The mean difference is significant at the .05 level.

b. Adjustment for multiple comparisons: Bonferroni.

Fig. 12.85 Post hoc multiple comparisons output from repeated-measures ANOVA in SPSS

12.10 Correlation Analysis

Correlation analysis is used to examine the relationship between two variables, x and y. These variables must be continuous, like height and weight. Suppose we draw a scatterplot of two variables x and y. Conventionally, x is plotted along the horizontal axis and y along the vertical axis.

1. *Pearson Correlation Coefficient*

When the plotted points on the scatterplot form a pattern that resembles a straight line, we say there is a linear relationship between the two variables (Fig. 12.86). The degree to which the points approximate a straight line is measured by the Pearson product-moment correlation coefficient, commonly referred to simply as the correlation coefficient. The population correlation coefficient is denoted by the Greek letter ρ (rho), while the sample correlation coefficient is denoted by r.

The formula for calculating the correlation coefficient r is as follows:

$$r = \frac{\Sigma(x-\bar{x})(y-\bar{y})}{\sqrt{\Sigma(x-\bar{x})^2\,\Sigma(y-\bar{y})^2}} \text{ or } \frac{n\Sigma XY-(\Sigma X)(\Sigma Y)}{\sqrt{\left[n\Sigma X^2-(\Sigma X)^2\right]\left[n\Sigma Y^2-(\Sigma Y)^2\right]}}$$

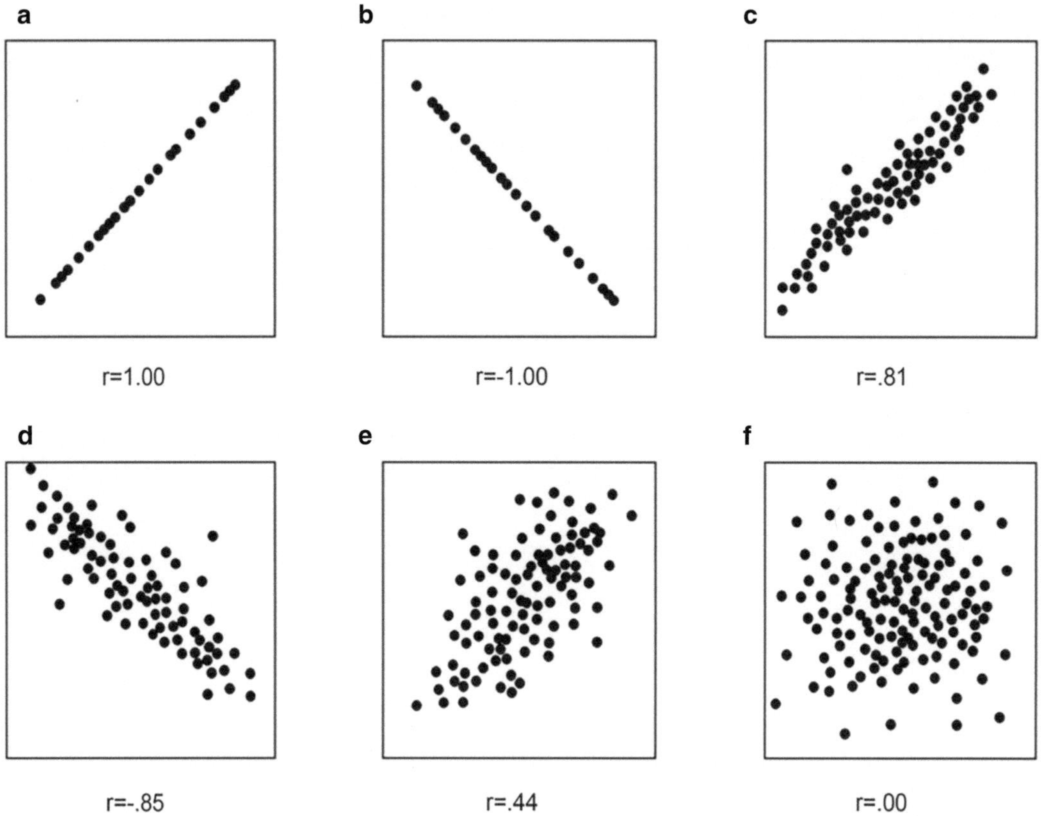

Fig. 12.86 Scatterplot and correlation coefficient

The correlation coefficient r has the following characteristics:

First, it ranges between -1 and $+1$.

Second, a positive sign (+) indicates that as one variable increases, the other variable also increases. A negative sign (−) indicates that as one variable increases, the other decreases.

Third, the magnitude of the correlation coefficient reflects how closely the data points cluster around the best-fitting straight line in the scatterplot. A value of $r = +1$ or $r = -1$ means that all data points lie exactly on a straight line. A value of $r = 0$ indicates that there is no linear relationship between the variables. The closer the absolute value of r is to 1, the stronger the linear relationship.

Fourth, the correlation coefficient is unitless—it has no unit of measurement.

Fifth, the correlation coefficient is meaningful only within the range of values observed in the sample. It cannot be assumed that the same r will apply to values outside the sample range.

Sixth, the value of r does not change if the roles of x and y are switched.

Seventh, a correlation between x and y does not imply causation.

Eighth, the value of r^2 represents the proportion of variance explained by the correlation. For example, if $r = 0.40$ and $p < 0.05$, then variable x explains 16% (= $0.40^2 \times 100$) of the variance in variable y.

Using a correlation coefficient in situations where it is not appropriate can lead to misleading interpretations. The correlation coefficient should not be used in the following cases:

First, when there is no linear relationship between the two variables, but rather a curvilinear relationship.
Second, when outliers are present in the data.
Third, when the scatterplot reveals multiple subgroup distributions, as illustrated in Fig. 12.87.

It is also important to note that the value of the correlation coefficient can vary significantly depending on how the range of data is restricted or how subgroups are combined. For example, suppose the correlation between plastic surgery resident exam scores and IQ is calculated and found to be $r = 0.8$. However, if the correlation is recalculated using only examinees who scored above 80 on the exam, the value might drop to $r = 0.2$. In general, restricting the range of data tends to lower the correlation coefficient (Fig. 12.88).

The correlation between variables can also differ significantly depending on which group is being analyzed. For instance, if the total sample is divided into younger and older patients, younger patients may show faster and more noticeable skin regeneration after a scar revision procedure, which may result in a moderately strong positive correlation between the extent of the procedure and the degree of skin improvement (Fig. 12.89). In contrast, older patients may exhibit reduced regenerative capacity or increased risk of pigmentation changes, potentially leading to a strong negative correlation. If the correlation coefficient is calculated by combining both younger and older patients, the overall correlation could approach zero, despite meaningful relationships existing within each subgroup. Thus, drawing the conclusion that "there is no correlation between procedure intensity and

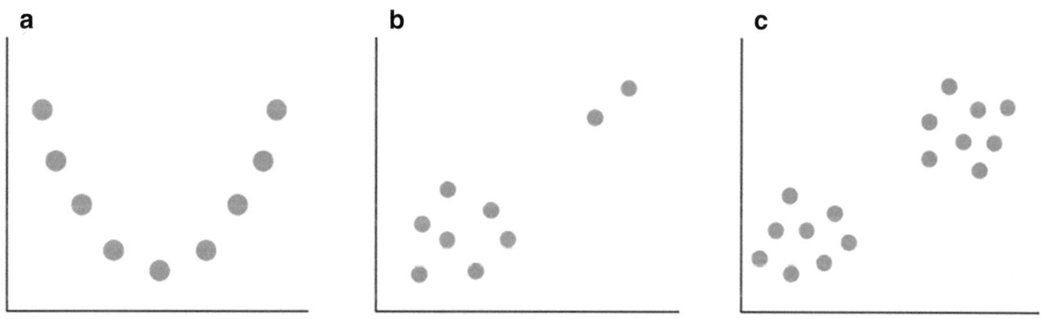

Fig. 12.87 A scatterplot inappropriate for interpreting the Pearson correlation coefficient

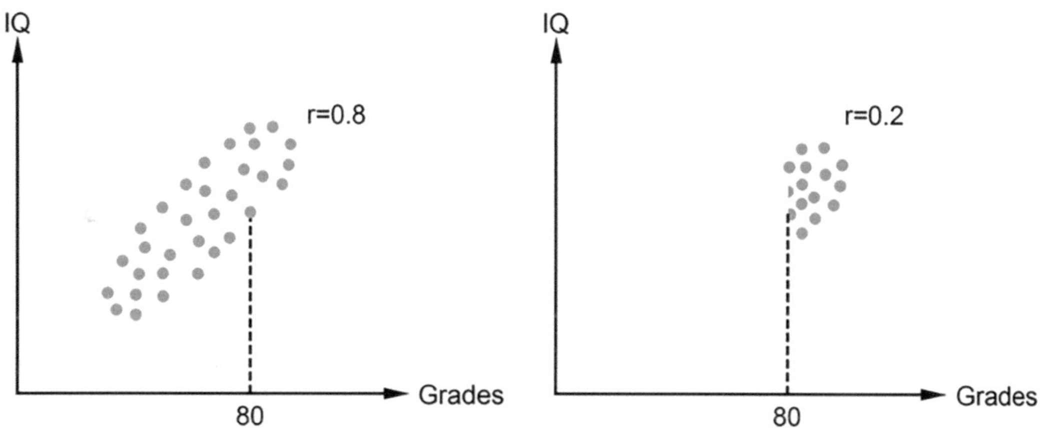

Fig. 12.88 Example of an inappropriate correlation coefficient

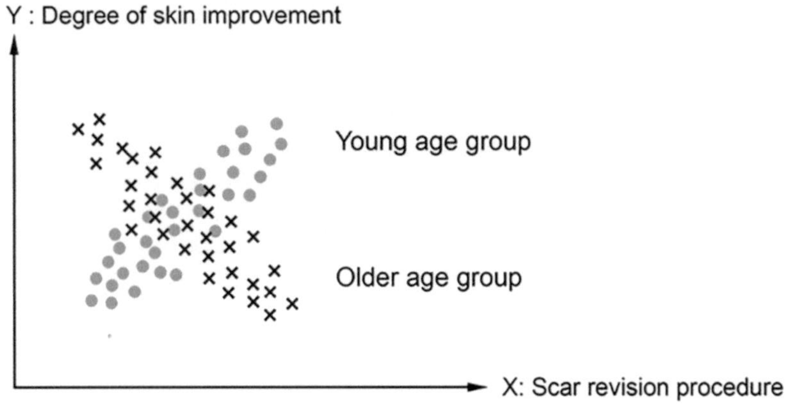

Fig. 12.89 Example of an inappropriate correlation coefficient

degree of skin improvement" based on this overall coefficient would be misleading and potentially dangerous. In such cases, it is more appropriate to analyze the correlation within each subgroup separately.

Once a correlation has been calculated, it is important to determine the probability of obtaining such a coefficient under the null hypothesis. To estimate this probability, a t-distribution is used, with degrees of freedom (df) equal to $n - 2$. To test the significance of the correlation, the sample correlation coefficient r is used to examine whether the population correlation coefficient (ρ) significantly differs from zero at a given significance level. In other words, one tests the null hypothesis H_0: $\rho = 0$, using the following test statistic formula.

$$t = \frac{r - 0}{\sqrt{\frac{1 - r^2}{n - 2}}} = \frac{r\sqrt{n - 2}}{\sqrt{1 - r^2}}$$

The statement "$r = 0.65$ with $p < 0.05$" means that if the true population correlation were 0, then in no more than 5 out of 100 repetitions of the study, a sample correlation as large as $r = 0.65$ would occur purely by sampling error. Even when a correlation coefficient is found to be statistically significant, its magnitude and direction must still be considered. Rejecting the null hypothesis and accepting the alternative hypothesis only tells us that a linear relationship exists; it does not imply causality between the two variables.

In hypothesis testing, the Type I error rate (i.e., the probability of rejecting a true null hypothesis) is typically controlled at 0.05. When performing a single test, we can compare the p-value to 0.05 directly. However, when multiple hypotheses are tested within the same study, the probability of obtaining at least one significant result by chance increases. This is similar to performing multiple t-tests on the same dataset, which also increases the likelihood of false positives. To address this problem, the Bonferroni correction is often used: the significance level ($\alpha = 0.05$) is divided by the number of comparisons to control the overall Type I error rate.

In correlation analysis, the null hypothesis typically states that there is no correlation (i.e., the population correlation coefficient $\rho = 0$). If multiple correlation tests are performed in the same study, even if each test uses a 0.05 significance level, the overall Type I error rate increases. To correct for this, divide the alpha level by the number of comparisons. For example, if you are calculating correlations among three assessment tools, there are three possible pairwise comparisons, so you would set your significance level to $0.05 / 3 = 0.017$ when evaluating statistical significance (Huang et al. 2015).

One important characteristic of the correlation coefficient is that the value of r has the properties of an ordinal scale. This means that an r value of 0.40 cannot be interpreted as representing twice the strength of association compared to an r of 0.20. Similarly, the difference between $r = 0.50$

and $r = 0.60$ is not equivalent to the difference between $r = 0.80$ and $r = 0.90$. Each correlation coefficient should be understood in terms of relative rank, not as an interval measurement. The correlation coefficient is not a direct measure of an underlying quantity, but rather an index used for convenience. There is no universally agreed-upon guideline for interpreting the strength of correlation coefficients, as interpretations may vary among researchers. According to Blesh (1974), the strength of correlation can be described as follows:

- 0.90 to 0.99: High correlation (*high reliability*)
- 0.80 to 0.89: Good correlation (*good reliability*)
- 0.70 to 0.79: Fair correlation (*fair reliability*)
- 0.69 or below: Low correlation (*poor reliability*)

2. *An Example of Pearson Correlation Analysis Using SPSS*

The following data are hypothetical measurements of skin thickness taken from 19 individuals undergoing laser treatment (Table 12.9). Skin thickness (in mm) was measured using a digital caliper before and after the procedure to assess post-treatment changes in dermal swelling.

Table 12.9 Changes in skin thickness before and after treatment before treatment (unit: mm)

Before treatment (changes in dermal swelling (unit:mm))	After treatment (changes in dermal swelling (unit:mm))
36.0	36.0
18.0	17.0
22.0	22.0
17.0	16.0
24.0	24.0
20.0	23.0
20.0	18.0
8.0	10.4
12.0	16.6
14.0	15.6
13.0	12.8
22.0	24.0
16.5	15.0
17.2	16.4
10.4	10.0
22.8	19.6
15.0	16.0
10.4	10.4
9.8	10.0

$$\sum X = 328.10 \sum Y = 332.80$$

$$\sum X^2 = 6451.29 \sum XY = 6475.82 \sum Y^2 = 6563.20$$

$$\left(\sum X\right)^2 = 107{,}649.61 \left(\sum Y\right)^2 = 110{,}755.84$$

$$r = \frac{n\sum XY - \left(\sum X\right)\left(\sum Y\right)}{\sqrt{\left[n\sum X^2 - \left(\sum X\right)^2\right]\left[n\sum Y^2 - \left(\sum Y\right)^2\right]}}$$

$$= \frac{19 \times 6475.82 - 328.10 \times 332.80}{\sqrt{\left[19 \times 6451.29 - 328.10^2\right]\left[19 \times 6563.20 - 332.80^2\right]}} = \frac{13{,}848.90}{\sqrt{14{,}924.90 \times 13{,}944.96}}$$

$$= \frac{13{,}848.90}{14{,}426.61} = 0.95995 = 0.96$$

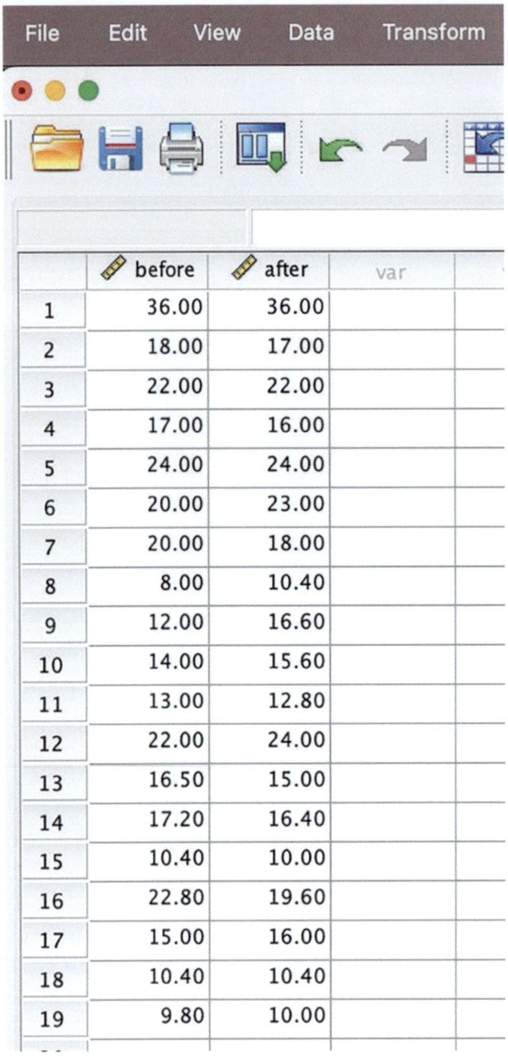

Fig. 12.90 Example dataset for conducting Pearson correlation analysis using SPSS

Let's analyze this dataset using SPSS. Launch SPSS and enter the data as shown in Fig. 12.90.

Click Analyze → Correlate → Bivariate (Fig. 12.91).

Select the variables "before" and "after" by highlighting both with your mouse, and then click the center arrow to move them to the Variables box (Fig. 12.92). Since the measurement values are on a ratio scale, make sure the checkbox for Pearson is selected.

Click OK when the following dialog box appears (Fig. 12.93). You will obtain a results table like the one below.

According to the output (Fig. 12.94), the Pearson correlation coefficient between the pre- and post-treatment skin thickness values is $r = 0.960$ ($p = 0.000$), indicating a strong positive correlation. This suggests a high likelihood and degree of association between the two variables. However, if, for instance, the simple correlation between serum cholesterol levels and skin thickness were $r = 0.08$, $p < 0.01$, this would indicate that although there is a statistically significant relationship ($p < 0.01$), the strength of the association is weak due to the low r value.

3. *Spearman's Rank Correlation Coefficient*

The nonparametric statistical method corresponding to Pearson's correlation coefficient is the Spearman's rank correlation coefficient, often referred to simply as the Spearman correlation. This method is used when at least one of the variables, either x or y, is measured at the ordinal level, when x or y does not follow a normal distribution, when the sample size is small, or when a linear relationship cannot be assumed. The Spearman correlation coefficient in the population is denoted as ρ_s, and the sample Spearman correlation coefficient is denoted as r_s. The formula for calculating the Spearman correlation coefficient from a sample is as follows:

$$r_s = 1 - \frac{6\sum d^2}{n\left(n^2 - 1\right)}$$

Spearman's rank correlation coefficient does not use r_s^2. An example of manually calculating Spearman's rank correlation coefficient is presented in Table 12.10. This example compares the relationship between theoretical course grades and practical skill performance scores among 10 students majoring in cosmetic dermatology.

$$\rho = 1 - \frac{6\left(37.00\right)}{10\left(100 - 1\right)} = 1 - \frac{220.00}{990.00}$$
$$= 1 - 0.22 = 0.78$$

To conduct Spearman correlation analysis using a nonparametric test method in SPSS, follow the same procedure as when calculating the Pearson

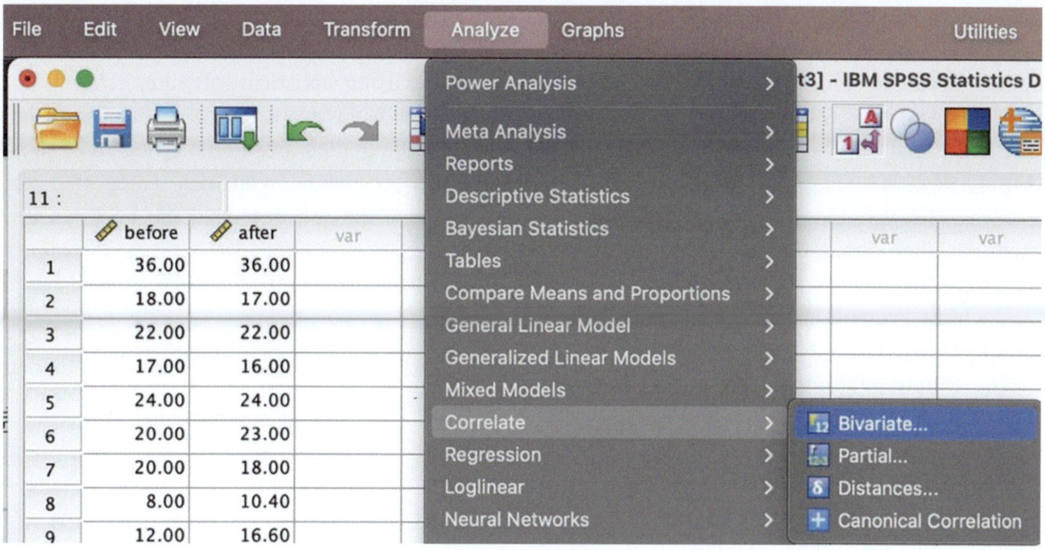

Fig. 12.91 Menu path for performing Pearson correlation analysis

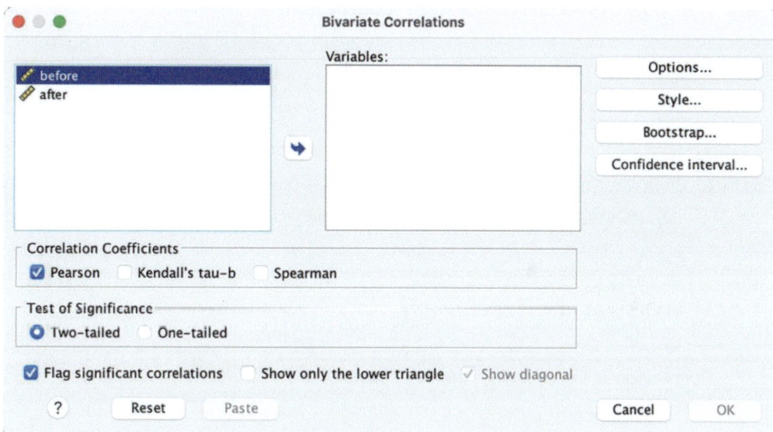

Fig. 12.92 Bivariate correlations dialog box for selecting variables and correlation options

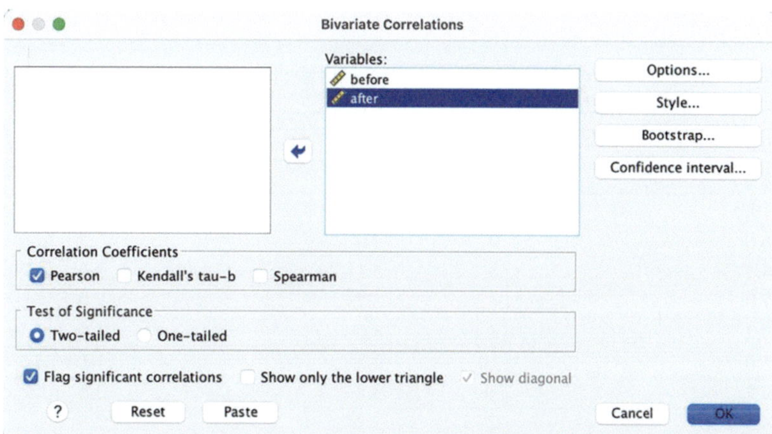

Fig. 12.93 Variables selected for Pearson correlation analysis in the bivariate correlations dialog box

correlation coefficient, but check the box for Spearman under the correlation coefficient options before clicking OK.

Enter the data as follows (Fig. 12.95).

Click Analyze → Correlate → Bivariate (Fig. 12.96).

Move the variables for which you want to examine the correlation to the right box (Fig. 12.97).

Uncheck Pearson and check Spearman, then click OK (Fig. 12.98).

The output table will appear as shown in Fig. 12.99.

4. *Point-Biserial Correlation Coefficient*

If variable *X* is a binary variable (e.g., Yes or No) and variable *Y* is a continuous variable, the relationship between the two can be examined using the point-biserial correlation coefficient.

Correlations

		before	after
before	Pearson Correlation	1	.960**
	Sig. (2-tailed)		<.001
	N	19	19
after	Pearson Correlation	.960**	1
	Sig. (2-tailed)	<.001	
	N	19	19

**. Correlation is significant at the 0.01 level (2-tailed).

Fig. 12.94 SPSS output showing the results of Pearson correlation analysis

The method of calculation is the same as that for the Pearson correlation coefficient, so it can be computed using statistical software.

If you want to examine the relationship between the treated area and the degree of post-treatment erythema, you can categorize the treated area into the face and the neck. In this

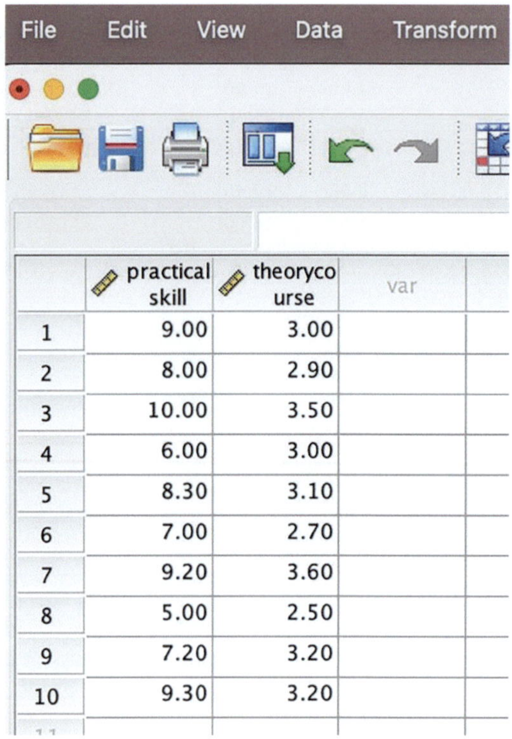

Fig. 12.95 Example dataset in SPSS for conducting Spearman's rank correlation coefficient analysis

Table 12.10 Rank correlation between theoretical course grades and practical skill performance scores

X (practical skill score)	Rank	*Y* (theory course grade)	Rank	(*X* – *Y*)	d^2
9.0	4	3.0	6.5	−2.5	6.25
8.0	6	2.9	8.0	−2.0	4.00
10.0	1	3.5	2.0	−1.0	1.00
6.0	9	3.0	6.5	2.5	6.25
8.3	5	3.1	5.0	0	0
7.0	8	2.7	9.0	−1.0	1.00
9.2	3	3.6	1.0	2.0	4.00
5.0	10	2.5	10.0	0	0
7.2	7	3.2	3.5	3.5	12.25
9.3	2	3.2	3.5	−1.5	2.25
					37

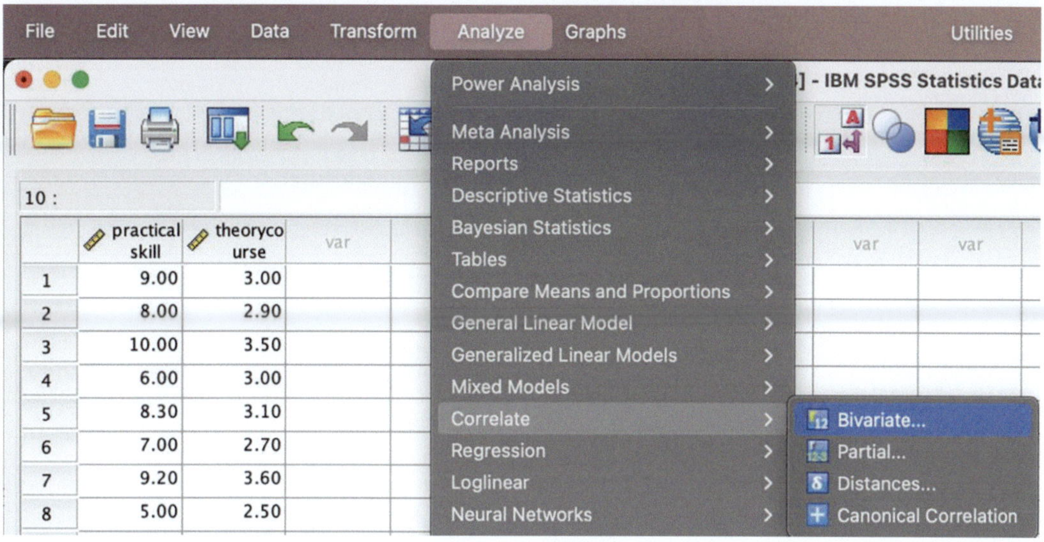

Fig. 12.96 Menu path for conducting Spearman's rank correlation

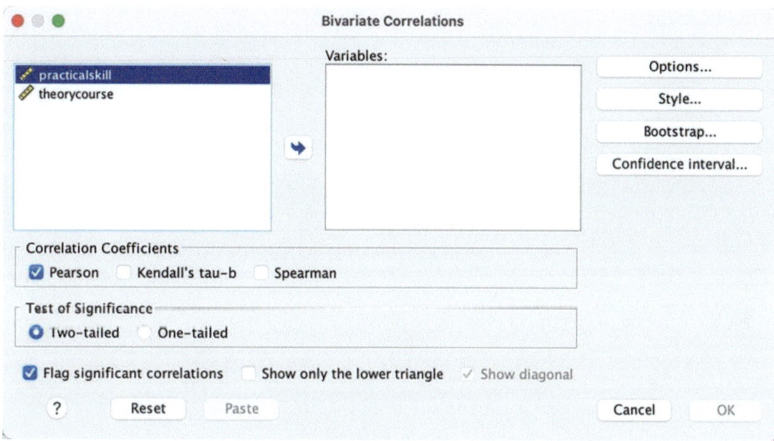

Fig. 12.97 Bivariate correlations dialog box in SPSS for conducting Spearman's rank correlation analysis

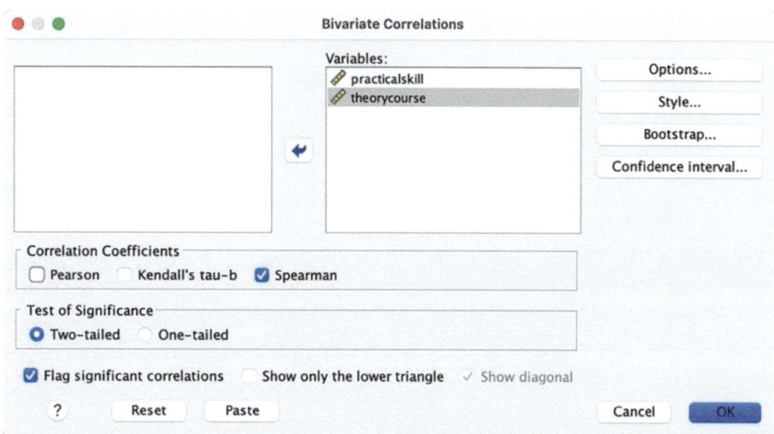

Fig. 12.98 Variables selected and Spearman correlation option checked in the bivariate correlations dialog box

Fig. 12.99 Output table showing results of Spearman's rank correlation analysis in SPSS

Correlations

			practicalskill	theorycourse
Spearman's rho	practicalskill	Correlation Coefficient	1.000	.774**
		Sig. (2-tailed)	.	.009
		N	10	10
	theorycourse	Correlation Coefficient	.774**	1.000
		Sig. (2-tailed)	.009	.
		N	10	10

**. Correlation is significant at the 0.01 level (2-tailed).

case, you may enter the data as shown in Fig. 12.100.

Click Analyze → Correlate → Bivariate, then move the variables into the right-hand box using the arrow button (Fig. 12.101).

Check that the Pearson option is selected under Correlation Coefficients, then click OK (Fig. 12.102).

The following results will be displayed (Fig. 12.103).

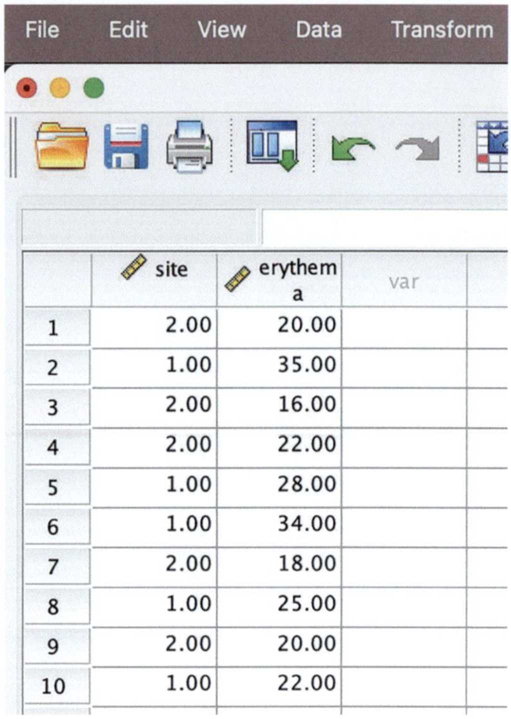

	site	erythema	var
1	2.00	20.00	
2	1.00	35.00	
3	2.00	16.00	
4	2.00	22.00	
5	1.00	28.00	
6	1.00	34.00	
7	2.00	18.00	
8	1.00	25.00	
9	2.00	20.00	
10	1.00	22.00	

Fig. 12.100 Example dataset for calculating the point-biserial correlation coefficient using SPSS

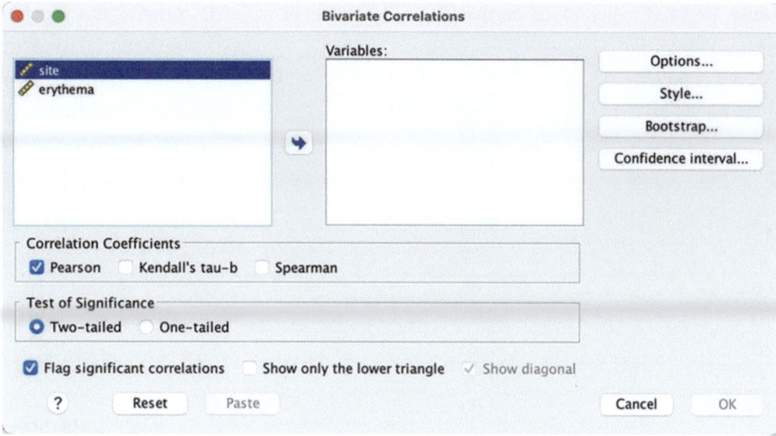

Fig. 12.101 Bivariate correlations dialog window after selecting "Bivariate" from the Analyze → Correlate menu in SPSS

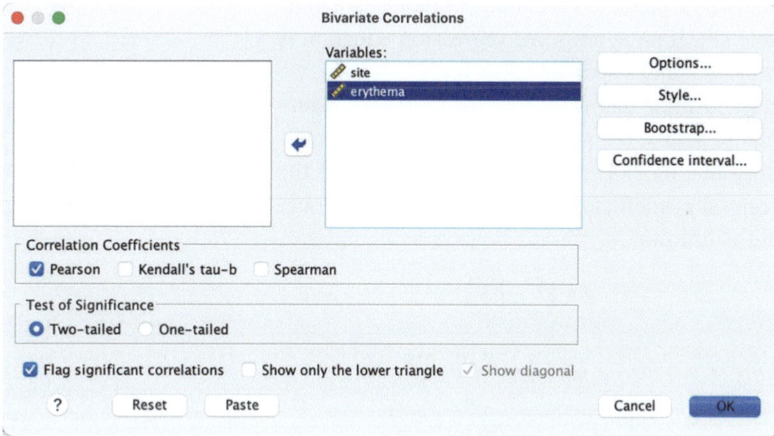

Fig. 12.102 Selection of the Pearson option and assignment of variables in the bivariate correlations dialog box in SPSS

Correlations

		site	erythema
site	Pearson Correlation	1	-.781**
	Sig. (2-tailed)		.008
	N	10	10
erythema	Pearson Correlation	-.781**	1
	Sig. (2-tailed)	.008	
	N	10	10

**. Correlation is significant at the 0.01 level (2-tailed).

Fig. 12.103 Output window displaying the results of the point-biserial correlation analysis using Pearson's r in SPSS

12.11 Regression Analysis

Sometimes, we want to predict the value of one variable using another. In such cases, we conduct a regression analysis. Regression is a statistical method that uses the relationship between variables to determine how one variable can predict another, based on the consistent patterns observed between them. While correlation treats both variables equally, regression analysis distinguishes between them: the variable used for prediction is called the independent variable (*X*), and the vari-

Table 12.11 Prediction of dermal response based on laser exposure time

X laser exposure time(seconds)	*Y* dermal response(RMS)
10	5.96
20	5.98
30	6.02
40	6.06
50	6.27
60	6.58
70	6.91
80	7.20
90	7.52
100	8.03

able being predicted is called the dependent variable (*Y*). If an appropriate regression equation is provided, and a specific value for *X* is known, we can substitute that value into the regression equation (e.g., $Y = bX + a$) to predict the corresponding value of *Y*. The formulas for calculating the regression coefficients *a* (intercept) and *b* (slope) are as follows:

$$a = \left(\bar{Y} - b\bar{X}\right)$$

$$b = \frac{\sum XY - \frac{(\sum X)(\sum Y)}{n}}{\sum X^2 - \frac{(\sum X)^2}{n}}$$

Table 12.11 shows the measured dermal response according to the laser exposure time. Based on this dataset, the predicted regression equation is $Y' = 5.380 + 0.023X$. For example, if the laser exposure time is 45 s, the predicted dermal response would be $Y' = 5.380 + 0.023 \times 45 = 6.420$ RMS (root mean square). Note that Y' is a predicted value, not an actual observed value—thus, a dermal response of exactly 6.420 RMS does not necessarily occur every time a 45-s laser exposure is applied. For instance, when the exposure time was 40 s, the regression model predicted a response of 6.30 RMS, but the actual observed value was 6.06 RMS, as seen in Table 12.11. Although there is a difference of 0.24 RMS between the predicted and actual values, the predicted value of 6.30 RMS represents the best estimate we can obtain without directly measuring the response during a 40-s laser treatment. The more data points we have when building a regression model, the more accurate our predictions become. A regression equation derived from 1000 data points will yield more reliable predictions than one based on just 10 or even 100 cases.

$$\sum X = 550 \qquad \sum Y = 66.53$$

$$\left(\sum X\right)^2 = 302{,}500 \qquad \left(\sum Y\right)^2 = 4426.24$$

$$\sum X^2 = 38{,}500 \qquad \sum Y^2 = 447.47$$

$$\sum XY = 3850$$

$$\bar{X} = 55.0 \quad \bar{Y} = 6.65 \quad r = .95$$

$$b = \frac{\sum XY - \frac{(\sum X)(\sum Y)}{n}}{\sum X^2 - \frac{(\sum X)^2}{n}} = \frac{3850 - \frac{(550)(66.53)}{10}}{38{,}500 - \frac{302{,}500}{10}}$$

$$= \frac{3850 - 3659.15}{38{,}500 - 30{,}250} = \frac{190.85}{8250} = 0.025$$

$$a = \left(\bar{Y} - b\bar{X}\right) = 6.65 - (0.023)55$$
$$= 6.65 - 1.27 = 5.38$$

$$Y' = 5.380 + 0.023X$$

Y' is the predicted of *Y* value

a is the intercept of *Y*

b is the slope of the line

X is the variable on which prediction is based

Correlation coefficients provide useful information before conducting a regression analysis because if the correlation is low, the regression equation will have limited predictive power. Caution is needed when using regression equations: the two variables must exhibit a linear relationship. That is, for example, as contraction time increases, the level of muscle activity should also increase. However, in practice, data rarely follow a perfect linear pattern when plotted as a scatter

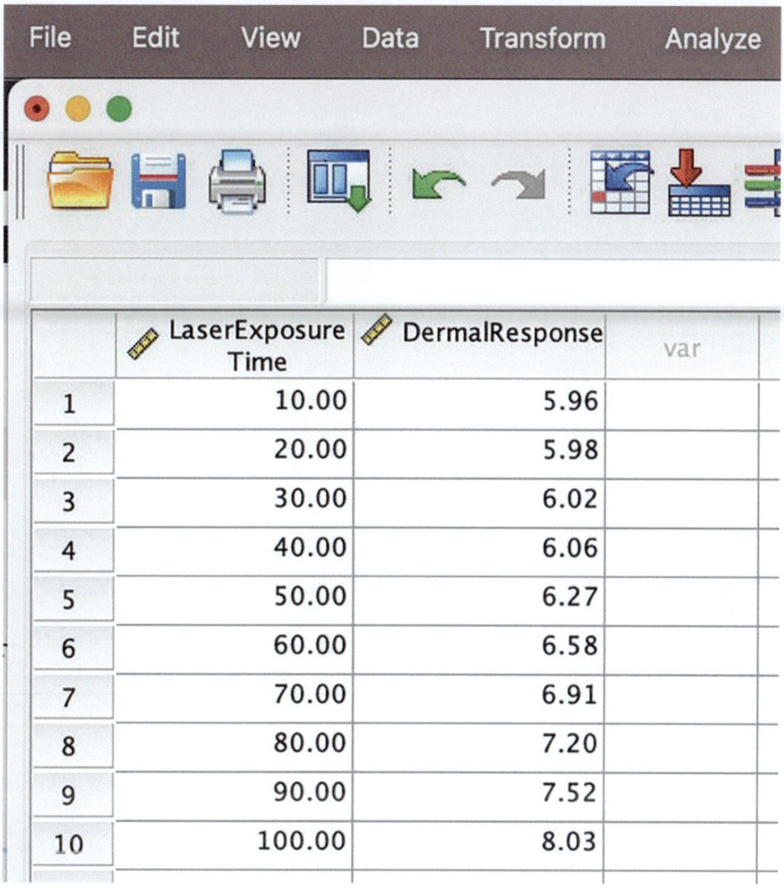

Fig. 12.104 Example dataset for conducting regression analysis in SPSS

diagram. Additionally, a high correlation does not necessarily imply causation. While it may be desirable to predict a subject's dermal reactivity level using a simple linear equation based on laser exposure time, dermal reactivity is not determined solely by exposure time. Many factors can influence the response, including age, gender, skin hydration, and baseline skin thickness. When all of these factors are incorporated into the model to estimate dermal reactivity, the analysis is referred to as multiple regression.

Let's analyze the example dataset using SPSS. Start SPSS and enter the data as shown in the previous table (Fig. 12.104).

Go to Analyze → Regression → Linear (Fig. 12.105).

Since the dependent variable is *dermal response*, move this variable to the Dependent field. Move *laser exposure time* to the Independent(s) field, as it is the independent variable (Fig. 12.106).

Click OK (Fig. 12.107).

A results table like the one below will be generated (Fig. 12.108). The correlation coefficient is $r = 0.954$, and the coefficient of determination is $R^2 = 0.910$. Furthermore, the regression model $Y' = 5.38 + 0.023X$ is shown to be statistically significant based on the F-test result.

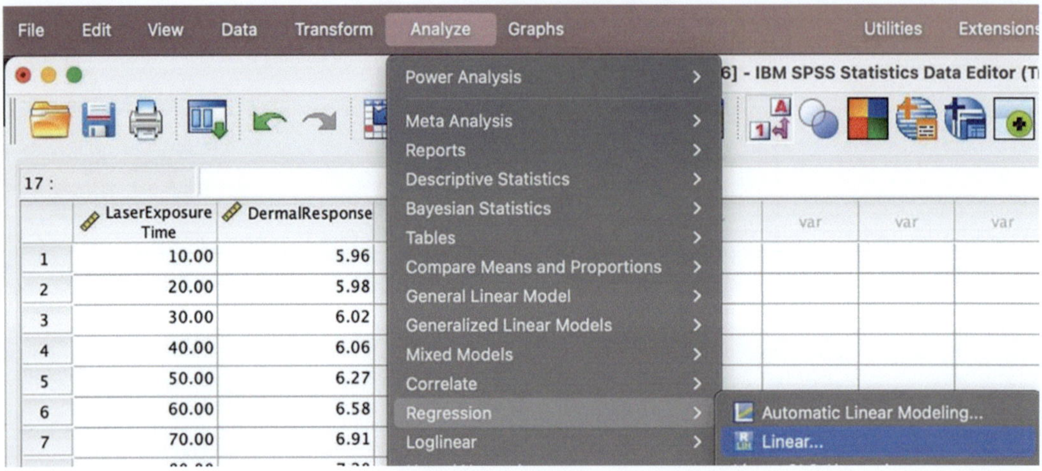

Fig. 12.105 Navigation path for linear regression analysis

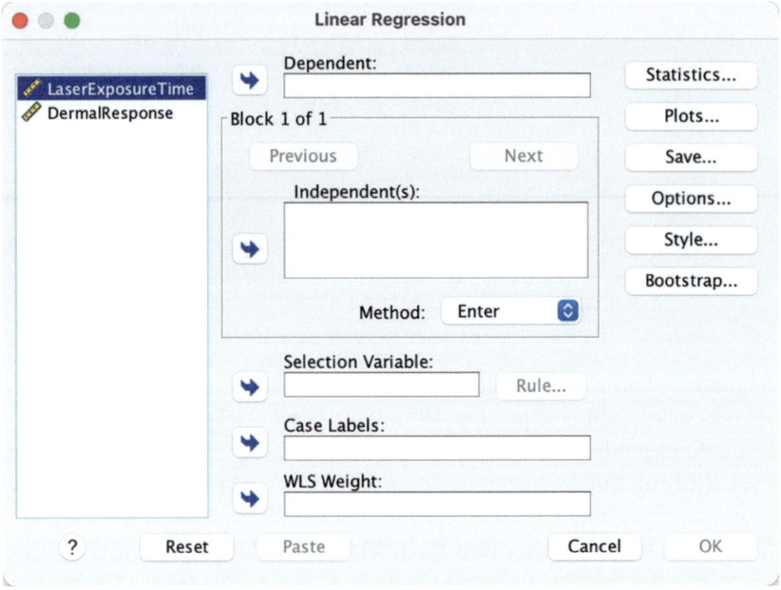

Fig. 12.106 Linear Regression dialog box displayed after selecting Analyze → Regression → Linear

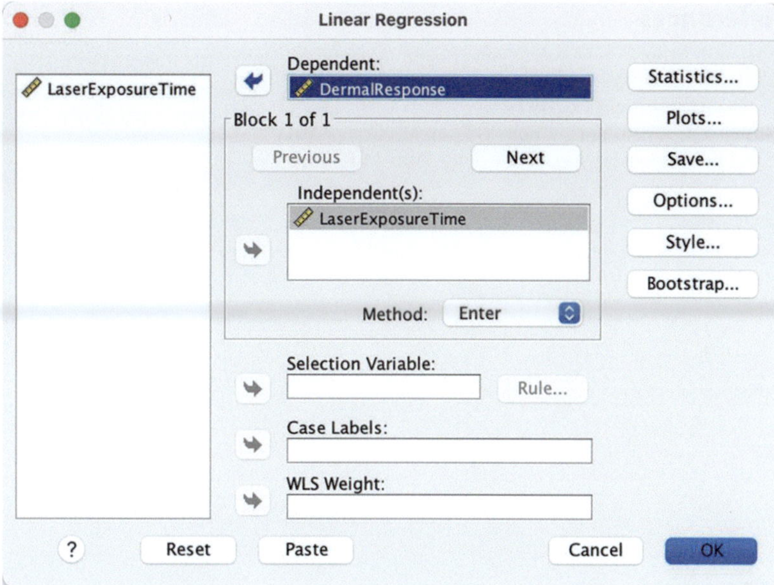

Fig. 12.107 Assignment of the dependent and independent variables in the linear regression dialog box

Model Summary

Model	R	R Square	Adjusted R Square	Std. Error of the Estimate
1	.954[a]	.910	.899	.23335

a. Predictors: (Constant), LaserExposureTime

ANOVA[a]

Model		Sum of Squares	df	Mean Square	F	Sig.
1	Regression	4.415	1	4.415	81.081	<.001[b]
	Residual	.436	8	.054		
	Total	4.851	9			

a. Dependent Variable: DermalResponse

b. Predictors: (Constant), LaserExposureTime

Coefficients[a]

Model		Unstandardized Coefficients B	Unstandardized Coefficients Std. Error	Standardized Coefficients Beta	t	Sig.
1	(Constant)	5.381	.159		33.754	<.001
	LaserExposureTime	.023	.003	.954	9.004	<.001

a. Dependent Variable: DermalResponse

Fig. 12.108 Output window displaying the results of the linear regression analysis, including coefficients and model summary

References

Blesh TE. Measurement in physical education. New York. The Ronald Press Co., 1974.

Huang Y-J, Chen K-L, Chou Y-T, et al. Comparison of the responsiveness of the long-form and simplified stroke rehabilitation assessment of movement: group- and individual-level analysis. Phys Ther 2015;95(8):1172–1183.

Norton BJ, Strube MJ. Understanding statistical power. J Orthop Sports Phys Ther 2001;31:307–315

13 Nonparametric Statistics

In general, statistics is broadly classified into parametric statistics and nonparametric statistics. The term metric refers to the measurement procedure, while para indicates the assumptions made about the population from which the data are drawn. Parametric tests are based on the following assumptions:

First, the samples are randomly selected.
Second, the scores are independent of each other.
Third, the data are normally distributed.
Fourth, the samples have equal variances.

One drawback of parametric statistical methods is that they often require time-consuming calculations when done manually, and they can be difficult to understand for individuals without a strong background in mathematics. All parametric tests require that these assumptions be met. In contrast, nonparametric tests do not require strict adherence to the same assumptions as parametric tests. For this reason, nonparametric methods are sometimes referred to as distribution-free methods. However, nonparametric tests have a higher probability of committing Type II errors. Parametric tests are more suitable for analyzing data measured on interval or ratio scales, whereas nonparametric tests are appropriate for data measured on nominal or ordinal scales. Compared to parametric tests, which can be complex and difficult to compute, nonparametric tests are simpler and easier to perform. Nonparametric methods are applied when the assumptions of parametric tests are difficult to satisfy, when the sample size is small, or when the distribution of the data cannot be assumed. Nevertheless, if the data meet the assumptions of parametric tests, it is preferable to use them instead of nonparametric tests, as parametric methods generally have higher statistical power.

Nonparametric test methods can be summarized as shown in Table 13.1.

Table 13.1 Summary of nonparametric test methods

Sample characteristics	Nominal scale	Ordinal scale
One sample (univariate)	Chi-square test	Kolmogorov–Smirnov test
Two related samples	McNemar test	Sign test, Wilcoxon signed-rank test
K related samples	Cochran's Q test	Friedman test
Two independent samples	Crosstab analysis	Median test, Mann–Whitney U test
K independent samples		Kruskal–Wallis test, Extension of the median test

K.-H. Yi, *Statistical Research Methods for Dermatologists and Plastic Surgeons*,
https://doi.org/10.1007/978-981-95-5668-7_13

13.1 Chi-Square Test

The one-sample χ^2 analysis is used to test whether there is a difference between the observed and expected frequencies included in nominal or ordinal scales. It is used when conducting a goodness-of-fit test[1] and when testing the independence[2] between variables composed of nominal or ordinal scales.

1. *One-Sample χ^2 Test*

This test examines whether the frequency observed in each category differs significantly from the expected frequency. The null hypothesis is stated as:

H_0: There is no difference between the observed and expected frequencies.

The χ^2 statistic is calculated using the following formula:

$$\chi^2 = \sum_{i=1}^{k} \frac{(O_i - E_i)^2}{E_i}$$

Where:

O_i = Observed frequency in category i
E_i = Expected frequency in category i

In general,

$$E_i = \sum_{i=1}^{k} O_i / k, \qquad k = \text{number of categories}$$

In this case, the calculated χ^2 follows a chi-square distribution with degrees of freedom equal to $k - 1$. To determine whether there is a significant difference between expected and observed frequencies, compare the calculated χ^2 statistic with the critical value from the chi-square distribution table, using the predetermined significance level and degrees of freedom. If the calculated χ^2 is equal to or greater than the table value, it is concluded that there is a significant difference. The chi-square test is more appropriate when the sample size is sufficiently large.

For example, when the number of categories is 2, the expected frequency in each cell should be at least 5. If there are more than 2 categories and more than 20% of the expected frequencies are less than 5, or if even one expected frequency is less than 1, then the chi-square test may not be valid. To address this, one can reduce the number of categories or collect more data to increase the sample size. In such cases, rather than using the chi-square test, it is more appropriate to use Fisher's exact test. Fisher's exact test is recommended under the following conditions:

1. When the total sample size is less than 20, or
2. When the total sample size is between 20 and 40 and any expected frequency is less than 5.

Let us consider an example of a chi-square test. Suppose we want to determine clients' preferences among four types of facial rejuvenation devices commonly used in dermatology clinics. The data are shown in Table 13.2. As shown in Table 13.2, the calculated chi-square statistic is 18.88. The critical value at a significance level of 0.05 with 3 degrees of freedom is 7.82. Since the chi-square statistic exceeds the critical value, the null hypothesis is rejected. To determine whether the observed frequencies differ from the expected ones, 90 clients were asked about their preference among the four facial rejuvenation devices. The expected frequency for each device is 90 ÷ 4 = 22.5. Because the observed chi-square statistic exceeds the critical value, it is concluded that

Table 13.2 An example of χ^2 test

Types	O	E	$O - E$	$(O - E)^2$	$(O - E)^2/E$
A	10	22.5	−12.5	156.25	6.94
B	15	22.5	−7.5	56.25	2.50
C	30	22.5	7.5	56.25	2.50
D	35	22.5	12.5	156.25	6.94
					Σ = 18.88

[1] Goodness-of-fit test: This tests how well the observed distribution (sample distribution) matches the expected distribution (theoretical distribution) for a population.

[2] Test of independence in a contingency table: This test compares the expected frequencies, calculated from the row and column totals of the contingency table, with the actual observed values in each cell.

the observed frequencies are significantly different from the expected frequencies. Therefore, we conclude that client preferences are not equal across the four facial rejuvenation devices.

2. χ^2 *Test for Two Samples*

Let us consider a case involving two groups, commonly referred to as a 2 × 2 table. This test is used to determine whether there is a statistically significant difference between two independent samples. In this case, the degrees of freedom are (2 – 1)(2 – 1) = 1. Suppose we aim to investigate whether there is a difference in the successful performance of a fine skin procedure—such as microdermabrasion—between left-handed and right-handed skincare specialists. The null hypothesis (H_0) would be: "There is no difference in procedural success between left-handed and right-handed practitioners." The alternative hypothesis (H_1) would be: "Right-handed practitioners perform the procedure more successfully than left-handed ones." For the task, each participant was asked to complete a precision-based microdermabrasion procedure on a synthetic skin model. A total of 100 trainees participated—50 were right-handed, and 50 were left-handed. Their outcomes were recorded as either successful or unsuccessful. The significance level was set at 0.05, and the data were organized into the following 2 × 2 contingency table.

	Left-handed	Right-handed	Total
Success	$A = 20$	$B = 18$	$38 = (A + B)$
Fail	$C = 30$	$D = 32$	$62 = (C + D)$
	$50 = (A + C)$	$50 = (B + D)$	$N = 100$

The χ^2 test statistic is calculated using the following formula:

$$\chi^2 = N(AD - BC)^2 / (A+B)(C+D)(A+C)(B+D)$$

$$= 100(20 \times 32 - 18 \times 30)^2 / (38)(62)(50)(50)$$

$$= 1{,}000{,}000 / 5{,}890{,}000 = 0.17$$

According to the chi-square distribution table, with a significance level of 0.05 and degrees of freedom of 1, the critical value is 3.84. Since the calculated χ^2 value is less than the critical value, we fail to reject the null hypothesis. Therefore, it is concluded that there is no statistically significant difference between left-handed and right-handed practitioners in terms of mastering microdermabrasion technique.

In chi-square tests with 1 degree of freedom, Yates' continuity correction[3] is typically applied.

McNemar's chi-square test[4] is used when analyzing paired data to examine whether there is a significant difference in the distribution between two related samples. While a chi-square test indicates whether an association exists or does not exist, it does not provide information about the strength of the association. To assess the degree of association between nominal variables, additional statistical measures must be applied. Common indices based on the chi-square statistic include phi coefficient, contingency coefficient, and Cramér's V. For ordinal variables, measures of association include Kendall's tau-b, Kendall's tau-c, gamma, and Somers' d.

Let us now analyze the above data using SPSS. Launch SPSS and enter the data as shown in Fig. 13.1.

Click Data → Weight Cases in SPSS (Fig. 13.2).

Click Weight cases by to specify the weighting variable (Fig. 13.3).

[3] Yates' Continuity Correction Formula

$$\chi^2 = \sum_{i=1}^{k} \frac{(|O_i - E_i| - 0.5)^2}{E_i}$$

[4] McNemar Formula

$$\chi^2 = \sum_{A,D} \frac{(O_i - E_i)^2}{E_i} = \frac{\left(A - \frac{A+D}{2}\right)^2}{\frac{A+D}{2}} + \frac{\left(D - \frac{A+D}{2}\right)^2}{\frac{A+D}{2}}$$

$$= \frac{(A-D)^2}{A+D}, \quad df = 2$$

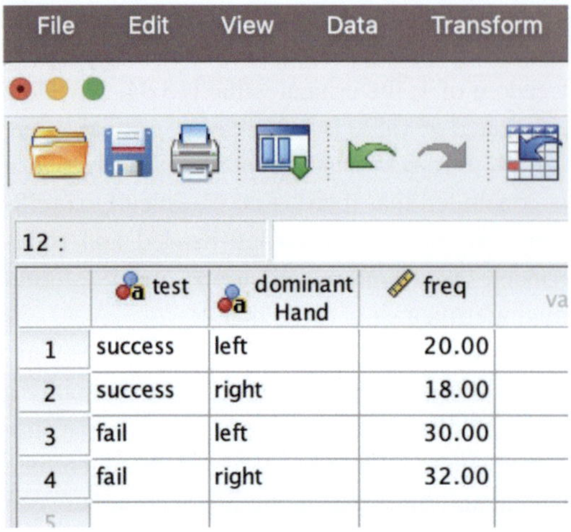

Fig. 13.1 Example dataset for conducting a chi-square test using SPSS

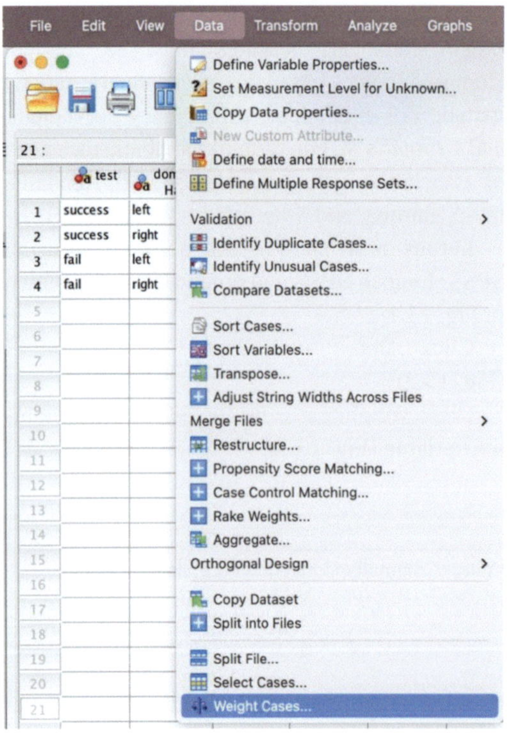

Fig. 13.2 Navigating to Weight Cases via Data → Weight Cases in SPSS

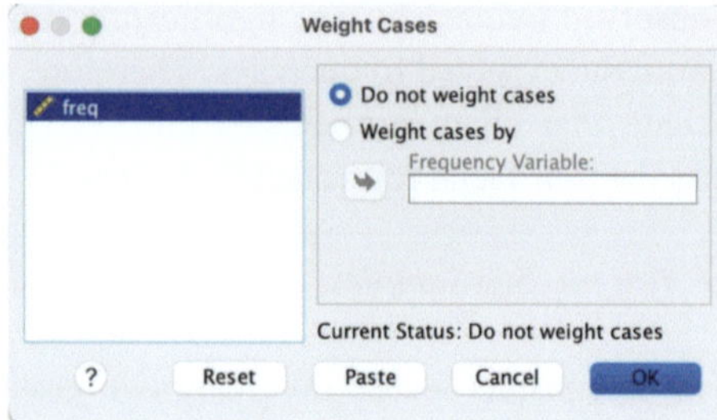

Fig. 13.3 Weight cases dialog box displayed after selecting the option in SPSS

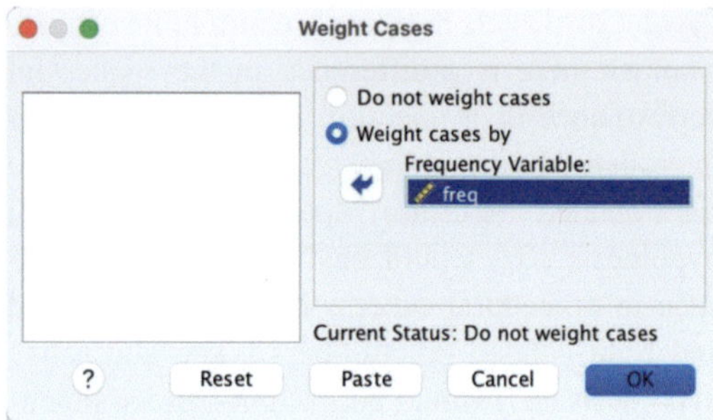

Fig. 13.4 Specifying a variable under "Weight cases by" in SPSS

Move the frequency variable to the box on the right, then click OK (Fig. 13.4).

Click Analyze → Descriptive Statistics → Crosstabs (Fig. 13.5).

Move the appropriate variables into the Row(s) and Column(s) fields, then click on Statistics (Fig. 13.6).

Check Chi-square, then click Continue. Finally, click OK to run the analysis (Figs. 13.7 and 13.8).

The following output table is displayed (Fig. 13.9).

In the output table, the chi-square statistic is 0.17 with a p-value of 0.680, indicating that there is no significant association between the two variables.

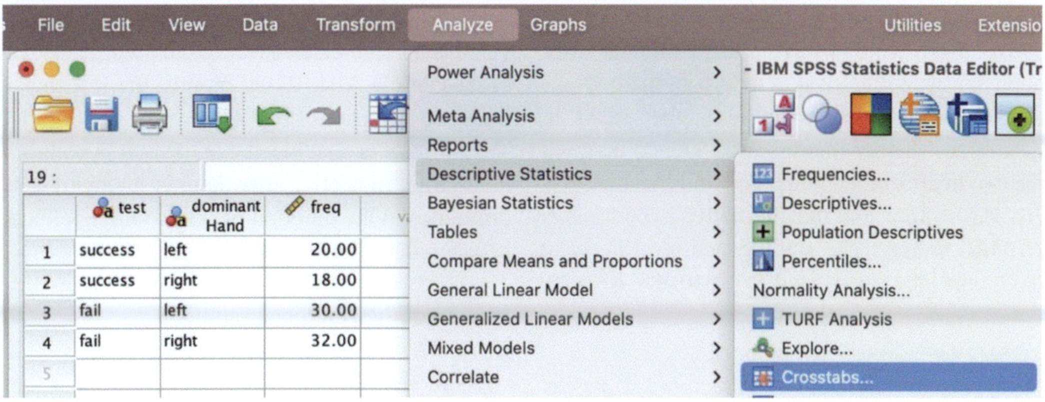

Fig. 13.5 Pathway to conduct a chi-square test

Fig. 13.6 Crosstabs dialog window displayed after selecting Analyze → Descriptive Statistics → Crosstabs in SPSS

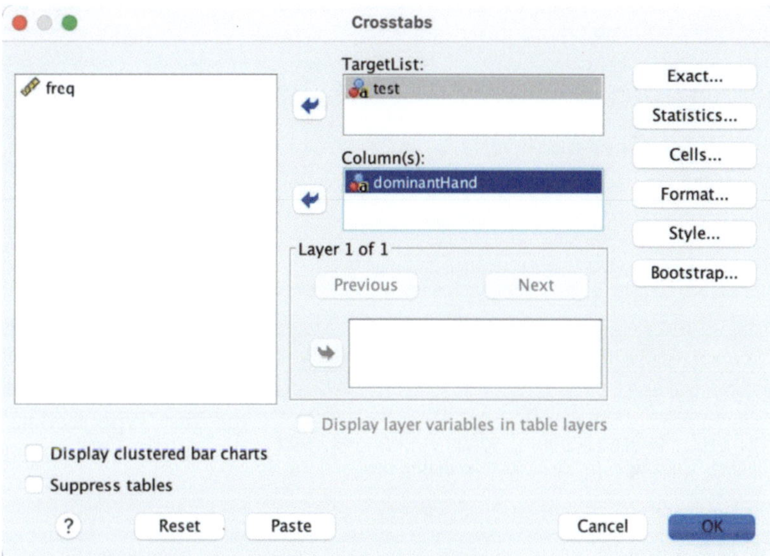

13.2 Median Test

In the median test, two independent samples are combined and ranked together to determine the overall median. Then, for each group, the number of values greater than, equal to, or less than the median is counted. The degrees of freedom for this test are 1, and the null hypothesis is H_0: $Md_A = Md_B$, meaning the two populations have the same median value. The alternative hypothesis is H_1: $Md_A \neq Md_B$, which indicates that the populations do not share the same median. This can be presented in a contingency table as follows:

	>	≤	
Method A	A	B	$A + B$
Method B	C	D	$C + D$
	$A + C$	$B + D$	N

This can be expressed using the chi-square formula as follows:

$$\chi^2 = N\left(AD - BC\right)^2 / \left(A + B\right)\left(C + D\right)\left(A + C\right)\left(B + D\right)$$

For example, suppose that the duration of skin-soothing effects was measured in minutes after applying two different skin treatment methods, as shown in Table 13.3. The researcher seeks to determine whether there is a difference between the two treatment methods. The null hypothesis is H_0: $Md_A = Md_B$, and the alternative hypothesis is H_1: $Md_A \neq Md_B$. The significance level is set at 0.05, and the calculated χ^2 statistic is 0.20. According to the χ^2 distribution table, the critical value at a significance level of 0.05 with 1 degree of freedom is 3.84. Based on this, the researcher finds no reason to reject the null hypothesis. Therefore, it is concluded that the null hypothesis holds true, indicating that there is no significant difference in the duration of skin-soothing effects between the two treatment methods.

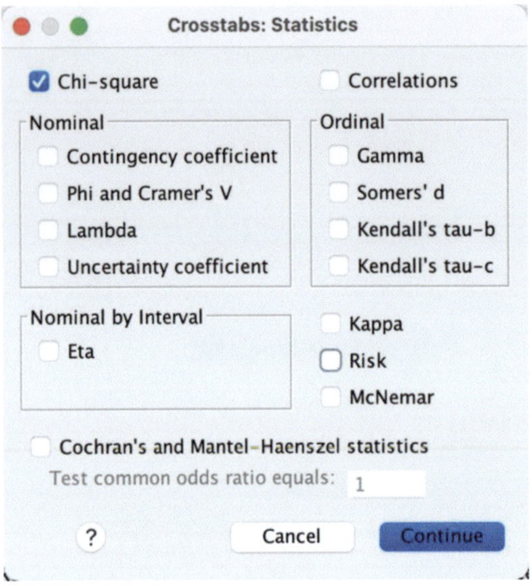

Fig. 13.7 Statistics options window displayed after clicking "Statistics" in the Crosstabs dialog box

Median of the combined sample = 7

$\chi^2 = 20(20–30)^2 / (10)(10)(9)(11) = 2000 / 9900 = 0.202$

	>	≤	
Method A	4^A	6^B	10
Method B	5^C	5^D	10
	9	11	20

Let's analyze the above data using SPSS. Launch SPSS and enter the data as follows (Fig. 13.10).

Go to Analyze → Nonparametric Tests → Legacy Dialogs → K Independent Samples and click it (Fig. 13.11).

Move the duration variable into the Test Variable List box, and move the method variable into the Grouping Variable box (Fig. 13.12). In the Test Type section, uncheck Kruskal–Wallis H, and check Median instead.

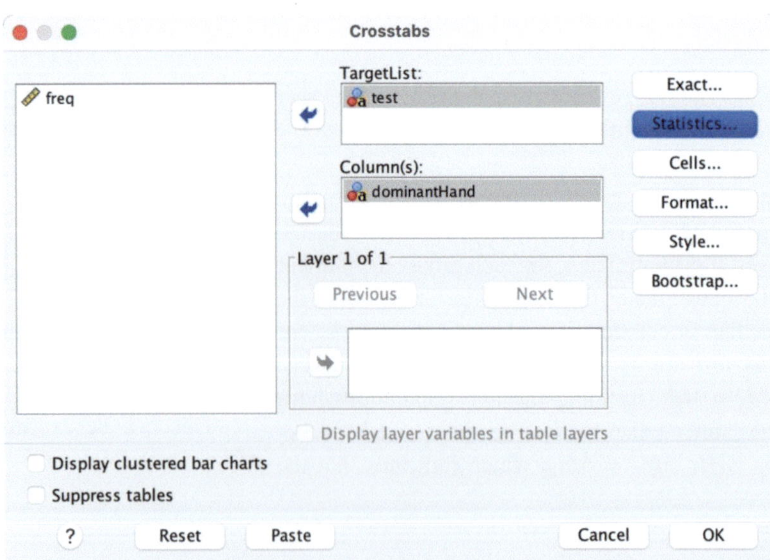

Fig. 13.8 Crosstabs dialog box in SPSS after selecting statistical options

test * dominantHand Crosstabulation

Count

		dominantHand left	dominantHand right	Total
test	fail	30	32	62
	success	20	18	38
Total		50	50	100

Chi-Square Tests

	Value	df	Asymptotic Significance (2-sided)	Exact Sig. (2-sided)	Exact Sig. (1-sided)
Pearson Chi-Square	.170[a]	1	.680		
Continuity Correction[b]	.042	1	.837		
Likelihood Ratio	.170	1	.680		
Fisher's Exact Test				.837	.418
N of Valid Cases	100				

a. 0 cells (0.0%) have expected count less than 5. The minimum expected count is 19.00.

b. Computed only for a 2x2 table

Fig. 13.9 Chi-square test output results in SPSS

Table 13.3 Comparison of two skin-soothing treatment methods

Method A (duration of skin soothing, in minutes)	Method B (duration of skin soothing, in minutes)
1	2
4	1
6	8
10	6
8	12
7	5
6	9
7	10
17	15
13	5

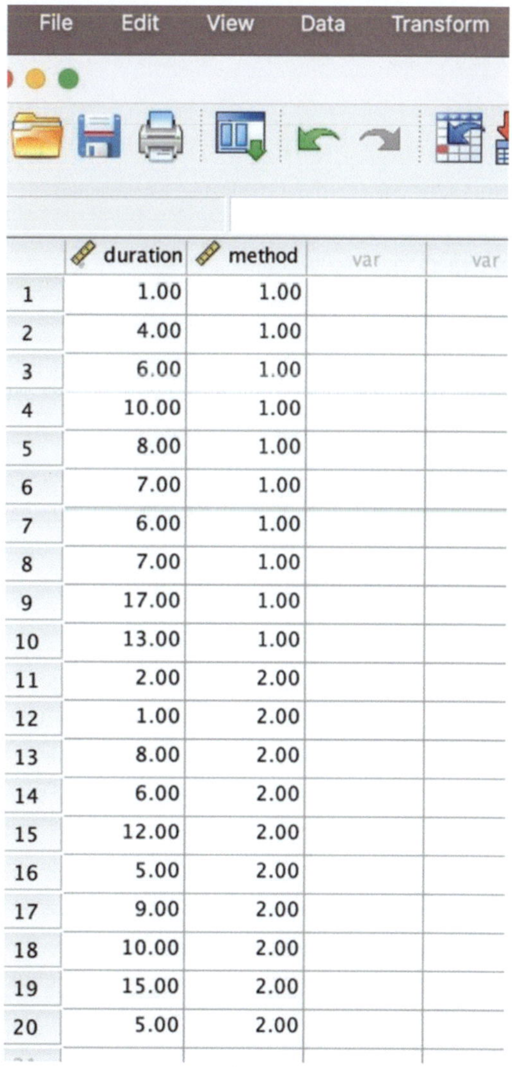

	duration	method	var	var
1	1.00	1.00		
2	4.00	1.00		
3	6.00	1.00		
4	10.00	1.00		
5	8.00	1.00		
6	7.00	1.00		
7	6.00	1.00		
8	7.00	1.00		
9	17.00	1.00		
10	13.00	1.00		
11	2.00	2.00		
12	1.00	2.00		
13	8.00	2.00		
14	6.00	2.00		
15	12.00	2.00		
16	5.00	2.00		
17	9.00	2.00		
18	10.00	2.00		
19	15.00	2.00		
20	5.00	2.00		

Fig. 13.10 Example dataset for median test analysis in SPSS

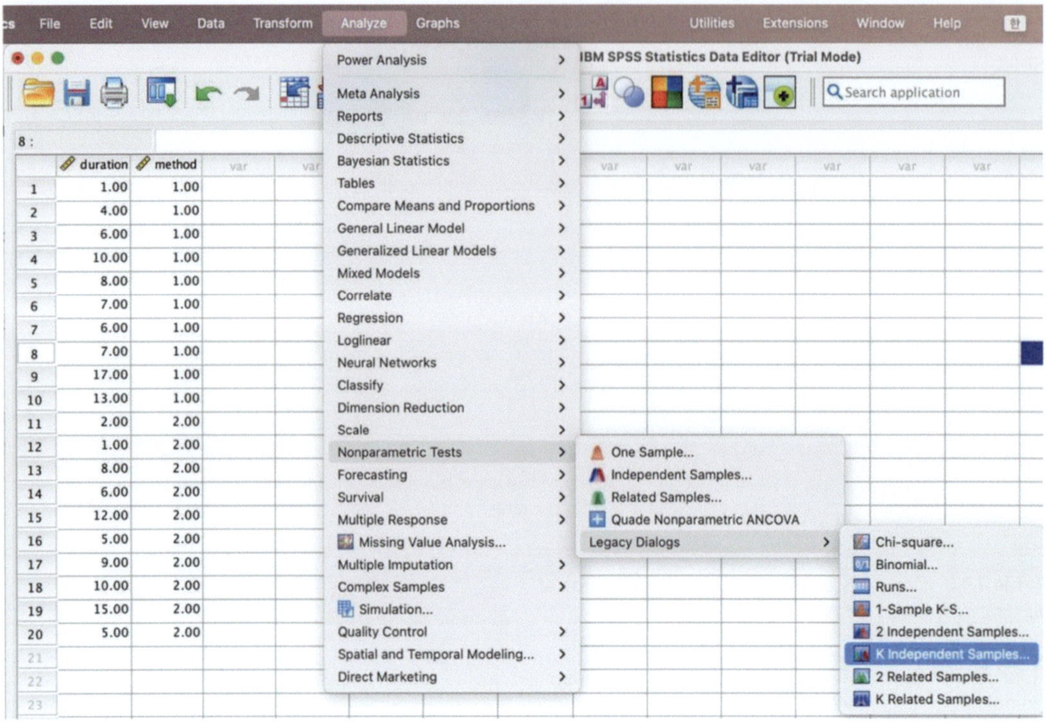

Fig. 13.11 Menu path for conducting a median test

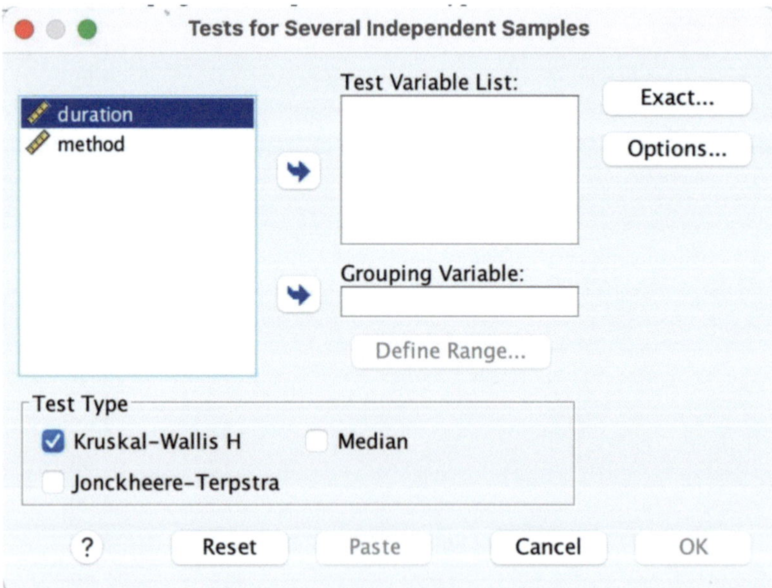

Fig. 13.12 Tests for several independent samples dialog window in SPSS

Click on "Define Range" (Fig. 13.13).

Enter 1 as the minimum value and 2 as the maximum value (Fig. 13.14). Then, click Continue.

Click OK (Fig. 13.15). Then, the output table will appear as shown in Fig. 13.16).

Fig. 13.13 Variables moved into the test fields before defining the group range in SPSS

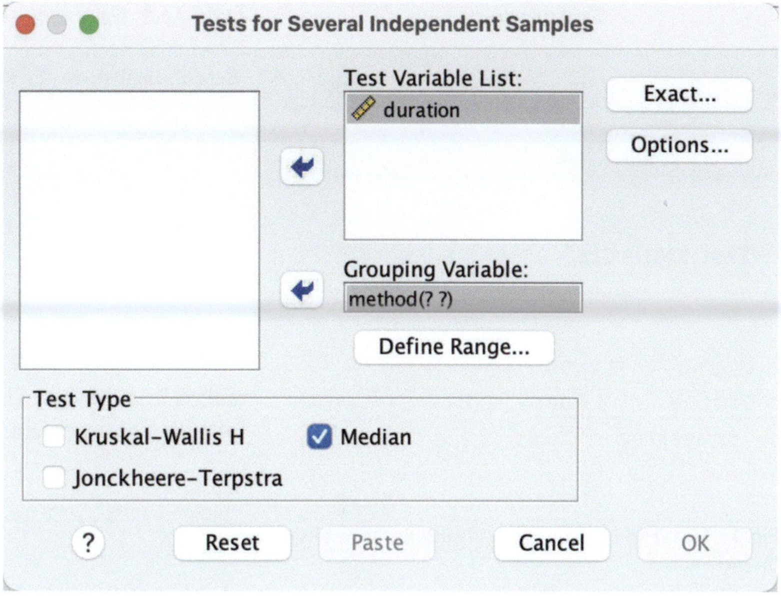

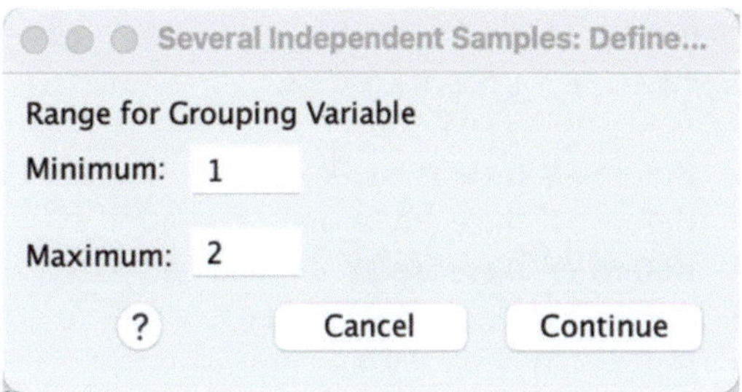

Fig. 13.14 Defining the grouping variable range in SPSS after selecting "Define Range"

Fig. 13.15 Dialog after defining the group range for the median test

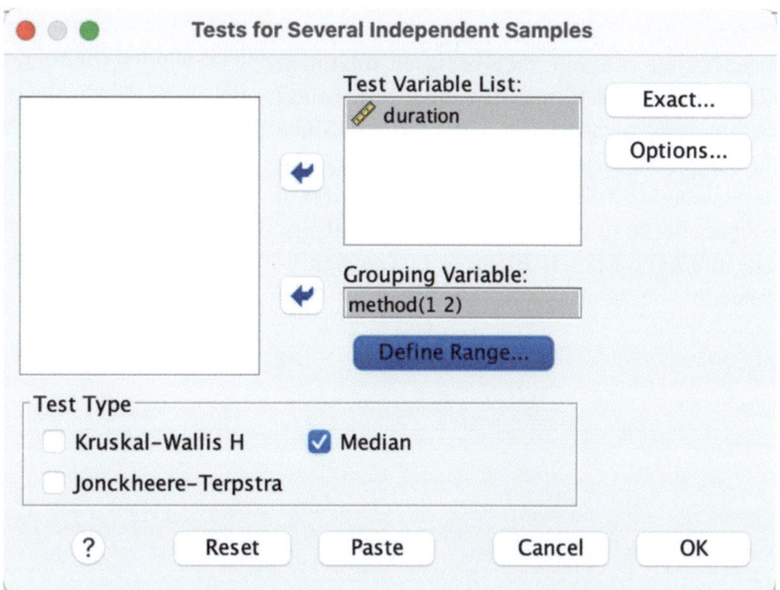

Frequencies

		method	
		1.00	2.00
duration	> Median	4	5
	<= Median	6	5

Test Statistics[a]

	duration
N	20
Median	7.0000
Exact Sig.	1.000

a. Grouping Variable: method

Fig. 13.16 SPSS output window displaying the results of the median test

13.3 Mann–Whitney U Test

The Mann–Whitney U test is a nonparametric method used to compare two independent samples, evaluating the equality of distributions based on mean ranks. It serves as a nonparametric alternative to the independent samples t-test used in parametric statistics.

For example, suppose that five rabbits received artificially induced wounds followed by laser treatment, and the healing time for each was recorded. A control group of seven rabbits also received artificially induced wounds but did not receive laser treatment (Table 13.4). The time required for wound healing was measured in both groups. Since the sample sizes are small and the data cannot be assumed to follow a normal distribution, a nonparametric test was chosen for analysis. The null hypothesis is H_0: $\mu_x = \mu_y$. The significance level is set at 0.05.

Table 13.4 Data comparing wound healing effects of laser treatment

Experimental group (X)	Rank	Control group (Y)	Rank
27	2	30	3
51	11	35	5
33	4	25	1
37	6	53	12
43	9	50	10
		38	7
		40	8

The data from both groups are combined and ranked from lowest to highest. This results in the following arrangement:

Rank	1	2	3	4	5	6	7	8	9	10	11	12
Group	*Y*	*X*	*Y*	*X*	*Y*	*X*	*Y*	*Y*	*X*	*Y*	*X*	*Y*

The U statistic is calculated by counting how many X values precede each Y value, and then summing those counts. In this case, $U = 1 + 2 + 3 + 3 + 4 + 5 = 18$.

- Before 3Y, there is one $X \rightarrow +1$
- Before 5Y, there are 2X and 4$X \rightarrow +2$
- Before 7Y, there are 2X, 4X, and 6$X \rightarrow +3$
- Before 8Y, there 2X, 4X, and 6$X \rightarrow +3$
- Before 10Y, four X values precede $\rightarrow +4$
- Before 12Y, five X values precede $\rightarrow +5$

In the Mann–Whitney U table, locate the U value of 18 when the cell corresponding to $n_y = 7$ (since the experimental group consists of 5 subjects and the control group consists of 7 subjects, the larger value, which is 7, is used).

To determine statistical significance, we consult the Mann–Whitney U distribution table using the larger of the two sample sizes $n_y = 7$ (since the experimental group consists of 5 subjects and the control group consists of 7 subjects, the larger value, which is 7, is used). When locating the

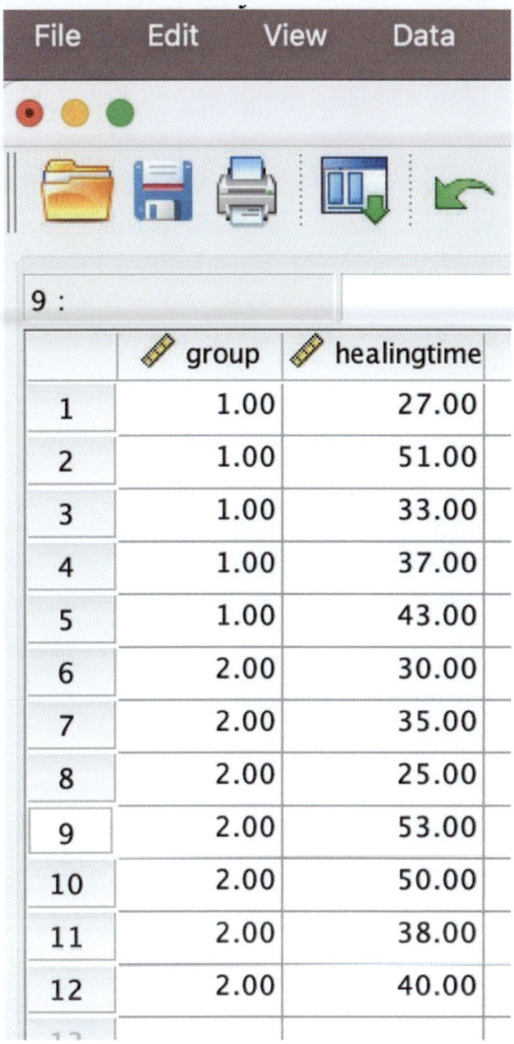

	group	healingtime
1	1.00	27.00
2	1.00	51.00
3	1.00	33.00
4	1.00	37.00
5	1.00	43.00
6	2.00	30.00
7	2.00	35.00
8	2.00	25.00
9	2.00	53.00
10	2.00	50.00
11	2.00	38.00
12	2.00	40.00

Fig. 13.17 Example dataset for conducting a Mann Whitney U test in SPSS

value for $n_x = 5$, the corresponding probability is 0.562. In this case, the null hypothesis is considered to be true, and it is concluded that there is no reason to reject the null hypothesis that there is no difference between the two groups.

The above procedure applies when the larger sample size of the two groups is 8 or less.

If the sample size falls between 9 and 20, or is greater than 20, a different procedure (formula) must be used accordingly.

Let us now analyze the above data using SPSS. Launch SPSS and enter the data as shown in Fig. 13.17.

Then, go to Analyze → Nonparametric Tests → Legacy Dialogs → 2 Independent Samples (Fig. 13.18).

Make sure that "Mann–Whitney U" is selected (Fig. 13.19).

Move the variable "healing time" into the Test Variable List box, and click Define Groups to specify the two groups (Figs. 13.20 and 13.21).

Click Continue, then click OK. The following output table will be generated (Fig. 13.22).

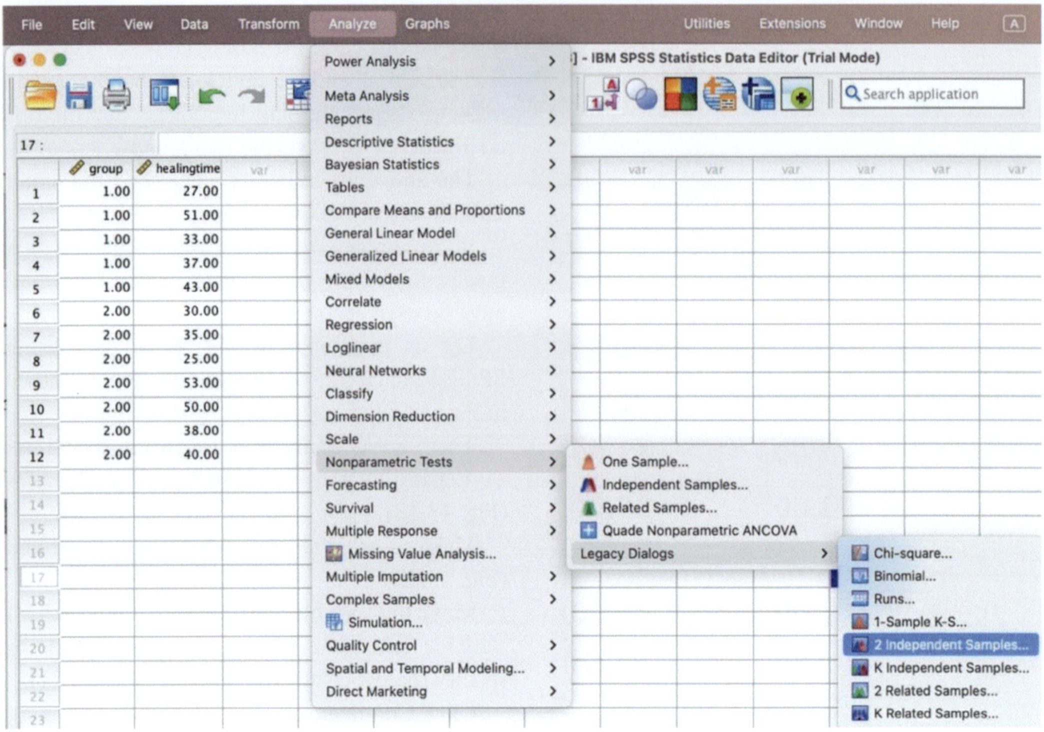

Fig. 13.18 Path to conduct the Mann–Whitney U test

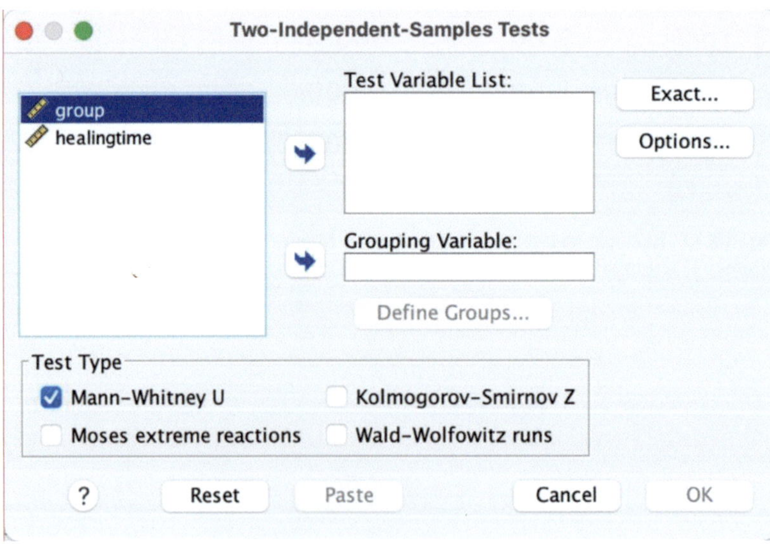

Fig. 13.19 Dialog box for two-independent-samples test in SPSS

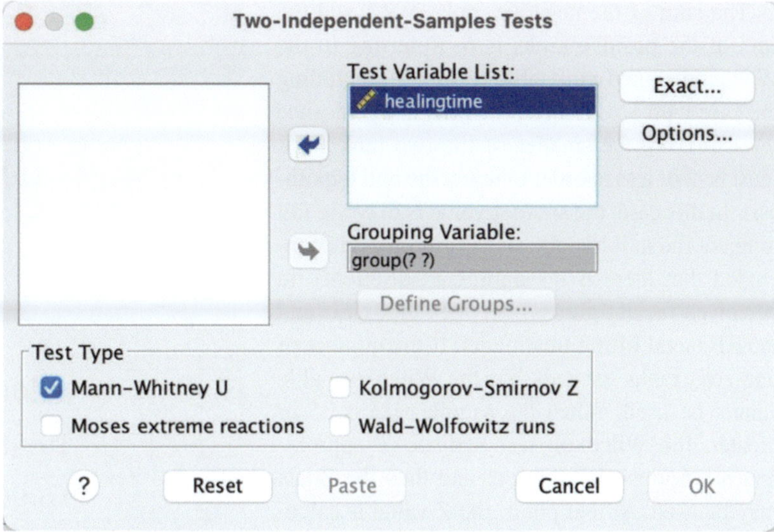

Fig. 13.20 Variable assignment screen before defining groups

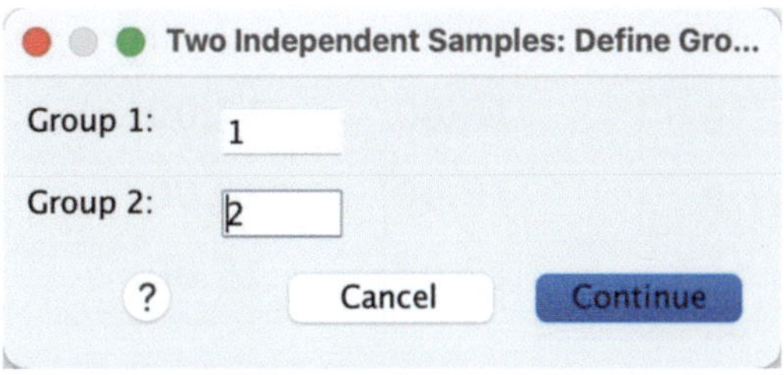

Fig. 13.21 Defining group values in the two-independent-samples test dialog

Ranks

	group	N	Mean Rank	Sum of Ranks
healingtime	1.00	5	6.40	32.00
	2.00	7	6.57	46.00
	Total	12		

Test Statistics[a]

	healingtime
Mann-Whitney U	17.000
Wilcoxon W	32.000
Z	-.081
Asymp. Sig. (2-tailed)	.935
Exact Sig. [2*(1-tailed Sig.)]	1.000[b]

a. Grouping Variable: group

b. Not corrected for ties.

Fig. 13.22 SPSS output window displaying results of the Mann–Whitney U Test

13.4 Wilcoxon Signed-Ranks Test

The Wilcoxon signed-ranks (matched-pairs) test is used to compare two related (paired) measurements. The procedure begins by calculating the difference between each pair, then assigning ranks based on the absolute values of the differences. Each rank is assigned a positive or negative sign(+, −) according to the direction of the difference. If there is no difference between a pair, it is excluded from the analysis. When two or more differences are equal, the average of their ranks (i.e., the midrank) is assigned.

Eight subjects underwent both high-intensity focused ultrasound (HIFU) and radiofrequency (RF) facial lifting treatments, spaced 1 week apart. After each treatment, participants rated their perceived facial tightness on a 0 to 20-point scale, where higher scores indicate stronger sensations of skin tightening. The paired data are shown below:

HIFU (X)	RF (Y)	Difference (d)	Rank
15	18	−3	−4.5
19	17	2	2.5
16	19	−3	−4.5
14	20	−6	−7
17	17	0	0
18	17	1	1
16	20	−4	−6
17	15	2	2.5

The sum of the negative ranks is 22, and the sum of the positive ranks is 6. Referring to the Wilcoxon signed-rank table for $n = 7$ (excluding the case with a zero difference), at a significance level of 0.05, the smaller of the two rank sums must be 2 or less in order to reject the null hypothesis. In this case, the smaller value is 6, so we fail to reject the null hypothesis. Therefore, it is concluded that there is no significant difference in perceived facial tightness between the HIFU and the RF facial lifting treatments. If the number of non-zero ranks exceeds 25, the Wilcoxon table cannot be used. When the sample size is 25 or greater, the Wilcoxon test statistic T approximates a normal distribution, and thus the Z-test may be used. At that point, the Z-value is calculated as follows:

$$Z = \frac{T - \frac{N(N+1)}{4}}{\sqrt{\frac{N(N+1)(2N+1)}{24}}}$$

Let us now analyze the data using SPSS. Launch SPSS and enter the data as shown in Fig. 13.23.

Go to Analyze → Nonparametric Tests → Legacy Dialogs → 2 Related Samples (Fig. 13.24).

Move the variables into the test pairs as shown, and ensure that "Wilcoxon" is selected (Fig. 13.25).

Click OK, and the following output table will be displayed (Fig. 13.26).

The term "Wilcoxon test" is used to refer to several different statistical procedures. The Wilcoxon matched-pairs signed-rank test is a nonparametric test used to compare pre- and post-measurements or data from matched subjects. It is often referred to more simply as the Wilcoxon matched-pairs test. The Wilcoxon signed-rank test is also a nonparametric method, but it is used to compare a set of values to a hypothetical median.

Meanwhile, the Wilcoxon rank-sum test is a nonparametric test used to compare two independent groups, and it yields the same results as the Mann–Whitney test.

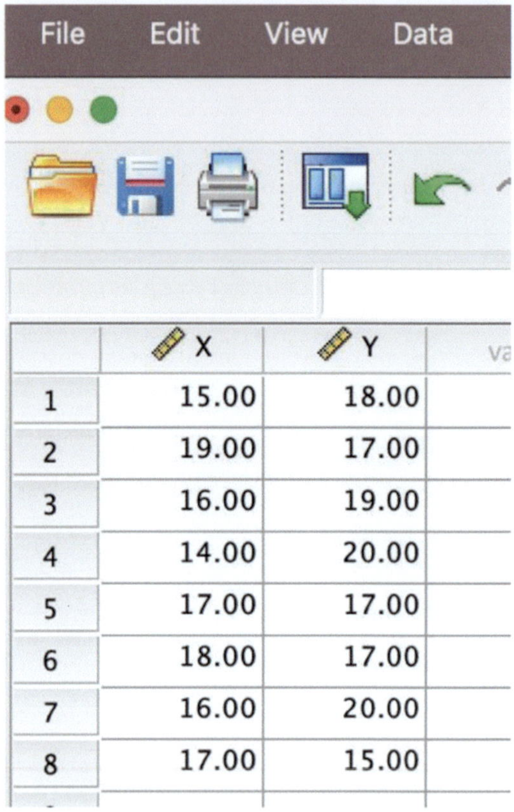

Fig. 13.23 Example dataset for the Wilcoxon signed-ranks test in SPSS

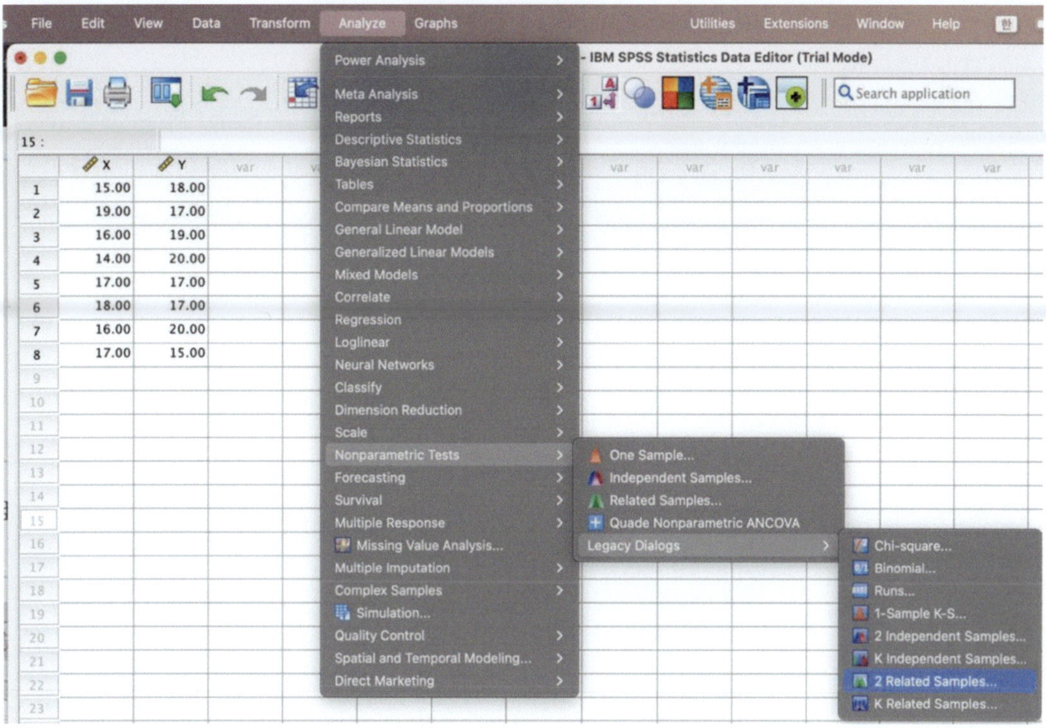

Fig. 13.24 Menu path for conducting a Wilcoxon signed-ranks test in SPSS

Fig. 13.25 Variables selected for the Wilcoxon signed-ranks Test after choosing "2 Related Samples" in SPSS

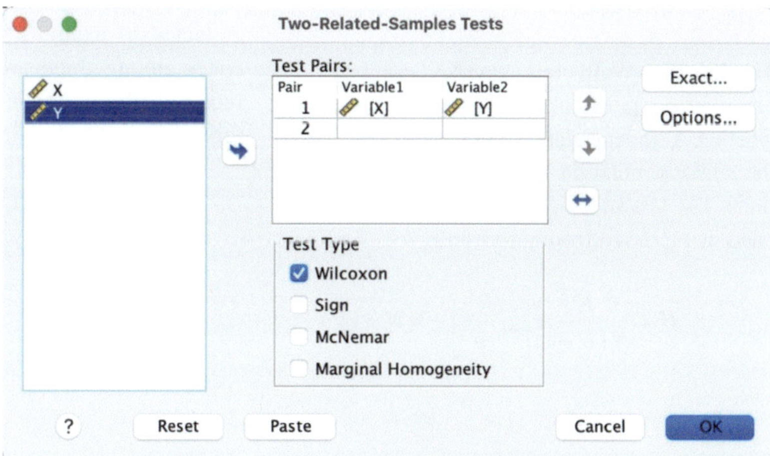

Fig. 13.26 SPSS output window showing the results of the Wilcoxon signed-ranks test

Wilcoxon Signed Ranks Test

Ranks

		N	Mean Rank	Sum of Ranks
Y – X	Negative Ranks	3[a]	2.00	6.00
	Positive Ranks	4[b]	5.50	22.00
	Ties	1[c]		
	Total	8		

a. Y < X
b. Y > X
c. Y = X

Test Statistics[a]

	Y – X
Z	-1.357[b]
Asymp. Sig. (2-tailed)	.175

a. Wilcoxon Signed Ranks Test

b. Based on negative ranks.

13.5 Kruskal–Wallis One-Way ANOVA

The Kruskal–Wallis one-way ANOVA is a nonparametric statistical test used to determine whether k independent samples originate from the same population or from different populations. The test statistic used is *H*, which is calculated using the following formula:

$$H = \frac{12}{N(N+1)}\left[\Sigma\frac{R^2}{n}\right] - 3(N+1)$$

This test requires that the level of measurement be at least ordinal. The following data were collected to examine whether there are differences among three groups of participants who received skin aesthetics training through one of three different instructional methods (Table 13.5).

$$T = t^3 - t, t: \text{tied ranks}$$

	3.5	6.5	9.5	11.5	13.5
t = the number of tied ranks	2	2	2	2	2
$T = (t^3 - t)$	6	6	6	6	6

Table 13.5 Exam scores based on skin aesthetic training method

Combined (textbook + practical)	Rank	Textbook only	Rank	Practical only	Rank
95	17	94	16	88	6.5
92	13.5	88	6.5	92	13.5
86	3.5	90	9.5	97	18
91	11.5	84	1	97	18
93	15	86	3.5	91	11.5
89	8	90	9.5	85	2
	Σ = 68.5		**Σ = 46.0**		**Σ = 56.5**

$$H = \frac{\frac{12}{18(18+1)}\left[\frac{68.5^2}{6}+\frac{46.0^2}{6}+\frac{56.5^2}{6}\right]-3(18+1)}{1-\frac{30}{18^3-18}} = \frac{\frac{12}{342}[1666.75]-57}{0.995} = 1.34$$

The calculated test statistic was $\chi^2 = 1.34$, with 2 degrees of freedom. The null hypothesis (H_0: $R_1 = R_2 = R_3$) states that there is no difference among the three instructional methods. Since the obtained χ^2 value (1.34) is less than the critical value ($\chi^2 = 5.99$) at the 0.05 significance level, it is concluded that there is no significant difference in effectiveness among the three skin aesthetics training methods.

Let us now analyze the above data using SPSS. Launch SPSS and enter the data as shown in Fig. 13.27.

Go to Analyze → Nonparametric Tests → Legacy Dialogs → K Independent Samples (Fig. 13.28).

Ensure that "Kruskal–Wallis H" is selected. Move "ExamScores" to the Test Variable List, and move "TrainingMethod" to the Grouping Variable box (Fig. 13.29).

Click Define Range to specify the groups (Fig. 13.30).

Since there are three groups in this dataset, enter 1 as the minimum and 3 as the maximum (Figs. 13.31 and 13.32).

Click Continue, then click OK. The following output table will be generated (Fig. 13.33).

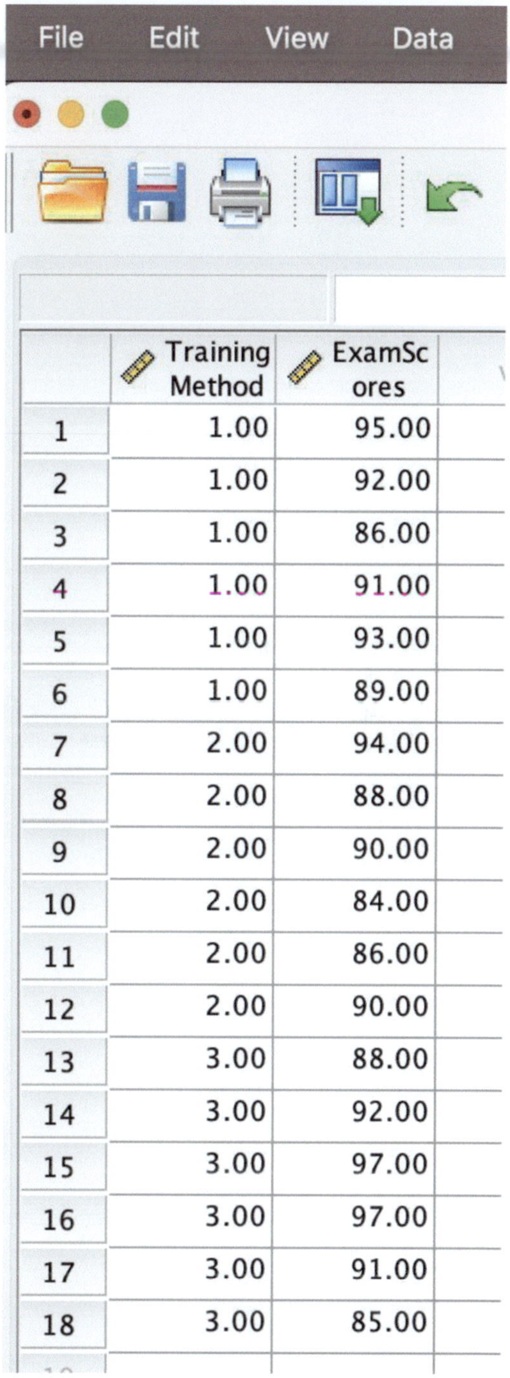

	TrainingMethod	ExamScores
1	1.00	95.00
2	1.00	92.00
3	1.00	86.00
4	1.00	91.00
5	1.00	93.00
6	1.00	89.00
7	2.00	94.00
8	2.00	88.00
9	2.00	90.00
10	2.00	84.00
11	2.00	86.00
12	2.00	90.00
13	3.00	88.00
14	3.00	92.00
15	3.00	97.00
16	3.00	97.00
17	3.00	91.00
18	3.00	85.00

Fig. 13.27 Example dataset for performing Kruskal–Wallis one-way ANOVA in SPSS

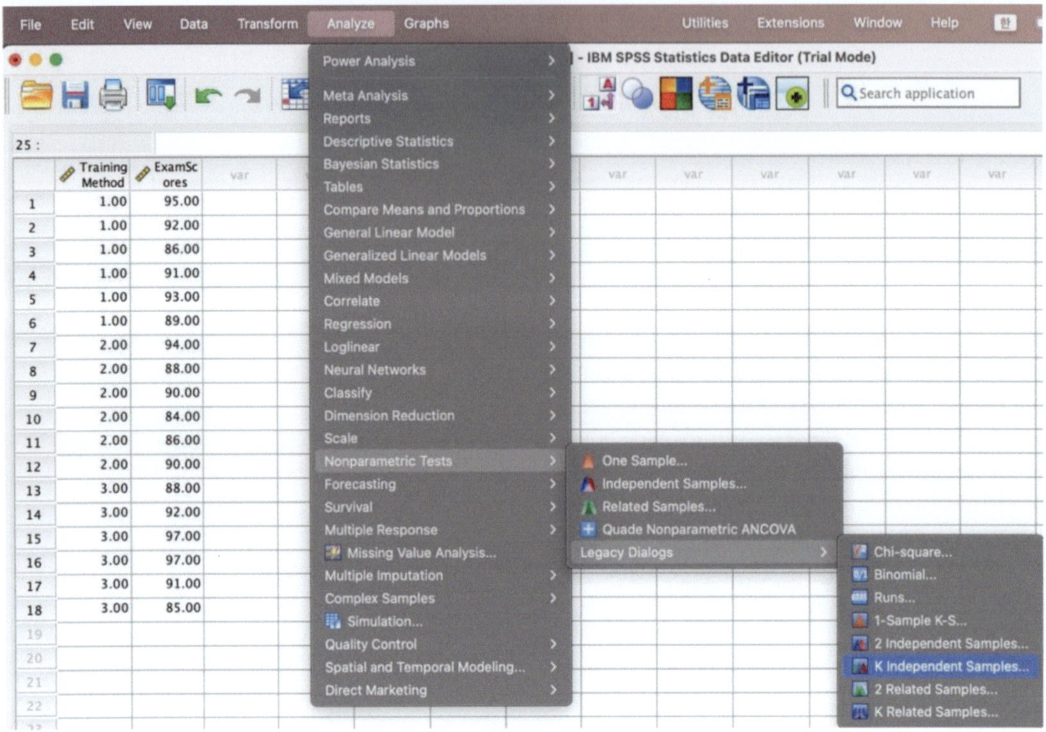

Fig. 13.28 Navigation path for Kruskal–Wallis one-way ANOVA

Fig. 13.29 Dialog window displayed after selecting "K Independent Samples" for Kruskal–Wallis analysis in SPSS

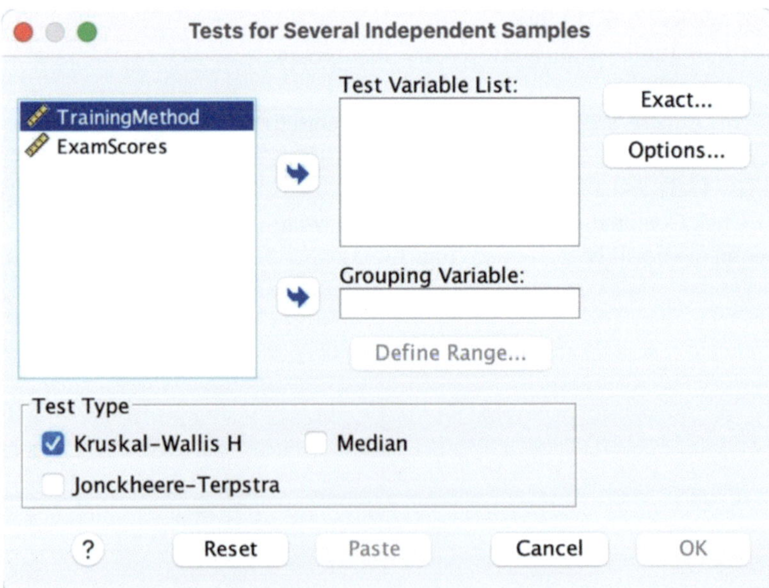

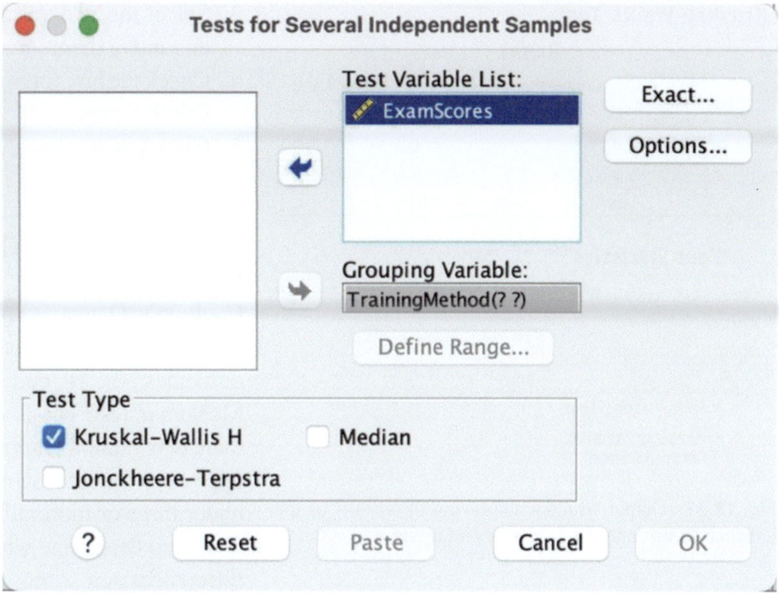

Fig. 13.30 Variables assigned to test fields prior to defining group range in the Kruskal–Wallis analysis dialog in SPSS

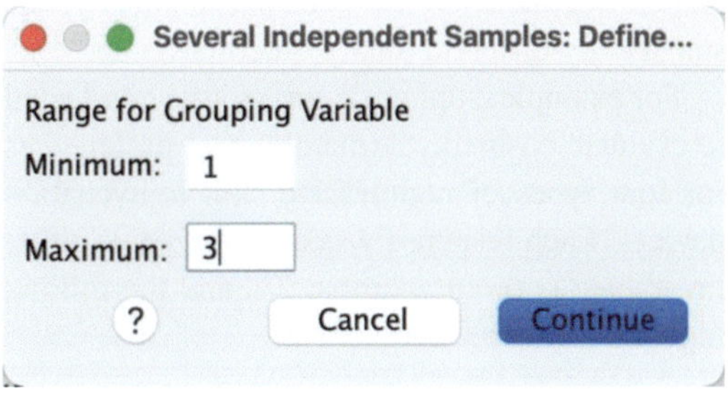

Fig. 13.31 Dialog box for defining the range of group values in the Kruskal–Wallis test setup in SPSS

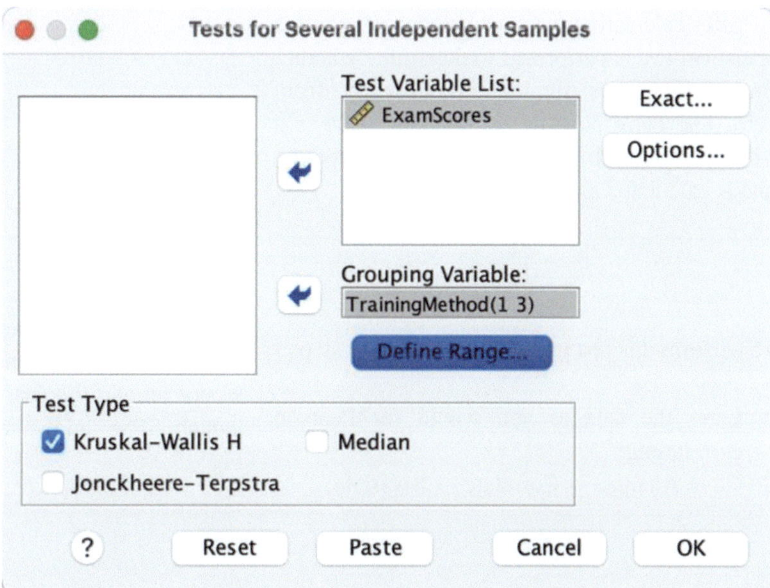

Fig. 13.32 Kruskal–Wallis test setup screen after defining the group range in SPSS

Kruskal–Wallis Test

Ranks

	TrainingMethod	N	Mean Rank
ExamScores	1.00	6	10.58
	2.00	6	7.00
	3.00	6	10.92
	Total	18	

Test Statistics[a,b]

	ExamScores
Kruskal-Wallis H	1.998
df	2
Asymp. Sig.	.368

a. Kruskal Wallis Test

b. Grouping Variable: TrainingMethod

Fig. 13.33 Output window displaying the results of the Kruskal–Wallis one-way ANOVA test in SPSS

13.6 Spearman's Rank Correlation Coefficient

Spearman's rank correlation coefficient is used to assess the correlation between two variables measured on an ordinal scale. The formula for calculating Spearman's rho is as follows:

$$r = 1 - \frac{6\sum_{i=1}^{n} d_i^2}{n\left(n^2 - 1\right)}$$

where n = number of observations, d_i = difference between the ranks of paired values.

After calculating the correlation coefficient, a statistical test is performed to determine whether the coefficient is significantly different from zero. The corresponding test statistic follows a t-distribution with $(n - 2)$ degrees of freedom, and is calculated as:

$$t = r_s \sqrt{\frac{n-2}{1-r_s^2}}$$

To perform this test in SPSS, follow these steps:

1. Enter the data as you would for Pearson correlation.
2. Go to Analyze → Correlate → Bivariate.
3. Select the two variables you wish to analyze and move them into the Variables box.
4. Check the box for Spearman under Correlation Coefficients.
5. Click OK to view the results.

13.7 Cochran's Q Test

Cochran's Q test is used to analyze K related variables that each have dichotomous (nominal) outcomes. It is conceptually similar to the McNemar test, but is extended to handle more than two related samples. This test is typically applied when the same subjects are evaluated under three or more different conditions, and the goal is to determine whether there are significant differences across those conditions. It can also be used to assess whether applying different experimental treatments to the same participants yields statistically different binary outcomes.

For example, suppose a survey was conducted to evaluate cosmetic dermatologists' preferences for four types of noninvasive skin rejuvenation devices. Each response was categorized as either favorable (1) or unfavorable (0), and the following data were obtained.

Dermatologists' preference ratings (1 = favorable, 0 = unfavorable) for four noninvasive skin rejuvenation devices

Dermatologist	IPL	RF	HIFU	LED
1	0	0	1	0
2	0	0	1	1
3	1	0	1	0
4	1	1	1	0
5	1	0	1	0
6	1	0	1	0
7	1	0	1	0
8	1	0	0	0
Total	6	1	7	1

In this case, the researcher aims to determine whether there are significant differences in preference among the four devices. To analyze this, launch SPSS and enter the data as shown in Fig. 13.34.

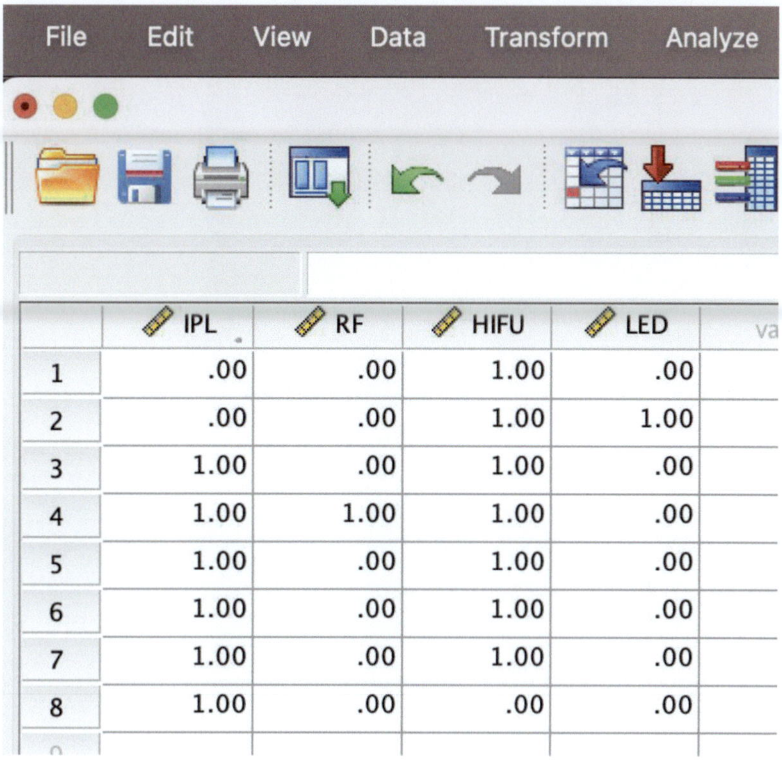

	IPL	RF	HIFU	LED
1	.00	.00	1.00	.00
2	.00	.00	1.00	1.00
3	1.00	.00	1.00	.00
4	1.00	1.00	1.00	.00
5	1.00	.00	1.00	.00
6	1.00	.00	1.00	.00
7	1.00	.00	1.00	.00
8	1.00	.00	.00	.00

Fig. 13.34 Example dataset for conducting Cochran's Q test using SPSS

Go to Analyze → Nonparametric Tests → Legacy Dialogs → K Related Samples (Fig. 13.35).

In the Test Type section, uncheck Friedman, and check Cochran's Q instead. Then, move the dependent variables to the box on the right (Fig. 13.36).

Click OK to run the test. The following output table will be generated (Fig. 13.37).

Based on the results, the *p*-value is less than the significance level of 0.05, indicating that there is a significant difference in preference among the four treatment methods.

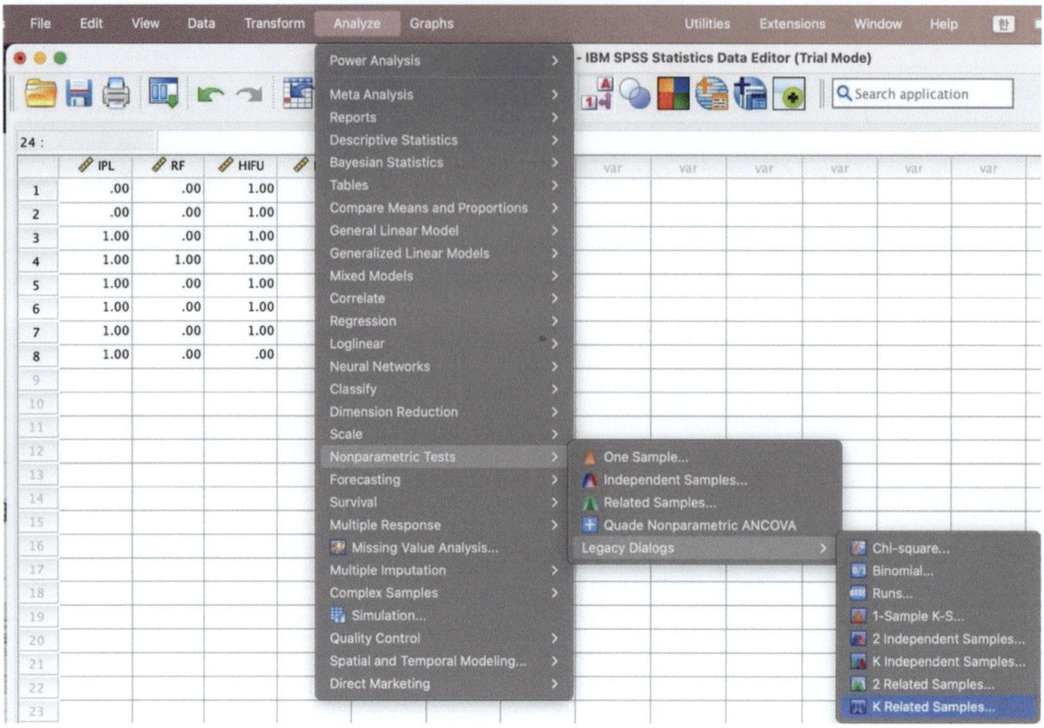

Fig. 13.35 Navigation path for Cochran's Q Test

Fig. 13.36 Dialog window displayed after selecting "K Related Samples" for Cochran's Q test in SPSS

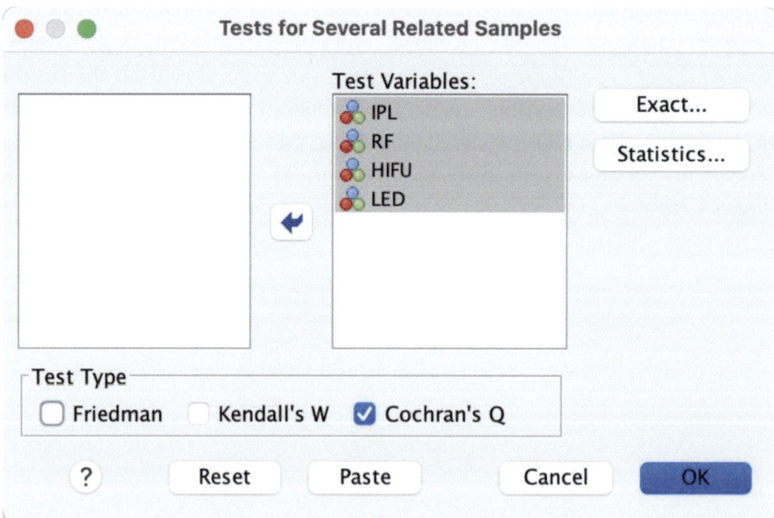

Cochran Test

Frequencies

	Value 0	1
IPL	2	6
RF	7	1
HIFU	1	7
LED	7	1

Test Statistics

N	8
Cochran's Q	12.724[a]
df	3
Asymp. Sig.	.005

a. 0 is treated as a success.

Fig. 13.37 SPSS output window showing the results of Cochran's Q test

13.8 Friedman Two-Way ANOVA

Friedman's two-way analysis of variance is used to determine whether K related samples originate from the same population. The level of measurement must be ordinal or higher. For example, suppose a study was conducted with eight patients, evaluating their preferences for four different treatment methods. Preferences were rated as Excellent, Good, Fair, or Poor, and the results were organized as shown in the following table.

Patient preferences for four treatment methods (1 = excellent, 2 = good, 3 = fair, 4 = poor)

Patient	Method 1	Method 2	Method 3	Method 4
1	3	2	1	4
2	4	3	1	2
3	2	4	1	3
4	1	3	2	4
5	2	3	1	4
6	1	4	2	3
7	2	3	1	4
8	1	4	2	3
Sum of ranks	16	26	11	27

If the researcher wishes to determine whether there are significant differences in preference among the treatment methods, the data should be entered into SPSS as shown in Fig. 13.38.

Go to Analyze → Nonparametric Tests → Legacy Dialogs → K Related Samples (Fig. 13.39).

Make sure that Friedman is checked, and move the dependent variables to the box on the right (Figs. 13.40 and 13.41).

Click OK to run the analysis. The following output table will be generated (Fig. 13.42).

Based on the results, the *p*-value is less than the 0.05 significance level, indicating that there are significant differences in preferences among the treatment methods. However, this test does not identify which specific methods differ from each other. In such cases, post-hoc analysis using the Wilcoxon signed-rank test is recommended, and significance should be determined using the Bonferroni correction. For example, if there are three pairwise comparisons, the adjusted significance level would be $0.05 / 3 \approx 0.017$.

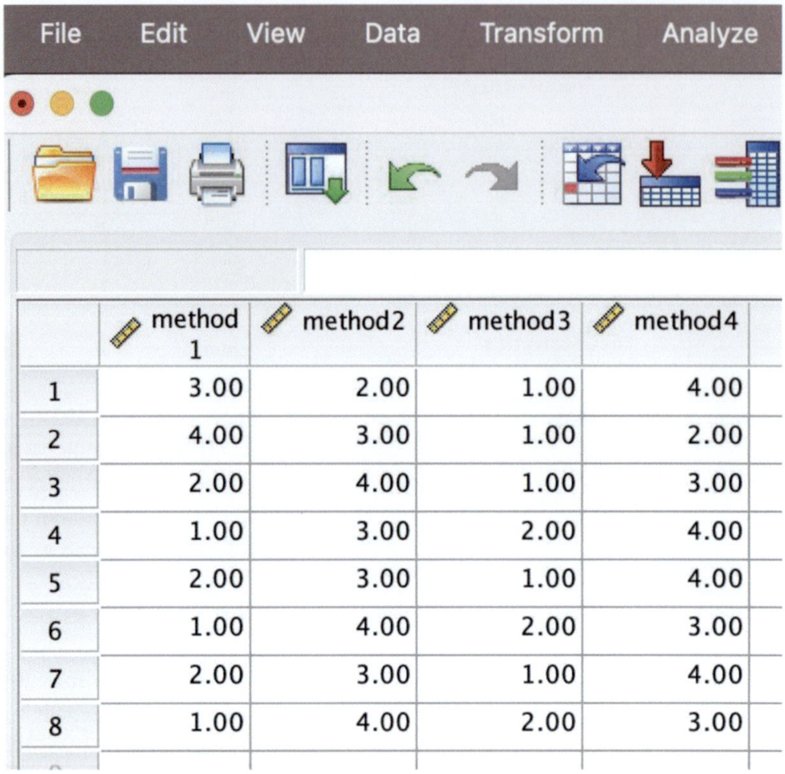

Fig. 13.38 Example dataset for performing Friedman two-way ANOVA in SPSS

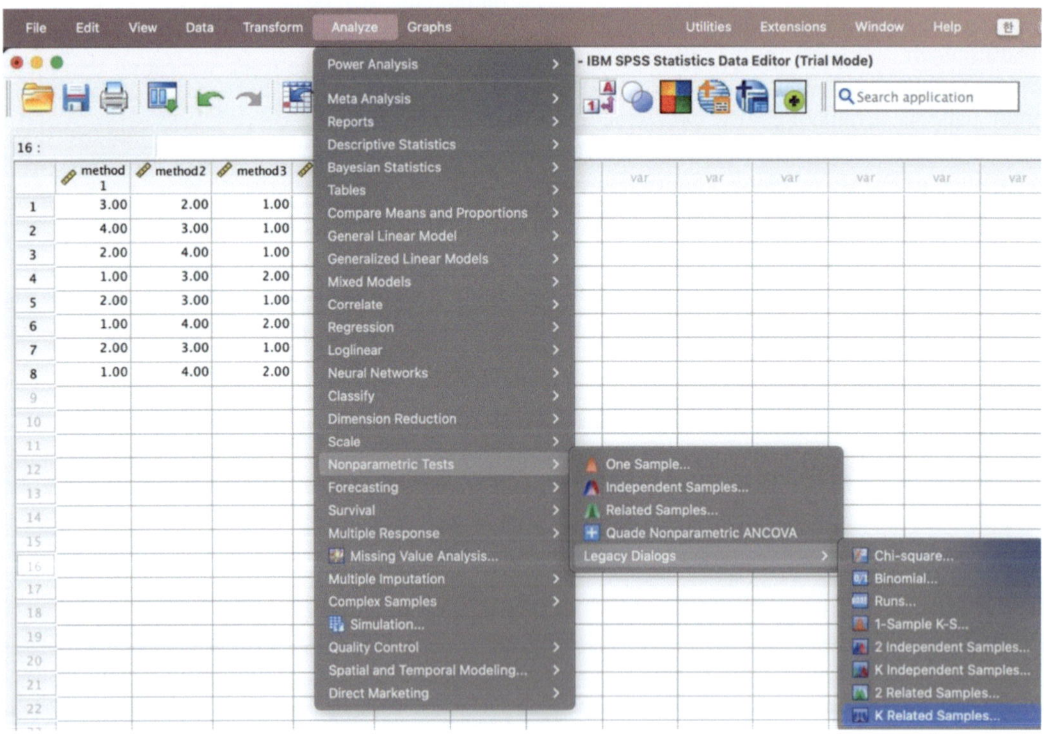

Fig. 13.39 Path to conduct Friedman two-way ANOVA

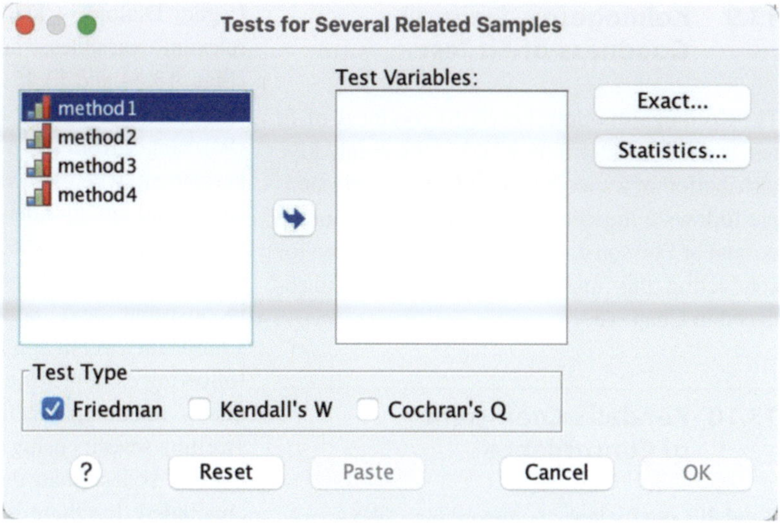

Fig. 13.40 K related samples dialog box used for conducting Friedman two-way ANOVA, Cochran's Q test

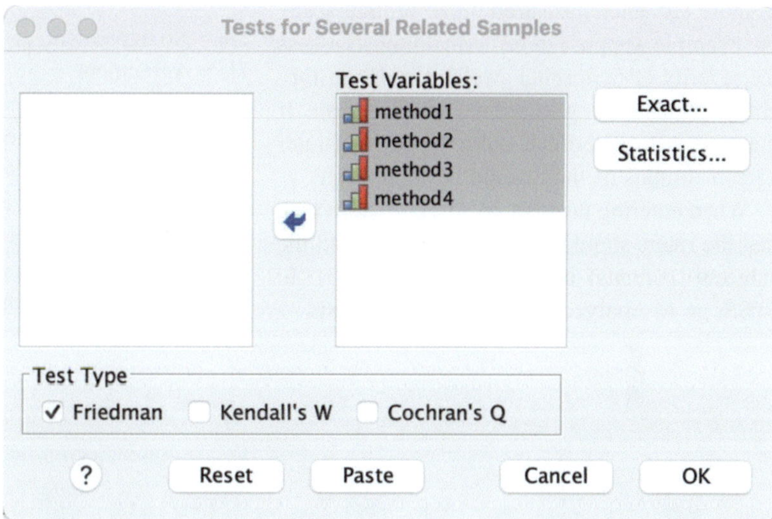

Fig. 13.41 All relevant variables moved into the "Test Variables" box in the K related samples dialog

Fig. 13.42 SPSS output screen displaying the results of the Friedman two-way ANOVA

Friedman Test

Ranks

	Mean Rank
method1	2.00
method2	3.25
method3	1.38
method4	3.38

Test Statistics[a]

N	8
Chi-Square	13.650
df	3
Asymp. Sig.	.003

a. Friedman Test

13.9 Kolmogorov–Smirnov Goodness-of-Fit Test

The Kolmogorov–Smirnov (K-S) goodness-of-fit test is used to determine whether the cumulative distribution of a specific variable in a single sample follows a theoretical distribution such as the normal or Poisson distribution. The procedure for conducting this analysis using SPSS is introduced in Chap. 15.

13.10 Kendall's Coefficient of Concordance

Kendall's coefficient of concordance (W) is used to evaluate the degree of agreement among three or more variables measured on an ordinal scale. For example, suppose three dermatologists assess the severity of periorbital swelling in 10 postoperative patients using an ordinal swelling scale. If the goal is to determine the level of inter-rater agreement, this method would be appropriate.

When entering the data, it is important to note that the raters should be placed in rows, and the subjects (patients) in columns (Fig. 13.43). In SPSS, go to Analyze → Nonparametric Tests → Legacy Dialogs → K Related Samples, select the relevant variables, and check Kendall's W (Figs. 13.44 and 13.45). Then click OK. The test statistic, Kendall's coefficient of concordance (W), ranges from 0 to 1. A value of 0 indicates no agreement, whereas a value of 1 indicates perfect agreement among raters. For example, if the significance level is 0.0053, which is less than 0.05, we reject the null hypothesis that the raters are inconsistent and conclude that there is a significant level of agreement among them. In the following example, four dermatologists independently rated eight patients on their periorbital swelling severity using an ordinal scale. Since the p-value is less than the significance level, it is concluded that there is a statistically significant agreement among the raters.

H_0 = No agreement
H_1 = Agreement

In the Test Type section, uncheck Friedman and check Kendall's W instead. Then, move all the variables from the left into the Test Variables box on the right (Fig. 13.46).

Click OK to run the analysis. The following output table will be generated (Fig. 13.47).

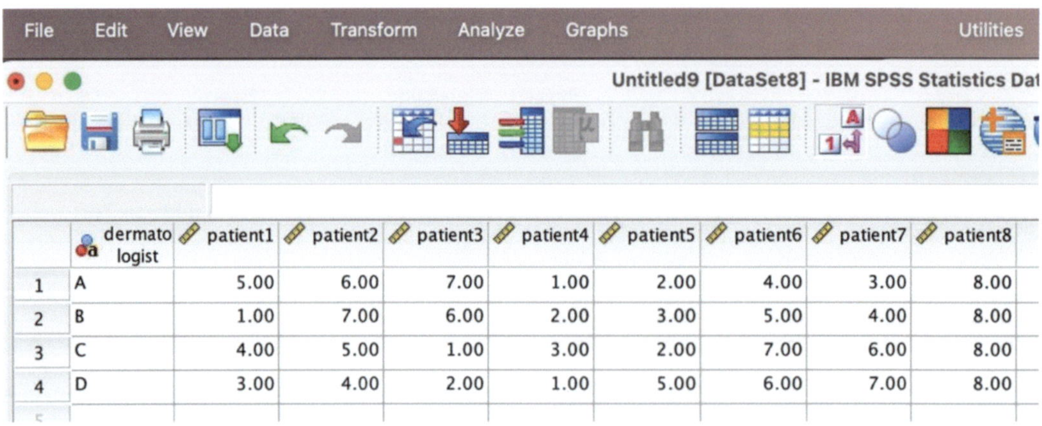

	dermatologist	patient1	patient2	patient3	patient4	patient5	patient6	patient7	patient8
1	A	5.00	6.00	7.00	1.00	2.00	4.00	3.00	8.00
2	B	1.00	7.00	6.00	2.00	3.00	5.00	4.00	8.00
3	C	4.00	5.00	1.00	3.00	2.00	7.00	6.00	8.00
4	D	3.00	4.00	2.00	1.00	5.00	6.00	7.00	8.00

Fig. 13.43 Example SPSS dataset for conducting Kendall's coefficient of concordance

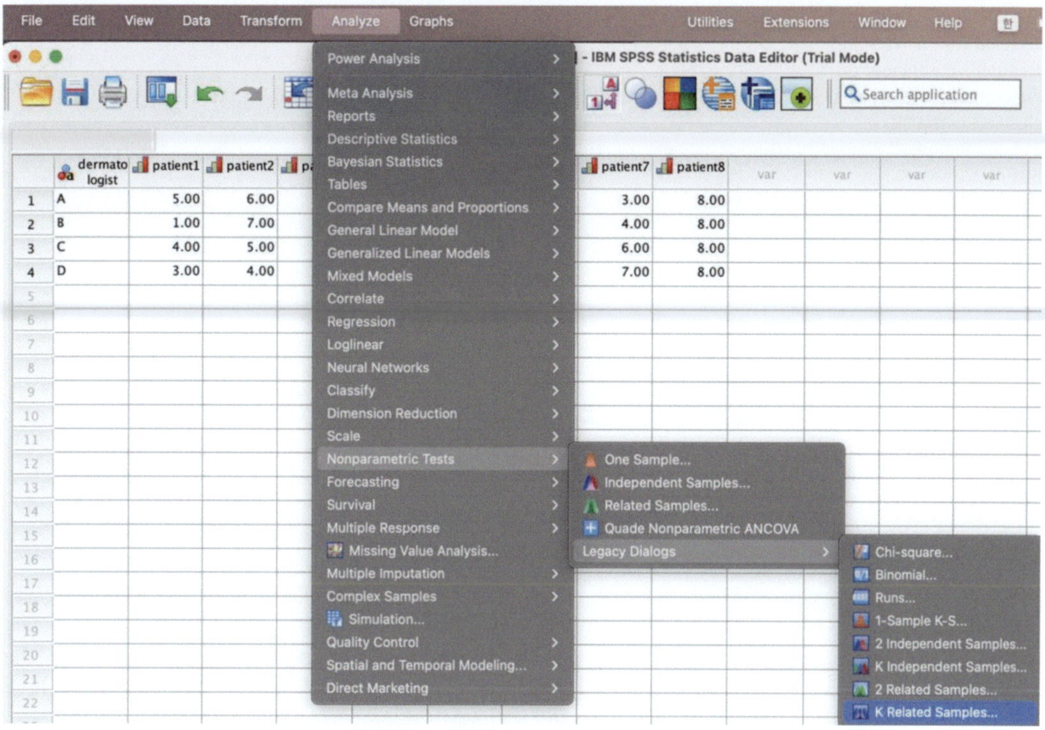

Fig. 13.44 Pathway to perform Kendall's coefficient of concordance in SPSS

Fig. 13.45 The "K Related Samples" dialog box in SPSS

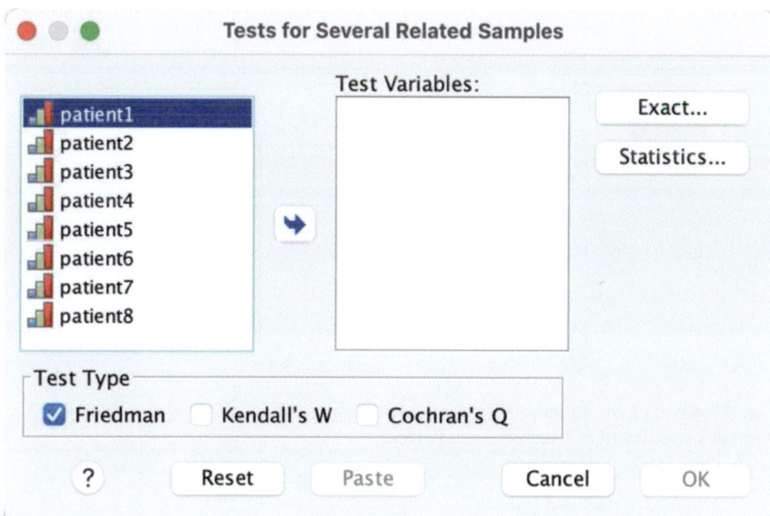

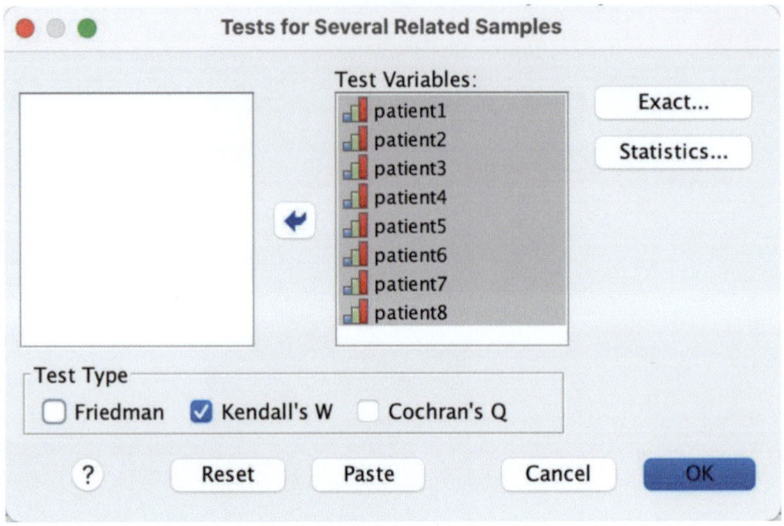

Fig. 13.46 Variables selected for analysis and Kendall's coefficient of concordance (W) option checked in the "K Related Samples" dialog box

Kendall's W Test

Ranks

	Mean Rank
patient1	3.25
patient2	5.50
patient3	4.00
patient4	1.75
patient5	3.00
patient6	5.50
patient7	5.00
patient8	8.00

Test Statistics

N	4
Kendall's W[a]	.622
Chi-Square	17.417
df	7
Asymp. Sig.	.015

a. Kendall's Coefficient of Concordance

Fig. 13.47 Output window displaying the results of Kendall's coefficient of concordance (W) test

13.11 McNemar Test

The McNemar test is used to analyze paired dichotomous data. For example, suppose we want to examine changes in patient attitudes toward the necessity of at-home LED therapy for skin rejuvenation before and after treatment in a sample of 20 cosmetic dermatology patients. The following is a hypothetical data table. In the table, 1 indicates a response that LED therapy at home is necessary, while 0 indicates a response that it is not necessary.

Patient attitudes toward at-home LED therapy before and after treatment (1 = necessary, 0 = not necessary)

Patient	Before treatment	After treatment
1	1	1
2	0	1
3	1	1
4	0	0
5	1	0
6	0	0
7	1	1
8	0	0
9	1	0
10	0	1
11	1	1
12	0	0
13	1	0
14	0	1
15	1	1
16	0	1
17	0	1
18	0	0
19	1	0
20	1	1

To determine whether there is a change in patient attitudes before and after treatment, the McNemar test should be used. For this dataset, the null hypothesis is stated as follows:

Null hypothesis (H_0): There is no change in patients' attitudes toward at-home LED therapy before and after treatment.

First, enter the data into SPSS as follows (Fig. 13.48).

In SPSS, go to Analyze → Nonparametric Tests → Legacy Dialogs → 2 Related Samples (Fig. 13.49).

Move the two variables to the box on the right, then uncheck Wilcoxon and check McNemar under Test Type (Figs. 13.50 and 13.51).

Click OK to run the test. The following output table will be generated (Fig. 13.52).

Since the *p*-value is greater than the 0.05 significance level, it is concluded that there is no significant change in patients' attitudes toward at-home LED therapy before and after treatment.

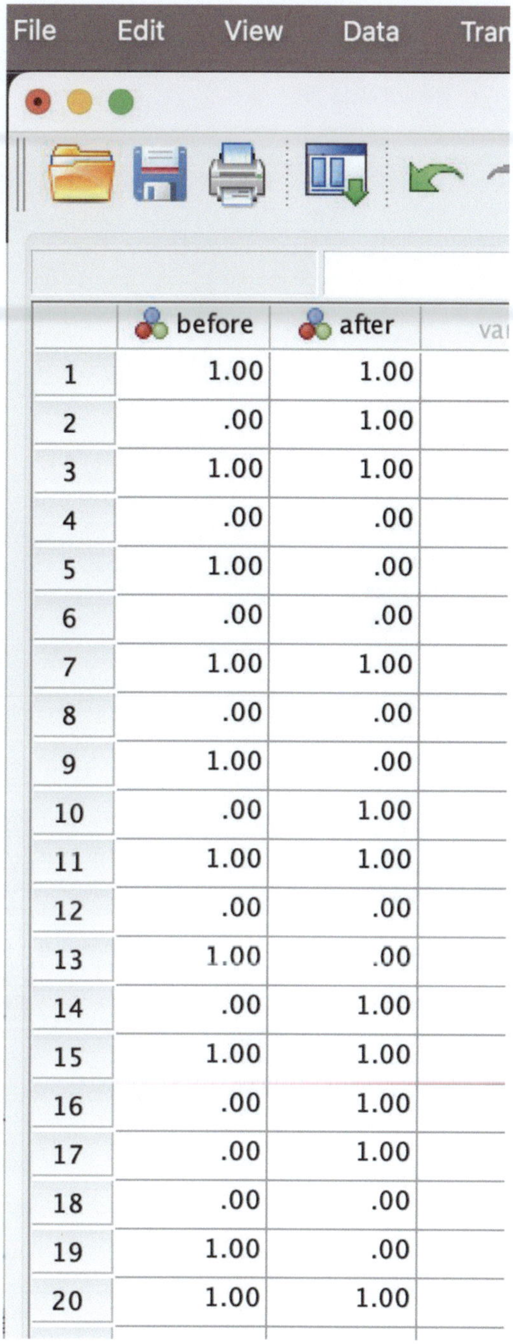

Fig. 13.48 Example dataset for conducting McNemar's test using SPSS

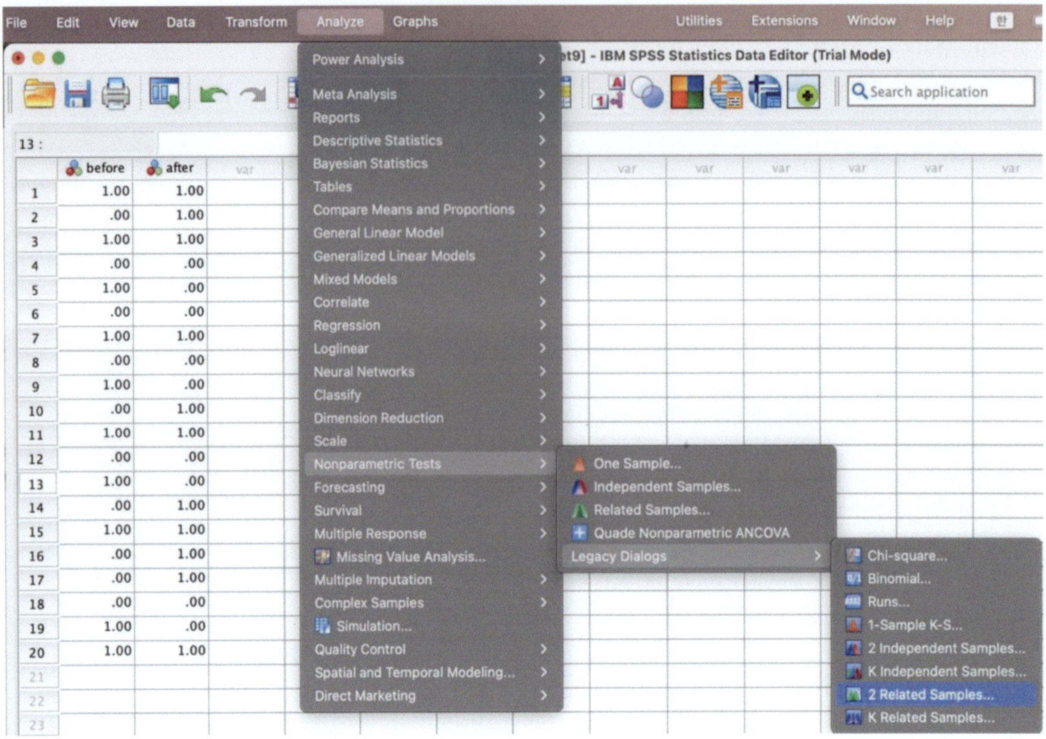

Fig. 13.49 Path to conduct McNemar's test in SPSS

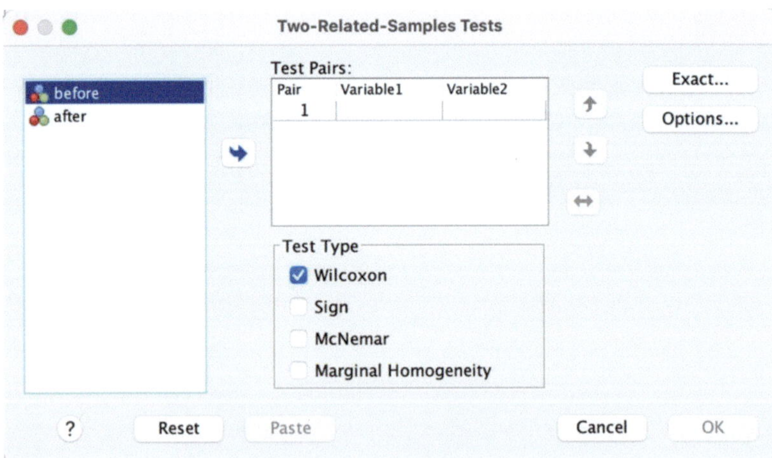

Fig. 13.50 Dialog box for McNemar's test after selecting Analyze → Nonparametric Tests → Legacy Dialogs → 2 Related Samples in SPSS

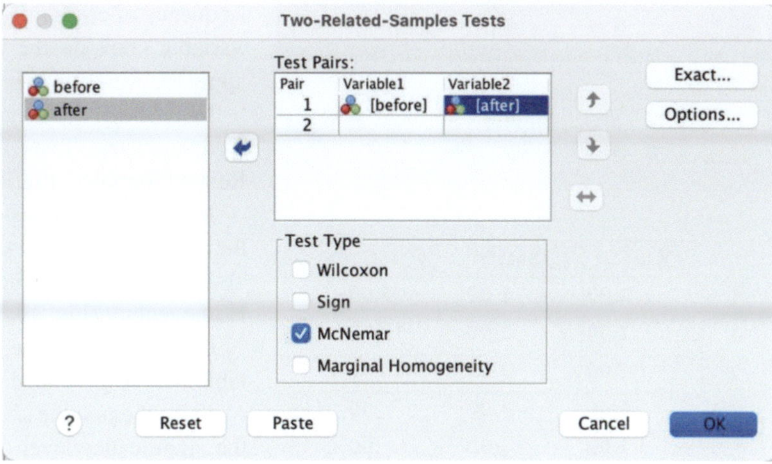

Fig. 13.51 Variables assigned for McNemar's Test, with the "McNemar" option selected in the two-related-samples dialog box in SPSS

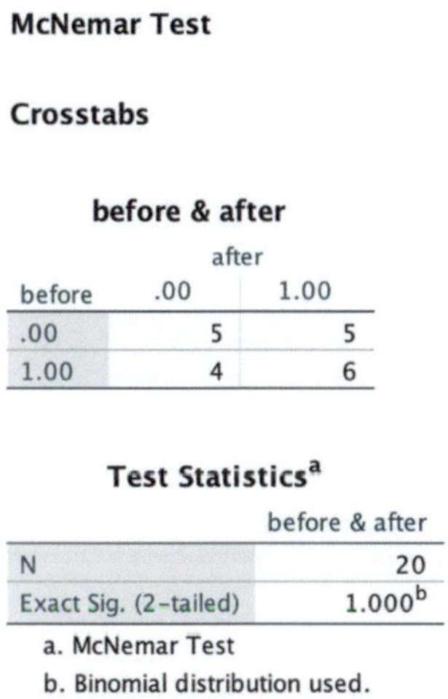

McNemar Test

Crosstabs

before & after

before	after .00	after 1.00
.00	5	5
1.00	4	6

Test Statistics[a]

	before & after
N	20
Exact Sig. (2-tailed)	1.000[b]

a. McNemar Test

b. Binomial distribution used.

Fig. 13.52 Output window showing the McNemar test results

13.12 Test of Marginal Homogeneity

The Marginal homogeneity test is used to analyze paired data when the level of measurement is ordinal. For example, suppose we assessed skin texture roughness in 178 patients before and after a fractional laser resurfacing procedure, using a 4-point ordinal scale adapted from a validated clinical grading system (e.g., 1 = smooth, 1+ = mildly rough, 2 = moderately rough, 3 = rough, 4 = very rough). The following is a hypothetical data matrix showing the distribution of skin texture scores before and after treatment:

Change in skin texture roughness (post-treatment vs. pre-treatment)

		Post-treatment				
		1	1+	2	3	4
Pre-treatment	1	8	12	10		
	1+	5	7	14		
	2		2	36	10	1
	3		1	3	13	7
	4			1	3	45

The researcher is interested in determining whether there is a change in skin texture grade before and after treatment. Accordingly, the hypotheses are set as follows:

Null hypothesis (H_0): There is no difference in skin texture roughness between pre- and post-treatment.

Alternative hypothesis (H_1): There is a difference in skin texture roughness between pre- and post-treatment.

Now, open SPSS and enter the data accordingly (Fig. 13.53).

To specify weighted cases in SPSS, follow these steps. Go to Data → Weight Cases (Fig. 13.54).

In the dialog box, select "Weight cases by" (Fig. 13.55). Move the variable representing the

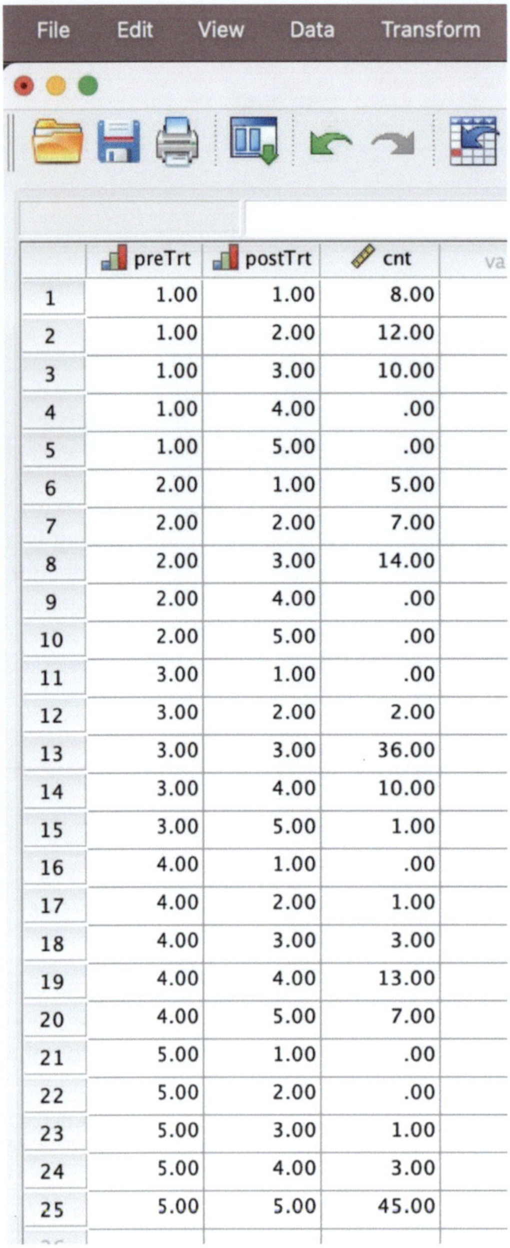

	preTrt	postTrt	cnt
1	1.00	1.00	8.00
2	1.00	2.00	12.00
3	1.00	3.00	10.00
4	1.00	4.00	.00
5	1.00	5.00	.00
6	2.00	1.00	5.00
7	2.00	2.00	7.00
8	2.00	3.00	14.00
9	2.00	4.00	.00
10	2.00	5.00	.00
11	3.00	1.00	.00
12	3.00	2.00	2.00
13	3.00	3.00	36.00
14	3.00	4.00	10.00
15	3.00	5.00	1.00
16	4.00	1.00	.00
17	4.00	2.00	1.00
18	4.00	3.00	3.00
19	4.00	4.00	13.00
20	4.00	5.00	7.00
21	5.00	1.00	.00
22	5.00	2.00	.00
23	5.00	3.00	1.00
24	5.00	4.00	3.00
25	5.00	5.00	45.00

Fig. 13.53 Example SPSS dataset for conducting the test of marginal homogeneity

frequency of cases (e.g., cnt) into the "Frequency Variable" box on the right. Then, click OK to apply the weighting (Fig. 13.56).

In SPSS, navigate to: Analyze → Nonparametric Tests → Legacy Dialogs → 2 Related Samples (Fig. 13.57).

Move the variables for preTrt and postTrt to the box on the right (Fig. 13.58). Then, under Test Type, uncheck Wilcoxon and check Marginal Homogeneity (Fig. 13.59).

Click OK to run the test. The following output table will be generated (Fig. 13.60).

Since the p-value is 0.000, which is well below the significance level of 0.05, the null hypothesis—that skin texture roughness remains unchanged before and after treatment—is rejected. Given that higher scores indicate rougher skin texture, the results suggest that skin texture worsened after fractional laser treatment compared to the pre-treatment condition.

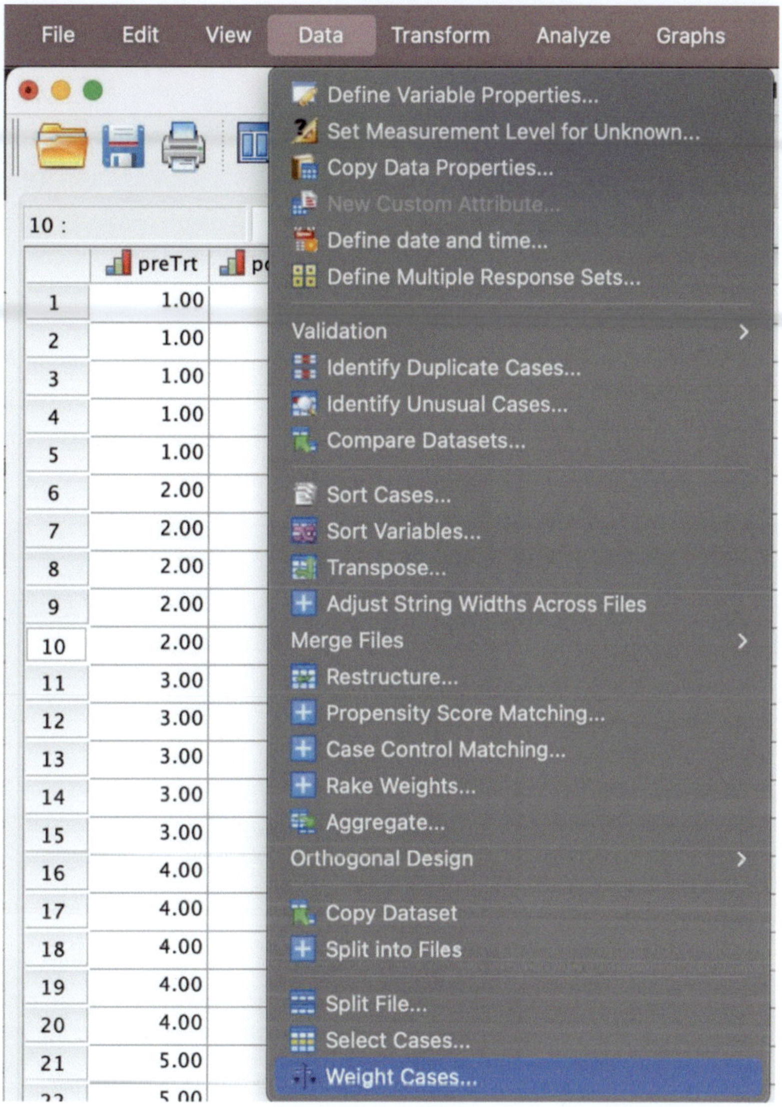

Fig. 13.54 Path to specify weighted cases: Data → Weight Cases

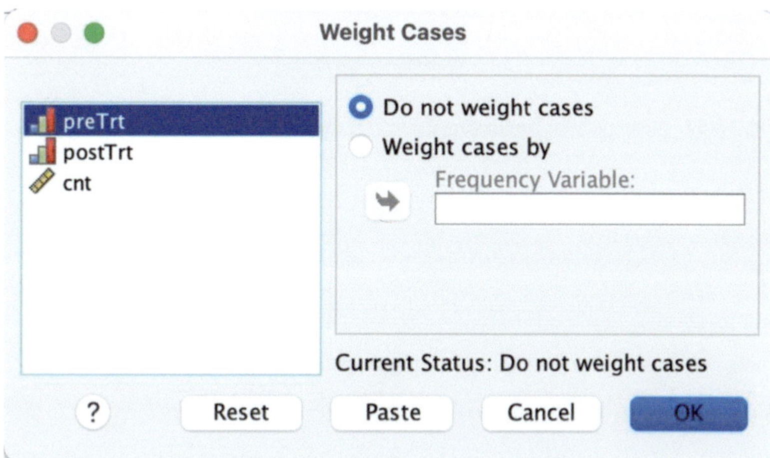

Fig. 13.55 Dialog box displayed after selecting "Weight Cases" in SPSS

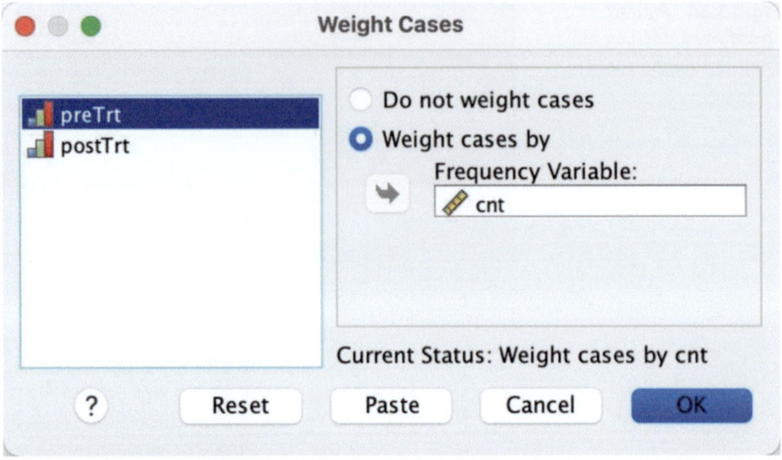

Fig. 13.56 Specifying a variable under "Weight cases by" in the weight cases dialog box in SPSS

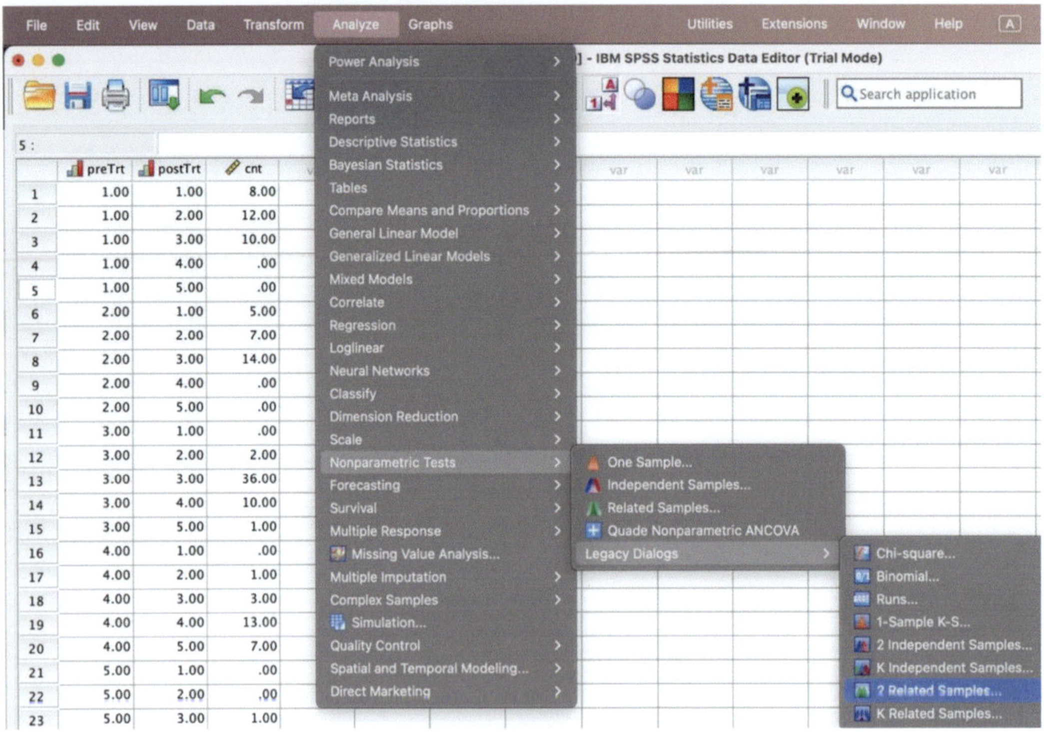

Fig. 13.57 Menu path for conducting the test of marginal homogeneity in SPSS

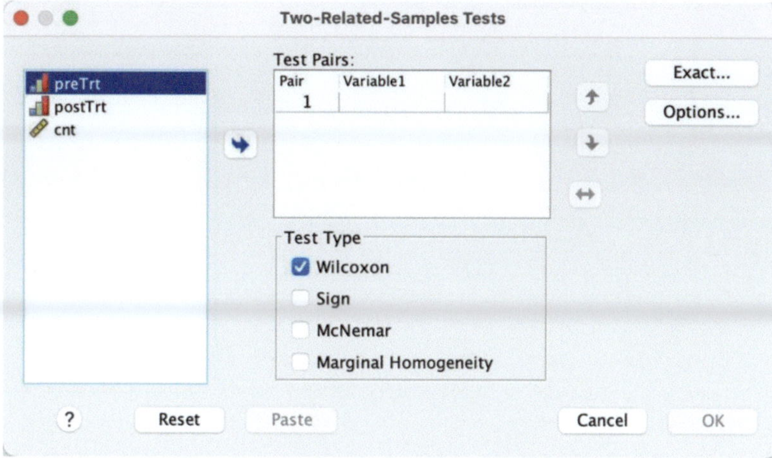

Fig. 13.58 Dialog box displayed after selecting "2 Related Samples" in SPSS

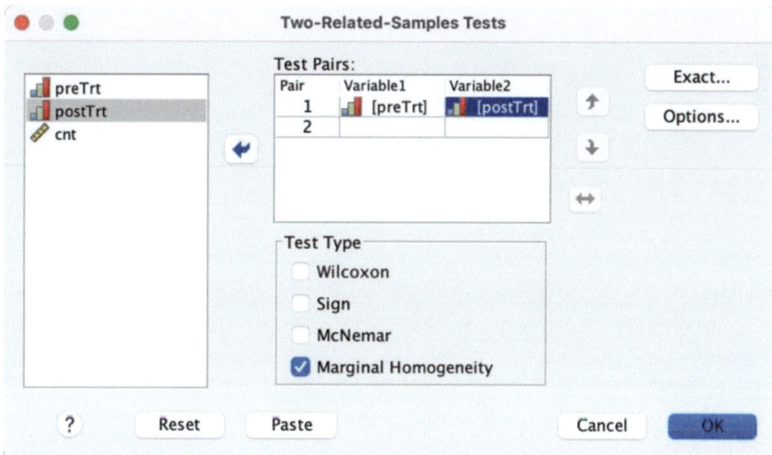

Fig. 13.59 SPSS dialog box for "2 Related Samples" after moving variables and selecting the "Marginal Homogeneity" test option

Marginal Homogeneity Test

	preTrt & postTrt
Distinct Values	5
Off-Diagonal Cases	69
Observed MH Statistic	163.000
Mean MH Statistic	187.000
Std. Deviation of MH Statistic	5.196
Std. MH Statistic	-4.619
Asymp. Sig. (2-tailed)	<.001

Fig. 13.60 SPSS output window displaying the results of the marginal homogeneity test

14 Multivariate Analysis

14.1 Partial Correlation

The Pearson product-moment correlation coefficient (r) is a commonly used statistic to indicate the relationship between two variables, X and Y. However, the r value has limitations, as it does not account for the influence of other variables that may affect the relationship. For example, suppose the correlation coefficient between patient age and hospital stay duration is 0.70. One might interpret this as older patients having longer hospital stays. However, this relationship could be more strongly influenced by the patient's functional status rather than age alone. To examine the pure relationship between age and hospital stay while controlling for functional status, we use a partial correlation coefficient.

Partial correlation analysis evaluates the relationship between two variables (X and Y) while statistically removing the influence of a third variable (Z):

1. Zero-order partial correlation: Measures the raw correlation between X and Y (i.e., standard Pearson correlation).
2. First-order partial correlation: Measures the correlation between X and Y controlling for one variable Z; denoted as $r_{xy.z}$.
3. Second-order partial correlation: Measures the correlation between X and Y controlling for two variables, Z_1 and Z_2; denoted as rxy.z1z2.

Partial correlation is a powerful tool for estimating the potential contribution of extraneous variables that may affect the observed relationship between two main variables.

14.2 Multiple Regression

Multiple regression analysis is used for a variety of purposes. First, to obtain a suitable equation that fits the available data. Second, to make inferences about the population that the sample data represent. In this case, the focus is more on the characteristics of the population than on the specific features of the sample. Third, to analyze data from carefully designed and conducted experiments, where the main interest lies not in the raw values themselves but in the relationships between variables.

Assumptions for Regression Inference:

1. The relationship between x and y in the population must be linear. That is, if we assume there is a mean y for each value of x, those means must lie on a straight line. This line can

K.-H. Yi, *Statistical Research Methods for Dermatologists and Plastic Surgeons*,
https://doi.org/10.1007/978-981-95-5668-7_14

be expressed as A + Bx, where A and B are fixed constants. For example, if $x = 1, 2, 3, \ldots$, the corresponding means of y should fall on a straight line—this is called the population regression line.

2. The variance of y for each value of x should be constant across the range of x values. This constant variance, or homoscedasticity, is often denoted as σ^2 (the variance of y relative to the regression line), and σ is the standard deviation.
3. For each x, the distribution of y-values should be approximately normal.
4. The observations of y must be independent of one another.

When there is only one independent and one dependent variable, correlation and regression yield similar insights, though regression explicitly defines one variable as the predictor (independent) and the other as the outcome (dependent). It's also important to note that correlation does not imply causation. In multiple regression, where several independent variables are used, the values of the regression coefficients can change each time a new variable is added or removed from the model. In a regression model, the regression coefficients are estimated by considering the influence of all independent variables simultaneously. For this reason, there are various methods of entering variables into the model, such as *forward selection*, *backward elimination*, *stepwise selection*, and *enter method*. If a researcher wants to examine the pure relationship between a single independent variable and the dependent variable—controlling for the effects of other variables—they should refer to the partial correlation coefficient.

When conducting multiple regression analysis using statistical software, it is often observed that, although several independent variables may appear related to the dependent variable in simple regression, only some of them are ultimately selected for inclusion in the final multiple regression model. There are various procedures for selecting variables from a large pool of potentially related predictors. Among the most commonly used are forward selection, backward elimination, and stepwise selection.

Forward selection begins by identifying the independent variable with the strongest explanatory power. Variables are added to the model one at a time, only if they significantly improve the model's explanatory ability. As selection progresses, the number of variables in the model increases.

Backward elimination starts with a full model containing all candidate variables. It then removes the variable with the least explanatory power, one at a time, as long as its removal does not significantly reduce the model's fit. As the elimination proceeds, fewer variables remain in the model.

Stepwise selection is a hybrid method that combines forward selection and backward elimination. The first step selects a variable using the forward method. After inclusion, the model checks whether removing that variable (using the backward method) significantly reduces explanatory power. If so, it is retained; otherwise, it is removed. This process is repeated iteratively, alternating between inclusion and exclusion at each stage.

These three methods do not always yield the same final regression equation. Among them, stepwise selection is the most widely used approach in practice (Bauer et al. 1991; Gowland 1984).

Multiple regression analysis is a statistical technique used to examine the relationship between one dependent variable and two or more independent variables. It is an extension of simple linear regression, where the predicted value of the dependent variable is denoted as $\hat{Y}$, and the predictor variables as X. The regression equation takes the form $\hat{Y} = a + bX$.

The primary objective of multiple regression analysis is to build a regression equation that calculates the predicted value $\hat{Y}$ based on multiple independent variables.

Regression Equation

The general form of a multiple regression equation is

$$\hat{Y} = a + b_1X_1 + b_2X_2 + b_3X_3 + \ldots + d_kX_k$$

Here, a is the regression constant (intercept) and $b_1, b_2, \ldots, b_k$ are the regression coefficients for each independent variable (X_1, X_2, …, X_k). k indicates the number of independent variables included in the model. Just like simple linear regression, multiple regression is based on the least squares method.

For example, if a person is 30 years old (AGE), weighs 60 kg (WT), has a systolic blood pressure (SBP) of 100 mmHg, and consumes 40 g of dietary fat per day (DIET), the predicted total cholesterol level would be

$$\hat{Y} = -80.0 + 1.64(\text{AGE}) + 0.6(\text{WT}) + 0.7(\text{SBP}) + 2.42(\text{DIET})$$

$$= -80.0 + 1.64(30) + 0.6(60) + 0.7(100) + 2.42(40) = 172\,\text{mg/dL}$$

Scatter plots are used to analyze residuals (also referred to as error terms) by displaying data points along the Y-axis and X-axis to examine predicted values. A residual scatter plot makes it easy to detect outliers. When the regression equation fits the data well in a linear fashion, the residuals tend to be very small. The Durbin–Watson statistic is used to assess whether autocorrelation exists among the residuals. If the Durbin–Watson value is close to 2, it suggests there is no correlation between the residuals, meaning that the assumption of independence among error terms in the regression model is satisfied. Conversely, if the Durbin–Watson value is close to 0 or 4, it indicates a correlation among residuals, suggesting that the regression model may be inappropriate for the data.

Standardized Regression Coefficients

Researchers often want to understand the relative importance of independent variables included in a regression equation. However, since each variable may have different units of measurement, it is not meaningful to directly compare their unstandardized coefficients (B values). To enable such comparisons, each variable is converted into its standardized form (Z-scores), and the resulting coefficient is referred to as β (beta), or the standardized regression coefficient. In regression analysis, the β coefficient represents the regression weight when all variables are standardized to have a standard deviation of 1. Because β values are free from the influence of differing units and variances, they allow for direct comparison of the relative effect of each independent variable within the model. The standardized regression coefficient β can thus be interpreted as the relative weight that each independent variable has on the predicted value $\hat{Y}$.

In the regression output, the t-value is used to test the null hypothesis that there is no association between the independent and dependent variables—in other words, that the regression coefficient is equal to zero. If the p-value corresponding to the t-test is less than 0.05 or 0.01, the variable is considered to make a statistically significant contribution to explaining the dependent variable.

Multicollinearity

One of the fundamental assumptions of regression analysis is that the independent variables should not be highly correlated with each other. When a significant correlation exists between two or more independent variables in a regression model, this condition is referred to as multicollinearity. If the tolerance value for the parameter estimate of a certain variable is close to 0, it indicates a high correlation with the variables already included in the regression model; if it is close to 1, it indicates little to no correlation.

Multiple Correlation and Coefficient of Determination

The overall correlation coefficient between the dependent variable Y and the set of independent variables is referred to as the multiple correlation coefficient. The value of the multiple correlation coefficient R lies between 0 and 1 ($0 \leq R \leq 1$). R represents the correlation between the observed value Y and the predicted value $\hat{Y}$. In the case of simple linear regression ($Y = a + bX_1$), the value of R is equivalent to the Pearson correlation coefficient. However, because the R value reflects the cumulative correlation from multiple variables, its interpretation can often be ambiguous. Therefore, to explain the relationship between the dependent variable Y and a set of independent variables, the coefficient of determination (R^2) is typically used. R^2 represents the proportion of the total variance in the dependent variable Y that can be explained by the set of independent variables. If the value of R^2 is high, it indicates a predictive model with strong explanatory power (i.e., high correlation). For example, if the coefficient of determination is found to be 0.454, it can be interpreted as the regression equation explaining approximately 45% of the variance in the dependent variable Y. Conversely, $1-R^2$ represents the portion of variance that cannot be explained by the regression model, including the independent variables. In multiple regression analysis, the adjusted coefficient of determination (adjusted R^2) is preferred over R^2 for evaluating the explanatory power of the model. This is because the value of R^2 tends to increase automatically as the number of independent variables increases. The adjusted R^2 takes into account the degrees of freedom (i.e., the number of independent variables included in the model) and provides a more accurate estimate of the model's explanatory power. When presenting the results of regression analysis in a table, the adjusted R^2 should be reported rather than the unadjusted R^2.

Analysis of Variance

In regression analysis, the appropriateness of the regression model is assessed using analysis of variance (ANOVA). ANOVA divides the total variance of the data into two parts: the variance that is explained by the regression model and the residual error (the portion not explained by the model). The degrees of freedom for the explained portion correspond to the number of independent variables included in the regression model, while the degrees of freedom for the total variance are equal to the number of total observations minus one. The null hypothesis (H_0) in ANOVA states that the slope of the population regression line is zero. If the p-value is less than 0.05 or 0.01, we reject the null hypothesis and conclude that the regression model is statistically significant—that is, the model is appropriate for explaining the relationship.

Standard Error of the Estimate

In many regression analysis programs, in addition to the coefficient of determination (R^2), the standard error of the estimate (SEE)—which is the standard deviation of the residuals—is also provided to indicate the accuracy of prediction. Residuals represent the difference between the actual observed values (y) and the predicted values obtained from the regression equation. A smaller SEE implies greater accuracy of the model.

Stepwise Multiple Regression

Multiple regression analysis is performed by entering independent variables into a regression equation. For example, consider a model analyzing how four independent variables influence cholesterol levels, the dependent variable. If the model explains 56% of the variance in cholesterol, this does not imply that each independent variable contributes equally to that explained variance. Stepwise multiple regression is advantageous in that it minimizes the number of predictors included in the model while maximizing the accuracy of prediction.

This method proceeds in sequential steps to assess the contribution of each independent variable. Forward selection starts by entering the single independent variable (X_1) that has the highest correlation with the dependent variable into the regression equation: $\hat{Y} = a + b_1X_1$. Next, among the remaining variables, the one that has the highest partial correlation with the dependent variable, controlling for X_1, is added: $\hat{Y} = a + b_1X_1 + b_2X_2$.

Backward elimination, in contrast, begins with all variables included in the model. Through partial correlation analysis, it sequentially removes the variable that contributes the least (i.e., has the smallest partial correlation with the dependent variable). Although backward elimination is used less frequently than forward selection, it can be helpful when aiming to simplify a complex model (Jones et al. 2003; Teseng and Chow 2000).

Dummy Variable

While regression analysis is typically used when independent variables are continuous and quantitative, nominal or categorical variables—such as sex, occupation, education level, race, behavioral traits, or smoker vs. non-smoker—are also often included as independent variables. In such cases, these qualitative nominal variables are converted into numerical form using *dummy coding*. For example, if we code the variable *sex* as male = 0 and female = 1, a regression equation predicting cholesterol levels by sex could be:

$$\hat{Y} = 220 - 27.5X$$

For females, $\hat{Y} = 220–27.5(1) = 194.5$. For males, $\hat{Y} = 220–27.5(0) = 220$. When a categorical variable has more than two categories (n categories), the number of dummy variables needed is $n - 1$. For instance, if the category "school grade" has 4 levels, then 3 dummy variables (X_1, X_2, X_3) are required. After coding, a multiple regression model might look like $\hat{Y} = 85–55X_1–25X_2–15X_3$. By inserting the corresponding values for each grade level into this equation, the predicted values for each grade can be calculated. The estimated values are: 30 for 1st grade, 60 for 2nd grade, 70 for 3rd grade, and 85 for 4th grade.

	X_1	X_2	X_3	
1st grade	1	0	0	$\hat{Y} = 85–55(1)–25(0)–15(0) = 30$
2nd grade	0	1	0	$\hat{Y} = 85–55(0)–25(1)–15(0) = 60$
3rd grade	0	0	1	$\hat{Y} = 85–55(0)–25(0)–15(1) = 70$
4th grade	0	0	0	$\hat{Y} = 85–55(0)–25(0)–15(0) = 85$

Because many variables of clinical interest are measured as nominal variables, the use of dummy variables is useful when analyzing clinical data using regression analysis methods. For example, let us consider a hypothetical example from the field of cosmetic dermatology. Suppose we aim to predict the cervicocephalic angle, which refers to the angle between the head and cervical spine and is often used to evaluate postural alignment in procedures involving the neck or jawline. In this example, the independent variables include age, height, weight, and sex, while the dependent variable is the cervicocephalic angle. Among the independent variables, age, height, and weight are continuous variables, whereas sex is a nominal variable with two categories (male and female). A dummy variable can be created for sex, coding male as 0 and female as 1. In this hypothetical dataset, stepwise multiple regression analysis was conducted, and sex was selected as the only independent variable in the final model. The resulting regression equation is as follows:

$$\text{Cervicocephalic angle} = 43.6 - 5.7 \times \text{Sex}\left(\text{Sex} : \text{male} = 0, \text{female} = 1\right)$$

From this result, it can be interpreted that female participants tend to exhibit a smaller cervicocephalic angle compared to male participants. When creating dummy variables in SPSS, go to the menu and click Transform → Recode into Different Variables. Move the variable you wish to recode into the Input Variable → Output Variable box. In the Name field for the output variable, assign a new name that clearly reflects the meaning of the dummy variable. After clicking Change, the selected variable will appear in the list as "variable → new dummy variable." Next, click Old and New Values to proceed with recoding. For example, if the original variable for sex was coded as 1 for male and 2 for female, you may recode it such that female = 1 and male = 0, to construct a binary dummy variable.

Using the previously described hypothetical study on cervicocephalic angle(cva) as an example, let us illustrate how to create a dummy variable in SPSS. In SPSS, the data would be entered as shown in Fig. 14.1.

If, for example, you want to name the dummy variable for sex as "Sex_Dummy," you can proceed as shown in Fig. 14.2.

Click on the variable "Sex" to move it to the right. In the Output Variable field, type in Sex_Dummy, and then click Change (Fig. 14.3).

Click on Old and New Values (Fig. 14.4). In the Old Value field, enter 2 (the original value representing female), and in the New Value field, enter 1 (the recoded value for female) (Fig. 14.5). Then click Add to apply this recoding.

The following screen will appear.

To recode the value 1 to 0 for the gender variable, enter 1 in the Old Value field and 0 in the New Value field, then click Add (Fig. 14.6).

Click Continue (Fig. 14.7).

In the Data View screen, a new variable named Sex_Dummy appears, and you can see that the values in the original Gender variable have been recoded—2 has been changed to 1, and 1 has been changed to 0 (Fig. 14.8).

Using this file, you can perform a multiple regression analysis by including the dummy variable Sex_Dummy instead of the originals sex variable as one of the independent variables. In SPSS, go to Analyze → Regression → Linear to proceed with the regression analysis using the dummy variable (Fig. 14.9).

Move the cva variable into the Dependent field and the height, weight, age, and Sex_Dummy variables into the Independent(s) field. Then click OK.

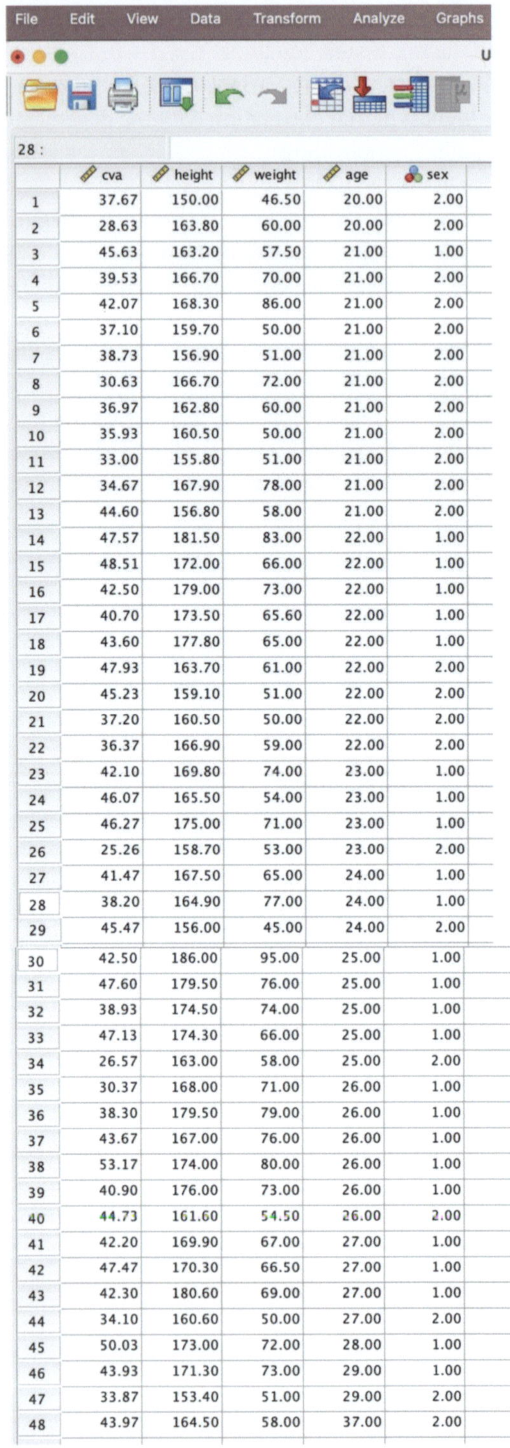

	cva	height	weight	age	sex
1	37.67	150.00	46.50	20.00	2.00
2	28.63	163.80	60.00	20.00	2.00
3	45.63	163.20	57.50	21.00	1.00
4	39.53	166.70	70.00	21.00	2.00
5	42.07	168.30	86.00	21.00	2.00
6	37.10	159.70	50.00	21.00	2.00
7	38.73	156.90	51.00	21.00	2.00
8	30.63	166.70	72.00	21.00	2.00
9	36.97	162.80	60.00	21.00	2.00
10	35.93	160.50	50.00	21.00	2.00
11	33.00	155.80	51.00	21.00	2.00
12	34.67	167.90	78.00	21.00	2.00
13	44.60	156.80	58.00	21.00	2.00
14	47.57	181.50	83.00	22.00	1.00
15	48.51	172.00	66.00	22.00	1.00
16	42.50	179.00	73.00	22.00	1.00
17	40.70	173.50	65.60	22.00	1.00
18	43.60	177.80	65.00	22.00	1.00
19	47.93	163.70	61.00	22.00	2.00
20	45.23	159.10	51.00	22.00	2.00
21	37.20	160.50	50.00	22.00	2.00
22	36.37	166.90	59.00	22.00	2.00
23	42.10	169.80	74.00	23.00	1.00
24	46.07	165.50	54.00	23.00	1.00
25	46.27	175.00	71.00	23.00	1.00
26	25.26	158.70	53.00	23.00	2.00
27	41.47	167.50	65.00	24.00	1.00
28	38.20	164.90	77.00	24.00	1.00
29	45.47	156.00	45.00	24.00	2.00
30	42.50	186.00	95.00	25.00	1.00
31	47.60	179.50	76.00	25.00	1.00
32	38.93	174.50	74.00	25.00	1.00
33	47.13	174.30	66.00	25.00	1.00
34	26.57	163.00	58.00	25.00	2.00
35	30.37	168.00	71.00	26.00	1.00
36	38.30	179.50	79.00	26.00	1.00
37	43.67	167.00	76.00	26.00	1.00
38	53.17	174.00	80.00	26.00	1.00
39	40.90	176.00	73.00	26.00	1.00
40	44.73	161.60	54.50	26.00	2.00
41	42.20	169.90	67.00	27.00	1.00
42	47.47	170.30	66.50	27.00	1.00
43	42.30	180.60	69.00	27.00	1.00
44	34.10	160.60	50.00	27.00	2.00
45	50.03	173.00	72.00	28.00	1.00
46	43.93	171.30	73.00	29.00	1.00
47	33.87	153.40	51.00	29.00	2.00
48	43.97	164.50	58.00	37.00	2.00

Fig. 14.1 Example dataset for regression analysis and dummy variable creation

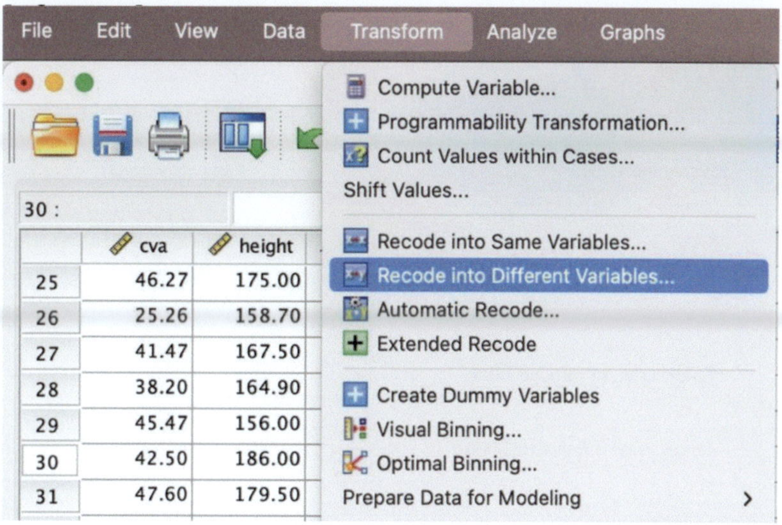

Fig. 14.2 Navigating to recoding: Transform → Recode into Different Variables in SPSS

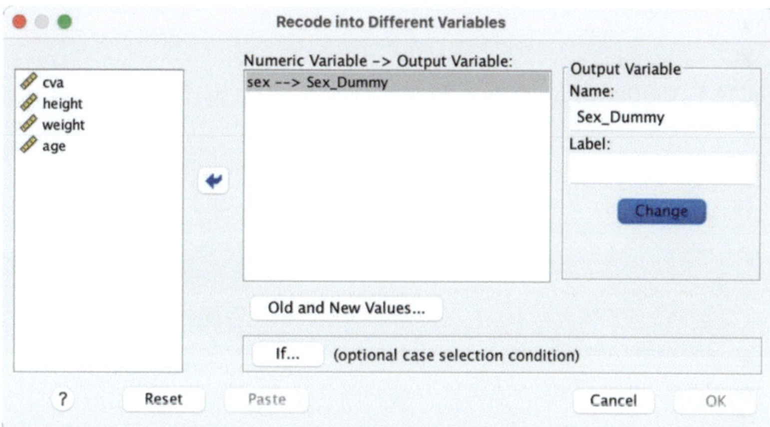

Fig. 14.3 Creating a dummy variable by specifying a new variable name in the Recode into Different Variables dialog box

The following results will be generated (Fig. 14.10):

In cases where a categorical variable like smoking status has three categories (e.g., 1 = smoker, 2 = non-smoker, 3 = former smoker), you only need to create two dummy variables (X_1 and X_2) to include them in a regression model. And in the case of smoking, it is coded as $X_1 \rightarrow 0$, $X_2 \rightarrow 0$; for non-smoking, it is coded as $X_1 \rightarrow 1$, $X_2 \rightarrow 0$; and for former smoking, it is coded as $X_1 \rightarrow 0$, $X_2 \rightarrow 1$, so that these can be included in the regression model.

Example

Smoking = 1 $X1 \rightarrow 0, X2 \rightarrow 0$

Non-smoking = 1 $X1 \rightarrow 1, X2 \rightarrow 0$

Former smoking = 1 $X1 \rightarrow 0, X2 \rightarrow 1$

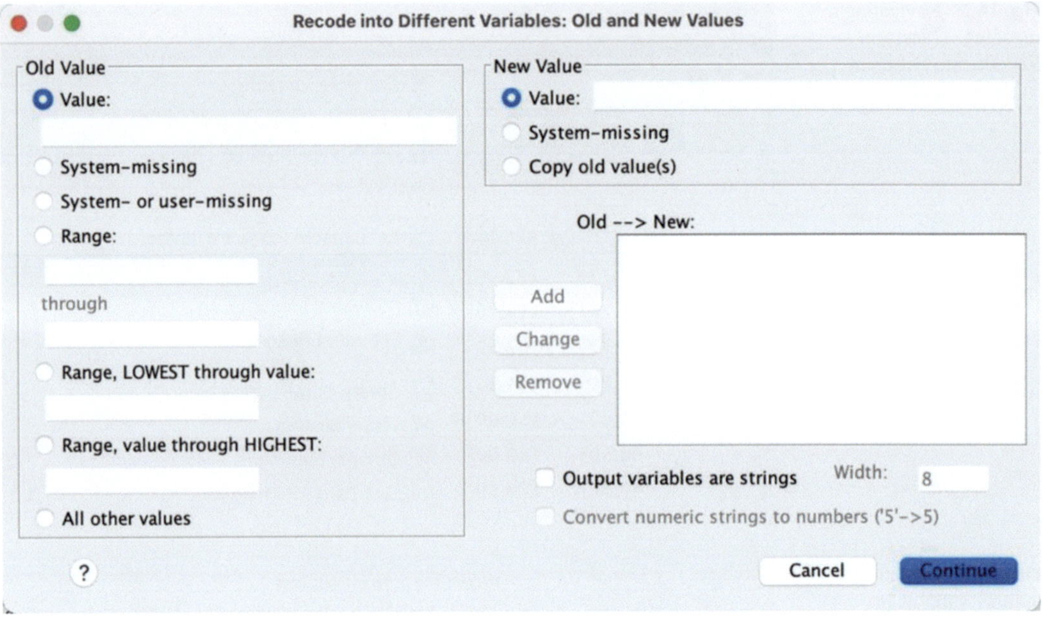

Fig. 14.4 The Old and New Values dialog box used to assign specific values for recoding dummy variables

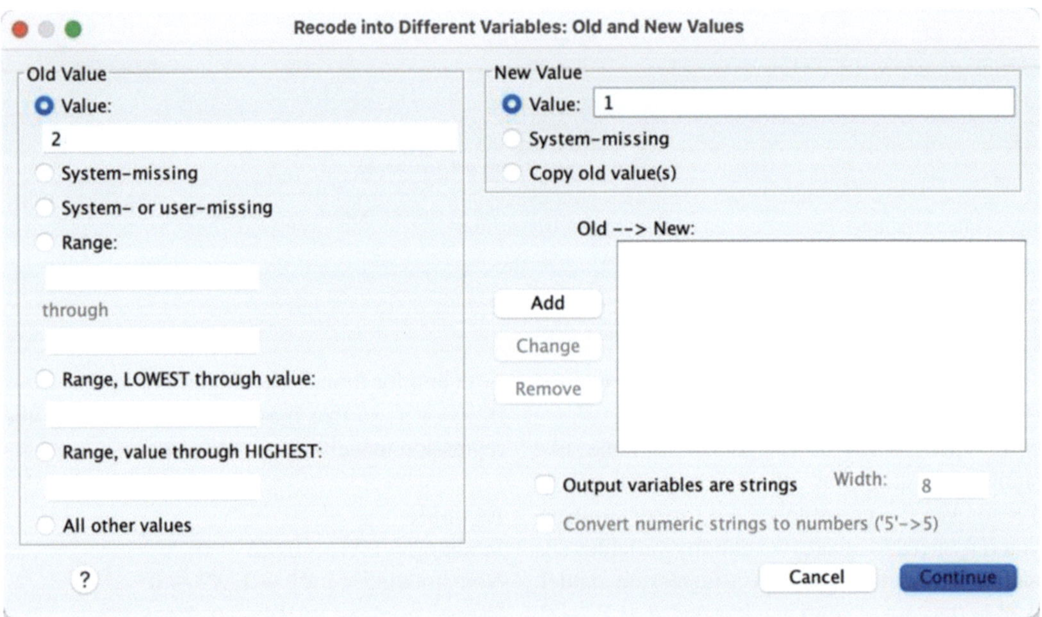

Fig. 14.5 Assigning new values to create dummy variables in the Old and New Values dialog box

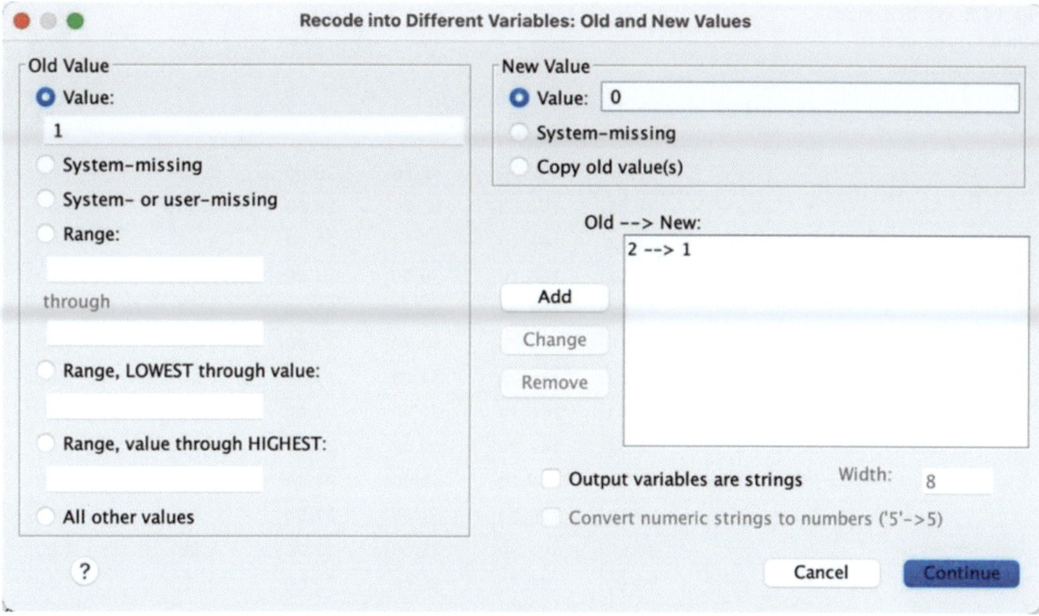

Fig. 14.6 New value assignment confirmed and added to the transformation rule list

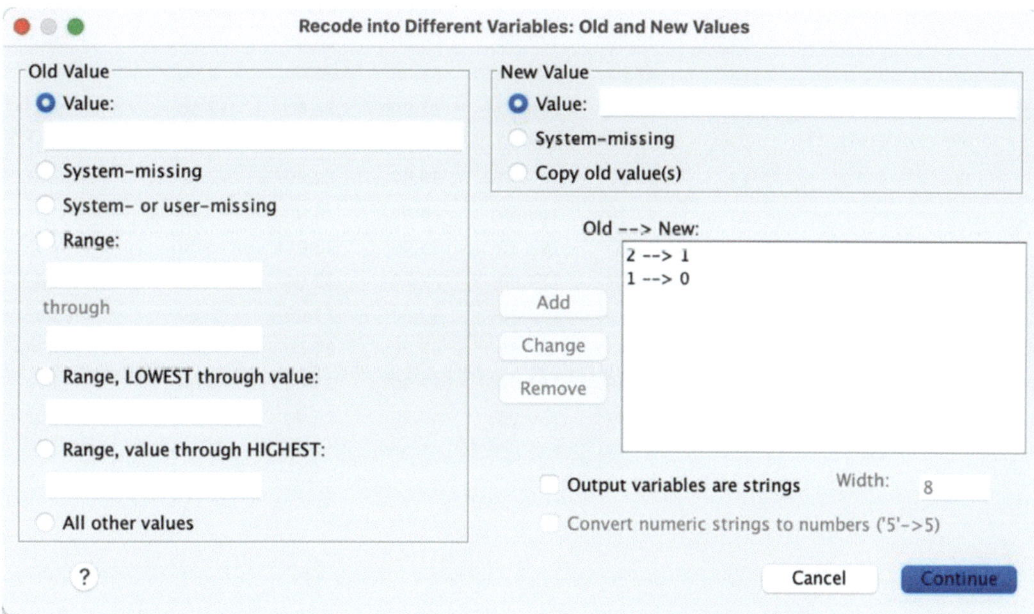

Fig. 14.7 Assigning additional dummy variable values using the Old and New Values dialog

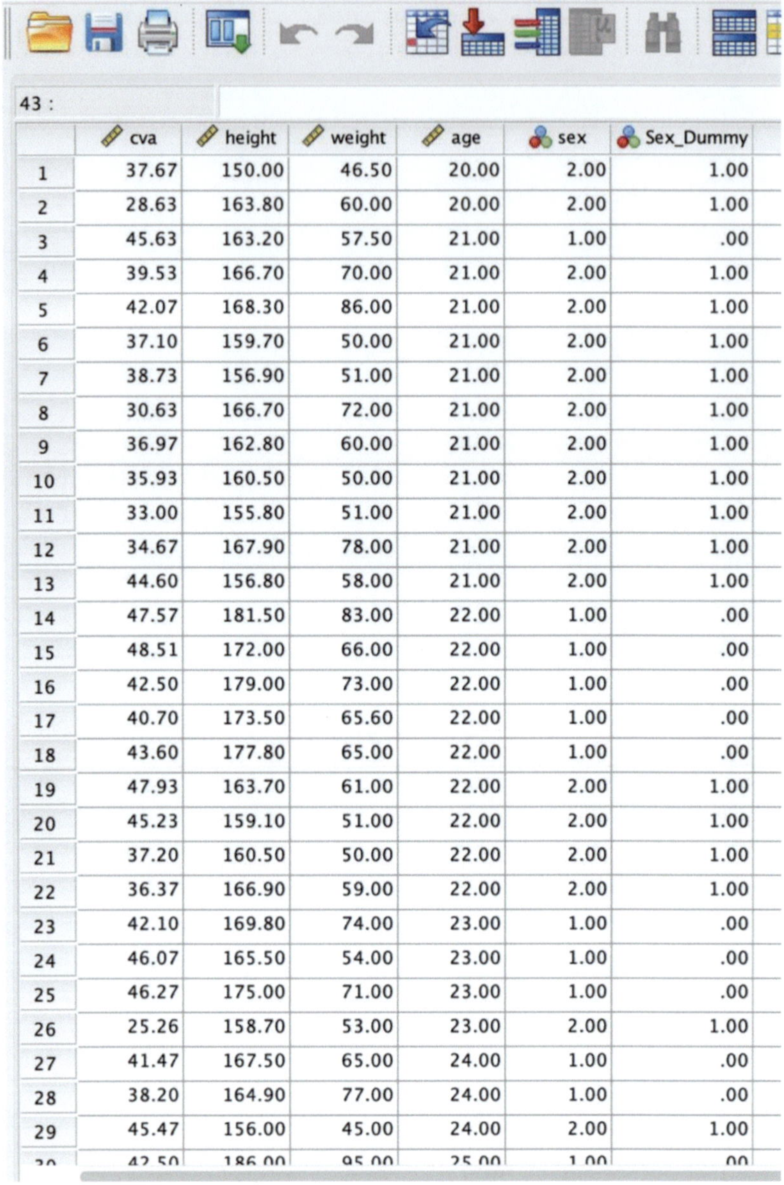

43 :

	cva	height	weight	age	sex	Sex_Dummy
1	37.67	150.00	46.50	20.00	2.00	1.00
2	28.63	163.80	60.00	20.00	2.00	1.00
3	45.63	163.20	57.50	21.00	1.00	.00
4	39.53	166.70	70.00	21.00	2.00	1.00
5	42.07	168.30	86.00	21.00	2.00	1.00
6	37.10	159.70	50.00	21.00	2.00	1.00
7	38.73	156.90	51.00	21.00	2.00	1.00
8	30.63	166.70	72.00	21.00	2.00	1.00
9	36.97	162.80	60.00	21.00	2.00	1.00
10	35.93	160.50	50.00	21.00	2.00	1.00
11	33.00	155.80	51.00	21.00	2.00	1.00
12	34.67	167.90	78.00	21.00	2.00	1.00
13	44.60	156.80	58.00	21.00	2.00	1.00
14	47.57	181.50	83.00	22.00	1.00	.00
15	48.51	172.00	66.00	22.00	1.00	.00
16	42.50	179.00	73.00	22.00	1.00	.00
17	40.70	173.50	65.60	22.00	1.00	.00
18	43.60	177.80	65.00	22.00	1.00	.00
19	47.93	163.70	61.00	22.00	2.00	1.00
20	45.23	159.10	51.00	22.00	2.00	1.00
21	37.20	160.50	50.00	22.00	2.00	1.00
22	36.37	166.90	59.00	22.00	2.00	1.00
23	42.10	169.80	74.00	23.00	1.00	.00
24	46.07	165.50	54.00	23.00	1.00	.00
25	46.27	175.00	71.00	23.00	1.00	.00
26	25.26	158.70	53.00	23.00	2.00	1.00
27	41.47	167.50	65.00	24.00	1.00	.00
28	38.20	164.90	77.00	24.00	1.00	.00
29	45.47	156.00	45.00	24.00	2.00	1.00
30	42.50	186.00	95.00	25.00	1.00	.00

Fig. 14.8 SPSS dataset with newly created dummy variables displayed in the variable view

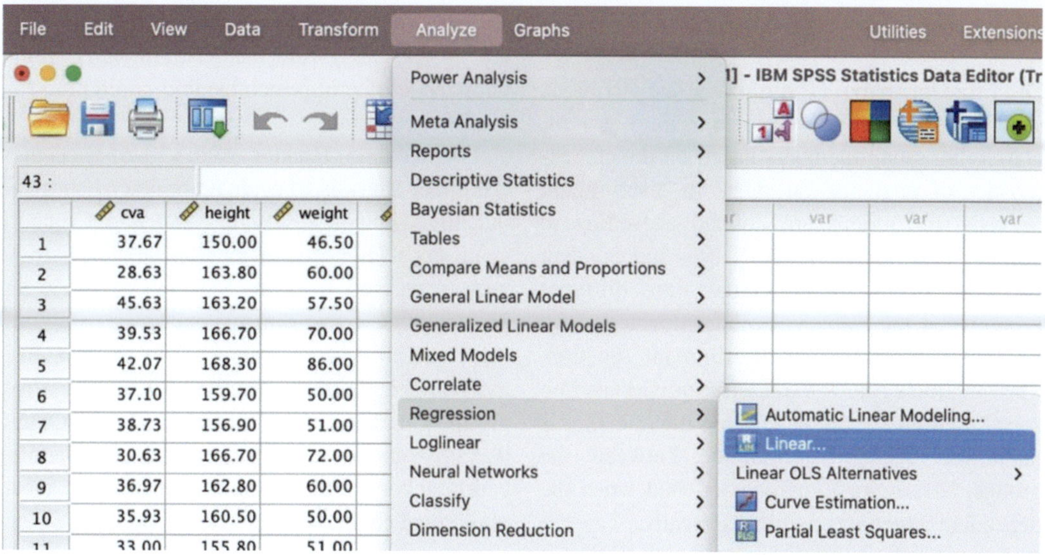

Fig. 14.9 Navigation path in SPSS to perform regression analysis using the dummy variable

Fig. 14.10 SPSS output window displaying the results of the linear regression analysis using the dummy variable

Variables Entered/Removed[a]

Model	Variables Entered	Variables Removed	Method
1	Sex_Dummy, age, weight, height[b]	.	Enter

a. Dependent Variable: cva

b. All requested variables entered.

Model Summary

Model	R	R Square	Adjusted R Square	Std. Error of the Estimate
1	.515[a]	.265	.196	5.60652

a. Predictors: (Constant), Sex_Dummy, age, weight, height

ANOVA[a]

Model		Sum of Squares	df	Mean Square	F	Sig.
1	Regression	486.989	4	121.747	3.873	.009[b]
	Residual	1351.624	43	31.433		
	Total	1838.613	47			

a. Dependent Variable: cva

b. Predictors: (Constant), Sex_Dummy, age, weight, height

Coefficients[a]

Model		Unstandardized Coefficients		Standardized Coefficients		
		B	Std. Error	Beta	t	Sig.
1	(Constant)	24.931	32.114		.776	.442
	height	.114	.214	.149	.534	.596
	weight	-.064	.123	-.118	-.519	.607
	age	.140	.268	.071	.522	.604
	Sex_Dummy	-5.502	2.536	-.444	-2.169	.036

a. Dependent Variable: cva

14.3 Discriminant Analysis

Discriminant analysis is a multivariate technique used to distinguish between two or more groups, classifying group members based on the characteristics of predictor variables. In discriminant analysis, the groups are defined according to specific criteria. The analysis uses independent variables to classify individuals into different groups, and the statistical model developed for this purpose is called a discriminant function. The function's role is to classify individuals into specific groups when their group membership is unknown, and to differentiate between the groups. Discriminant analysis is used when the dependent variable is nominal in scale.

For example, one can conduct a discriminant analysis to predict whether an emergency room patient is at risk of death using clinical data from past patients stored in the hospital's records. Discriminant analysis involves identifying discriminating variables that can best differentiate among two or more heterogeneous groups. Based on data collected for these variables by group, the analysis provides a classification rule that minimizes classification error.

This classification rule can also be used to predict the group membership of individuals whose actual group is unknown. For instance, if emergency patients are classified into two groups—survivors and non-survivors—discriminant analysis can determine which group a current patient most likely belongs to, based on physical examination results such as blood pressure and hemoglobin levels.

The discriminant function is expressed as:

$$D = d_1X_1 + d_2X_2 + d_3X_3 + \ldots + d_pX_p$$

where D is the discriminant score, $d_1, d_2, \ldots, d_p$ are the discriminant function coefficients (similar to beta weights), and p is the number of predictors. Discriminant analysis is used to classify individual cases into groups. It often involves first using independent samples t-tests or analysis of variance (ANOVA) to identify variables that significantly differentiate groups. Discriminant analysis is appropriate when the dependent variable is categorical and the independent variables are at least interval scale. Additionally, prior knowledge of group membership is required for model development.

For example, Rickart et al. (2025) used discriminant analysis to evaluate midfacial surgical outcomes in patients with Apert and Crouzon syndromes. High-dimensional facial morphology vectors derived from an SD-VAE model were projected into a two-dimensional space using linear discriminant analysis (LDA) to visualize morphological differences from a healthy control group. Quadratic discriminant analysis (QDA) was subsequently employed to assess the classification accuracy of pre- and postoperative morphological changes (Rickart et al. 2025).

14.4 Factor Analysis

Factor analysis is a method used to group together variables that are highly correlated with one another. Because it clusters variables based on strong correlations, it serves several purposes:

1. Summarizing data
2. Identifying the structure of variables
3. Eliminating unnecessary variables
4. Assessing the validity of measurement tools
5. Using factor scores for further analysis (e.g., scale construction)

Unlike methods that primarily aim to compare or predict, factor analysis is used to explore and verify the structure embedded within a large set of variables. Its main purpose is to examine the underlying structure by explaining the essence of inter-variable correlations. Although the method involves a degree of subjectivity, which can lead to more debate compared to other statistical techniques, it is particularly useful for identifying the essence of abstract or complex phenomena.

Through factor analysis, abstract components underlying a large group of variables can be extracted, thereby reducing and organizing the data into manageable sets based on conceptual similarity. The key interest lies in the conceptual interpretation of newly formed factors and the relative strength of association between each variable and its factor.

1. Factor: A small set of grouped variables that share high correlations with each other.
2. Factor loadings: The correlations between the variables and their respective factors, indicating the nature of each factor. The squared factor loading represents the proportion of variance in the variable explained by the factor. When the factors are independent, the correlations between the factors and observed variables are considered factor loadings. These are conceptually similar to standardized regression coefficients in regression analysis or path coefficients in path analysis.
3. Communality (hj^2): Represents how much of a variable's variance is accounted for by the extracted factors. It can be interpreted as the proportion of variance explained by common factors, conceptually similar to the coefficient of determination (R^2).
4. Eigenvalue: Indicates the amount of information (variance) in the data that is accounted for by each factor.
5. Factor analysis models:
   (i) Principal component analysis (PCA): Typically used when the goal is to condense as much information as possible into a few components for prediction purposes.
   (ii) Principal factor analysis (common factor analysis): Used when the aim is to uncover latent factors or dimensions that are not immediately apparent.

- Factor Rotation Methods
  (i) Orthogonal Rotation: In orthogonal rotation, the axes of the factors remain at 90 degrees to each other during extraction. This method assumes that the factors are independent of one another. It is commonly used when there is no specific theoretical reason to assume correlations among the factors.
  (ii) Oblique Rotation: Oblique rotation is used when it is assumed that the extracted factors are correlated with one another. This approach allows for more flexibility in identifying latent structures that may share underlying variance.

% of Variance Explained by Each

Total Variance Explained

Factor	Initial Eigenvalues			Extraction Sums of Squared Loadings			Rotation Sums Squared Loadings		
	Total	% of Variance	Cumulative %	Total	% of Variance	Cumulative %	Total	% of Variance	Cumulative %
1	3.647	36.473	36.473	3.647	36.473	36.473	2.472	24.717	24.717
2	1.315	13.148	49.621	1.315	13.148	49.621	2.049	20.495	45.212
3	1.223	12.229	61.850	1.223	12.229	61.850	1.664	16.638	61.850
4	.800	7.999	69.849						
5	.728	7.283	77.133						
6	.633	6.326	83.459						
7	.530	5.297	88.756						
8	.427	4.270	93.027						
9	.353	3.527	96.553						
10	.345	3.447	100.000						

Eigenvalues

Extracted Factors (Unrotated)

Extracted Factors (Rotated)

Items	Factors		
	1	2	3
Item 3	.553	-.455	.213
Item 7	.502	-.483	.025
Item 9	.555	-.523	-.033
Item 12	.908	-.152	.258
Item 11	.596	.372	-.082
Item 5	.488	.265	-.662
Item 4	.489	.233	-.663
Item 6	.534	.259	.321
Item 18	.153	.432	.455

Factor Extraction Method: Principal Component Analysis Number of Extracted Factors: 3

Factor Loadings: Each cell value represents the correlation between the factor and the item.

Eigenvalue of Factor 1 = the sum of the squared factor loadings in the first column

Eigenvalue of Factor 2 = the sum of the squared factor loadings in the second column

Eigenvalue of Factor 3 = the sum of the squared factor loadings in the third column

Communality: For example, Communality (Item 3) = $(.553)^2 + (-.455)^2 + (.213)^2$

Items	Factors		
	1	2	3
Item 3	.553	−.455	.213
Item 7	.502	−.483	.025
Item 9	.555	−.523	−.033
Item 12	.908	−.152	.258
Item 11	.596	.372	−.082
Item 5	.488	.265	−.662
Item 4	.489	.233	−.663
Item 6	.534	.259	.321
Item 18	.153	.432	.455

- Factor Extraction Method: Principal Component Analysis; Number of Extracted Factors: 3
- Factor Loadings: Each cell value represents the correlation between the factor and the item.
- Eigenvalue of Factor 1 = the sum of the squared factor loadings in the first column
- Eigenvalue of Factor 2 = the sum of the squared factor loadings in the second column
- Eigenvalue of Factor 3 = the sum of the

squared factor loadings in the third column

- Communality: For example, Communality (Item 3) = $(.553)^2 + (-.455)^2 + (.213)^2$

Extraction of Factors

The first step in factor analysis is to construct a correlation matrix of all the test items. Based on these intercorrelations, the principal components of the data are identified. This process involves identifying the linear relationships among the factors and grouping similar variables based on these relationships. In statistical terms, this corresponds to examining the data in a multidimensional space and clustering variables that exhibit strong correlations, thereby rearranging them according to similarity. These grouped variables are then restructured and extracted as factors or components, which is the essence of the factor extraction process.

Principal component analysis extracts factors from the data matrix by combining variables that exhibit strong linear relationships capable of explaining a large portion of the total variance in the data. The first factor is extracted to account for as much of the total variance as possible. The second factor is extracted and reordered from among the remaining variables, as the one that explains the next largest portion of the remaining total variance.

The most commonly used method for determining the number of factors is the eigenvalue criterion, which retains only those factors with eigenvalues greater than or equal to 1. Another widely used method is the scree plot (Fig. 14.11).

As a result of principal component analysis, the factor loadings representing variables on each factor are presented in the form of a factor matrix. When a factor loading is close to 1.00, the corresponding variable is interpreted as being associated with the first factor; when it is close to 0.00, it is considered to be associated with other factors. Factor loadings can be interpreted similarly to correlation coefficients, ranging from 0.00 to ±1.00. A factor loading greater than 0.30 or 0.40 indicates a meaningful level of correlation. When interpreting, only the absolute value of the factor loading is considered.

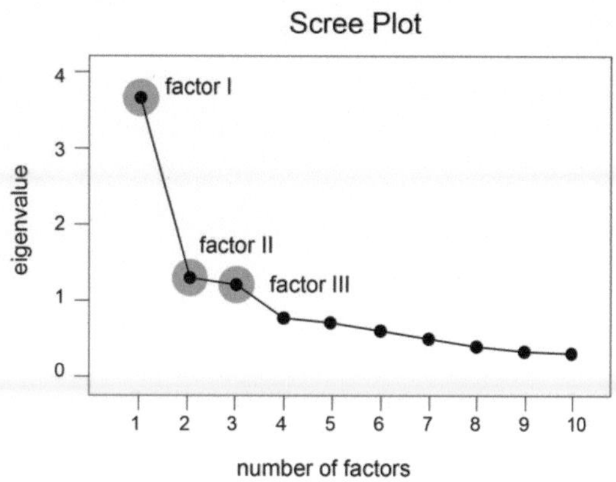

Fig. 14.11 Scree plot for determining the number of factors to retain

To assess the suitability of the data for factor analysis, the Kaiser–Meyer–Olkin (KMO) measure is used. According to Kaiser (1974), a KMO value above 0.9 is considered marvelous, 0.8 to 0.9 is meritorious, 0.7 to 0.8 is middling, 0.6 to 0.7 is mediocre, 0.5 to 0.6 is miserable, and below 0.5 is unacceptable. Generally, a KMO value of at least 0.6 is recommended.

Bartlett's Sphericity Test is used to determine whether the variables included in a factor analysis are correlated with one another. If there is no correlation among the variables used in factor analysis, then the variables grouped under each factor would not share meaningful associations, making it inappropriate to treat them as a common factor. The null hypothesis (H_0) of Bartlett's test is that "there is no correlation among the variables," while the alternative hypothesis (H_1) is that "there is correlation among the variables." Therefore, if the approximate chi-square test statistic is sufficiently large and the p-value is small, it can be used as evidence that the dataset is suitable for factor analysis.

If it is difficult to interpret the results because it is unclear which variable corresponds to which factor, the next step is to perform factor rotation.

Factor Rotation

Factor rotation is a complex and multidimensional concept (Fig. 14.12). It involves rotating two axes to rearrange the variables closer to each axis,

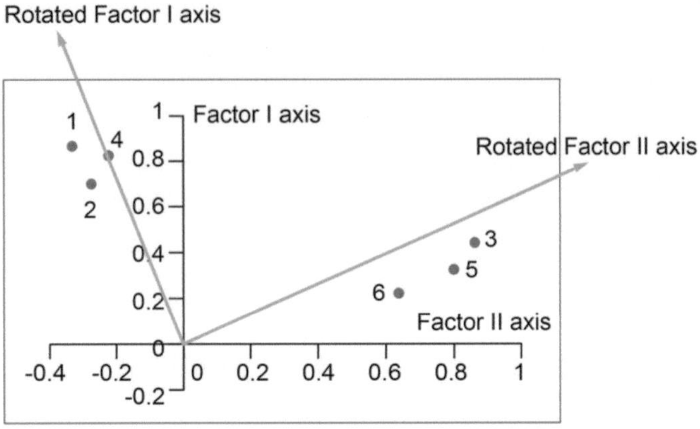

Fig. 14.12 Visualization of factor rotation: unrotated vs. rotated factor axes

thereby simplifying the factor structure. The most commonly used method is varimax rotation.

Orthogonal rotation maintains the right angles between the axes while rotating them, assuming that there is no correlation between the factors.

Oblique rotation, though less commonly used, can lead to factors becoming closely aligned, which increases the correlation between them and can make interpretation more difficult.

Naming Factors

The final step of factor analysis is to assign names to the factors based on the characteristics of the significant variables within each factor. This is done by considering the theoretical constructs and common themes shared by the grouped variables. Since this process is inherently subjective, it can at times be challenging.

Application of Factor Analysis

Exploratory Analysis

Factor analysis is used to explore different types of answers to the research question. In exploratory research approaches, it is often applied to identify latent constructs that were not previously evident.

Reduction of Data

Factor analysis simplifies tests by grouping individual items into unified concepts for evaluation. To reduce the number of items, a composite summary score for each concept can be developed. In principal component analysis, composite scores are used to reduce the number of factors, aiding in the simplification of complex data structures.

Limitations of Factor Analysis

One limitation of factor analysis is that the process of naming the extracted factors is inherently subjective, as it relies on the researcher's judgment. This subjectivity can lead to disagreement or controversy regarding the interpretation of the factors (Kaiser 1974).

14.5 Logistic Regression

Logistic regression is a specialized form of multiple regression in which the dependent variable (*Y*) is dichotomous—for example, survival vs. death or disease vs. no disease. It is commonly used in epidemiology to identify risk factors associated with disease within exposed populations. This method is appropriate when the independent variables are either categorical or continuous, and the dependent variable is categorical, typically representing the probability (odds) of a certain event, such as disease occurrence.

Let us briefly examine how to calculate the odds ratio. The odds of an event are defined as the number of times the event occurs divided by the number of times it does not occur. For example,

Table 14.1 Summary of ANOVA types

Type of analysis	Number of independent variables	Number of dependent variables	Number of covariates
One-way ANOVA	1	1	None
Multi-way ANOVA	2 or more	1	None
Multivariate ANOVA (MANOVA)	2 or more	2 or more	None
Analysis of Covariance (ANCOVA)	1	1	1 or more

if 51 out of every 100 births are male, the odds of a male birth occurring randomly is 51 to 49, or 1.04. This is equivalent to 0.51/0.49. An odds greater than 1 indicates a higher likelihood of the event occurring, whereas an odds less than 1 implies a lower likelihood. The odds ratio is the odds in the treatment group divided by the odds in the control group. In situations where events are rare, the odds ratio approximates the relative risk and is often interpreted as such, because saying that "the risk is doubled" or "halved" tends to be more intuitive than expressing a probability like 0.51. In logistic regression, it is customary to report the odds ratio along with a 95% confidence interval. A variable is considered statistically significant only if the confidence interval does not include 1 (Matsui et al. 2017; Rao et al. 2014; Hardy et al. 2014).

14.6 Multivariate Analysis of Variance (MANOVA)

In many clinical research designs, it is common to evaluate one or more dependent variables simultaneously. For instance, consider a study measuring changes in facial skin condition after a specific dermatologic treatment. Multiple skin parameters—such as skin hydration and transepidermal water loss (TEWL)—might be assessed at the same time using specialized equipment. If such types of data were analyzed using *t*-tests or ANOVA, each dependent variable would be examined separately. This results in two major issues.

First, performing multiple tests within a single experiment increases the risk of Type I error. Second, *t*-tests and ANOVA are designed to test only one outcome variable at a time and assume each test represents an independent event. However, in cases such as the above, the dependent variables are not independent of each other; one outcome may influence another. Therefore, in such situations, multivariate analysis of variance (MANOVA) is far more appropriate than simple ANOVA.

For example, if skin redness (erythema) and patient-reported discomfort are the dependent variables, and the independent variable is treatment type (e.g., topical agent, laser therapy, or microneedling), conducting a one-way ANOVA for erythema and a separate one-way ANOVA for discomfort increases the risk of Type I error. Instead, it is more appropriate to analyze both outcomes simultaneously using MANOVA to evaluate the effectiveness of the three treatment types (Table 14.1).

14.7 Analysis of Covariance (ANCOVA)

Concept of Analysis of Covariance

In an analysis of variance (ANOVA), suppose a significant difference in group means is observed, and the independent variable under consideration is the type of treatment. Furthermore, assume that there are inherent differences in baseline impairment levels (or timing of intervention) across groups, which are known to substantially influence functional outcomes in daily activities. Under such circumstances, it becomes problematic to attribute differences in functional performance solely to the treatment methods (e.g., Treatment A, B, or C). This is because the groups differ in their baseline impairment levels, which themselves could influence the outcome, independently of the treatment effect.

Consequently, the observed group differences may be attributable to the treatment type, to the baseline impairment, or to an interaction of both factors—thus making interpretation ambiguous. To obtain pure experimental results, it is essential that only the independent variable influences the dependent variable, while all confounding variables are adequately controlled.

The primary aim of experimental design is to isolate the effect of the independent variable on the dependent variable by controlling for other extraneous variables.

When such extraneous or confounding variables cannot be directly controlled through experimental procedures, their influence can be statistically adjusted using a method known as analysis of covariance (ANCOVA). ANCOVA is a statistical technique that combines elements of ANOVA and regression analysis to account for the effects of covariates—i.e., variables other than the primary independent variable that may influence the dependent variable. Rather than experimental control, ANCOVA provides post hoc statistical control of such covariates.

In ANCOVA, these uncontrolled influencing variables are referred to as covariates. The dependent variable is denoted by Y, the independent variable by X, and the influence of the covariate is removed using the linear regression method.

Example Ma'or and Voss (1997) conducted a study to compare the effects of two active skin treatments and one placebo control group. A total of 60 participants were randomly assigned to one of the three treatment groups ($n = 20$ per group). In order to evaluate post-treatment skin roughness, the researchers applied analysis of covariance (ANCOVA), using pre-treatment skin softness scores as a covariate. This statistical approach allowed them to control for baseline differences in skin condition, enabling a more accurate assessment of treatment efficacy (Ma'Or et al. 1997).

14.8 Cluster Analysis

Cluster analysis is a statistical method used to classify a large number of individuals (or cases) into several groups, or clusters, such that individuals within the same cluster are more similar to each other than to those in other clusters. The term "individual" here can refer to people, animals, or other units of analysis depending on the research context.

This method is distinct from discriminant analysis. In discriminant analysis, the groups to which individuals belong are clearly defined in advance. In contrast, cluster analysis does not start with predefined group structures. For example, patients with facial wrinkles might be categorized into mild, moderate, or severe groups based on wrinkle depth and distribution. This would be a form of discriminant analysis, as the classification criteria are clearly defined in advance.

However, in cluster analysis, patients with facial wrinkles would be grouped based on similarities without prior knowledge of the exact categories. As another example, consider a family shopping for all their vacation needs at a supermarket. At checkout, the clerk may separate items into different bags—meats and vegetables in one, frozen foods in another, and daily necessities in yet another. This kind of sorting can be viewed as an informal application of cluster analysis.

Let n represent the number of individuals (cases) and p the number of observed variables used to describe each individual. The number of clusters is denoted by c. In essence, cluster analysis involves using the data given in an $n \times p$ matrix to classify the n individuals into c clusters in such a way that individuals in the same cluster are similar to each other, and those in different clusters are dissimilar (Krywuczky et al. 2025; Tibble et al. 2020).

References

Bauer DM, Finch DC, McGough KP, et al. A comparative analysis of several crutch-length-estimation techniques. Phys Ther. 1991;17:294–300.

Gowland C. Predicting sensorimotor recovery following stroke rehabilitation. Physiother Can. 1984;36:313–320.

Jones CA, Voaklander DC, Suarez-Almazor ME. Determinants of function after total knee arthroplasty. Phys Ther. 2003;83(8):696–706.

Teseng MH, Chow SMK. Perceptual-motor function of school-age children with slow handwriting speed. Am J Occup Ther. 2000;54:83–89.

Rickart, Alexander J., Foti, Simone, van de Lande, Lara S., Wagner, Connor, Schievano, Silvia, Jeelani, Noorul Owase, Clarkson, Matthew J., Ong, Juling, Swanson, Jordan, Bartlett, Scott P., Taylor, Jesse A., Dunaway, David J. Using a Disentangled Neural Network to Objectively Assess the Outcomes of Midfacial Surgery in Syndromic Craniosynostosis. *Plastic and Reconstructive Surgery* 155(5):p 884e–892e, May 2025.

Kaiser HF. An index of factorial simplicity. Psychometrika. 1974;39: 31–36.

Matsui, Mary & Dela Cruz, Jomer & Tang, Jiawen & Deng, Bin & Xie, Xiaoyuan & Lei, Guan. (2017). Logistic regression analysis differentiates high from low computer users by facial skin conditions in a population of Chinese women. *Applied Informatics*. 4. https://doi.org/10.1186/s40535-016-0031-0.

Rao, S., Stolle, E., Sher, S., Lin, C., Momen, B., & Nahabedian, M. (2014). A multiple logistic regression analysis of complications following microsurgical breast reconstruction. *Gland Surgery, 3*(4), 226–231.

Hardy KL, Davis KE, Constantine RS, et al. The impact of operative time on complications after plastic surgery: a multivariate regression analysis of 1753 cases. *Aesthet Surg J*. 2014;34(4):614–622.

Ma'Or, Z., S. Yehuda, and W. Voss. 1997. "Skin Smoothing Effects of Dead Sea Minerals: Comparative Profilometric Evaluation of Skin Surface." *International Journal of Cosmetic Science* 19: 105–10.

Krywuczky, F., Kokkoris, M., Kleijnen, M. *et al.* A laypeople's typology of cosmetic surgeries using cluster analysis. *Sci Rep* 15, 13415 (2025).

Tibble, H. et al. A data-driven typology of asthma medication adherence using cluster analysis. *Sci. Rep.* 10 (1), 14999 (2020)

15 Selection of Statistical Methods

When analyzing data, the selection of appropriate statistical methods requires careful consideration of the purpose of the analysis, the level of measurement, the number of groups, and the number of variables involved. The objectives of data analysis can generally be classified into three categories: (1) comparison, (2) determination of association, and (3) prediction. In other words, it is necessary to first determine whether the goal is to describe the distribution of a particular group, to examine the existence and strength of relationships between variables, to assess the effect of an intervention, or to predict a certain phenomenon.

Variables can be categorized according to their level of measurement: nominal scale, ordinal scale, interval scale, or ratio scale. Each variable must be represented by one of these four levels. The choice of statistical method depends largely on the measurement level of the data col lected. If the variables are measured at the nominal or ordinal level, non-parametric tests should be applied. If the variables are measured at the interval or ratio level, parametric tests are appropriate. Traditional methods of statistical inference are applied when the probability distribution (or population) from which the sample is drawn is known (e.g., normal or binomial distribution), and are used to estimate or test the unknown parameters that define these distributions. When the form of the distribution is known but the specific parameters are not, the method of inference used is referred to in statistics as a parametric method. However, in some cases, it may be difficult to assume that the population distribution follows a normal distribution, or it may be entirely impossible to make any assumption about the form of the distribution. In such situations, how can statistical inference be conducted? These cases call for what are known as nonparametric methods or distribution-free methods.

15.1 Methods for Assessing Normality

To apply parametric statistical methods, it is assumed that the random sample has been drawn from a population that follows a normal distribution. If the sample does not originate from a normally distributed population, the application of such methods can lead to incorrect conclusions. For instance, constructing a 95% confidence

K.-H. Yi, *Statistical Research Methods for Dermatologists and Plastic Surgeons*,
https://doi.org/10.1007/978-981-95-5668-7_15

interval based on non-normally distributed data may result in an actual confidence level of only 91%. A more serious concern, however, lies in the issue of efficiency. An efficient method refers to one that yields better estimates or statistical tests with smaller sample sizes by making optimal use of the data. In cases where the population does not follow a normal distribution, various nonparametric methods tend to be more efficient than methods based on the normal distribution.

To determine whether the measured data follow a normal distribution, one may use the one-sample Kolmogorov–Smirnov test or the Shapiro–Wilk test. In this context, the null hypothesis (H_0) is "the data follow a normal distribution," and the alternative hypothesis (H_1) is "the data do not follow a normal distribution."

In SPSS, to test for normality, go to Analyze → Nonparametric Tests → Legacy Dialogs → 1-Sample K-S, move the relevant variable into the test field, and click OK (Figs. 15.1, 15.2, 15.3, and 15.4). In the following example, the normality of the variable cervicocephalic angle was tested, and the result was $p = 0.190$ (Fig. 15.5). Since this p-value exceeds the significance level of 0.05, the data are judged to satisfy the assumption of normality.

The one-sample Kolmogorov–Smirnov test is a method typically used when the sample size is very large, whereas the Shapiro–Wilk test is commonly applied to general datasets. The closer the Shapiro–Wilk value is to 1, the more likely it is that the data follow a normal distribution.

To view the Shapiro–Wilk value in SPSS, go to: Analyze → Descriptive Statistics → Explore (Fig. 15.6). Move the variable of interest to the Dependent List box and click Plots → check Normality plots with tests, then click Continue and OK (Figs. 15.7, 15.8, and 15.9).

The following results are obtained (Fig. 15.10).

Interpreting the results of the normality test, the null hypothesis is "H_0: Cervicocephalic angle measurements follow a normal distribution." The p-values are $p = 0.190$ and $p = 0.271$, both of which are greater than the significance level of 0.05. Therefore, the null hypothesis is not rejected, and it is interpreted that the data follow a normal distribution. In the normal Q–Q plot of the cervicocephalic angle, the closer the observed values are to the straight line, the more strongly it supports the interpretation that the data are normally distributed (Fig. 15.11).

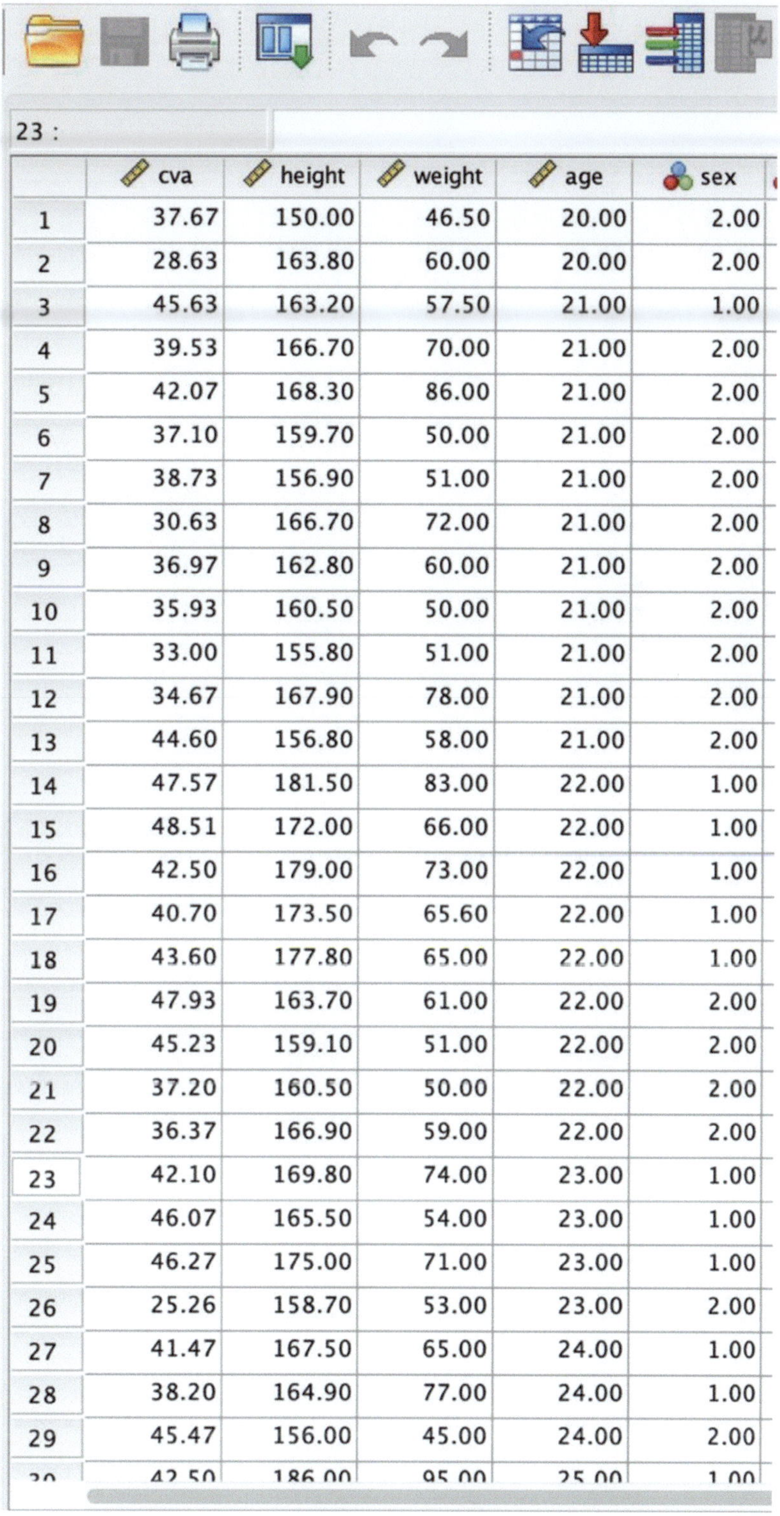

23 :

	cva	height	weight	age	sex
1	37.67	150.00	46.50	20.00	2.00
2	28.63	163.80	60.00	20.00	2.00
3	45.63	163.20	57.50	21.00	1.00
4	39.53	166.70	70.00	21.00	2.00
5	42.07	168.30	86.00	21.00	2.00
6	37.10	159.70	50.00	21.00	2.00
7	38.73	156.90	51.00	21.00	2.00
8	30.63	166.70	72.00	21.00	2.00
9	36.97	162.80	60.00	21.00	2.00
10	35.93	160.50	50.00	21.00	2.00
11	33.00	155.80	51.00	21.00	2.00
12	34.67	167.90	78.00	21.00	2.00
13	44.60	156.80	58.00	21.00	2.00
14	47.57	181.50	83.00	22.00	1.00
15	48.51	172.00	66.00	22.00	1.00
16	42.50	179.00	73.00	22.00	1.00
17	40.70	173.50	65.60	22.00	1.00
18	43.60	177.80	65.00	22.00	1.00
19	47.93	163.70	61.00	22.00	2.00
20	45.23	159.10	51.00	22.00	2.00
21	37.20	160.50	50.00	22.00	2.00
22	36.37	166.90	59.00	22.00	2.00
23	42.10	169.80	74.00	23.00	1.00
24	46.07	165.50	54.00	23.00	1.00
25	46.27	175.00	71.00	23.00	1.00
26	25.26	158.70	53.00	23.00	2.00
27	41.47	167.50	65.00	24.00	1.00
28	38.20	164.90	77.00	24.00	1.00
29	45.47	156.00	45.00	24.00	2.00
30	42.50	186.00	95.00	25.00	1.00

Fig. 15.1 Example dataset for assessing normality in SPSS

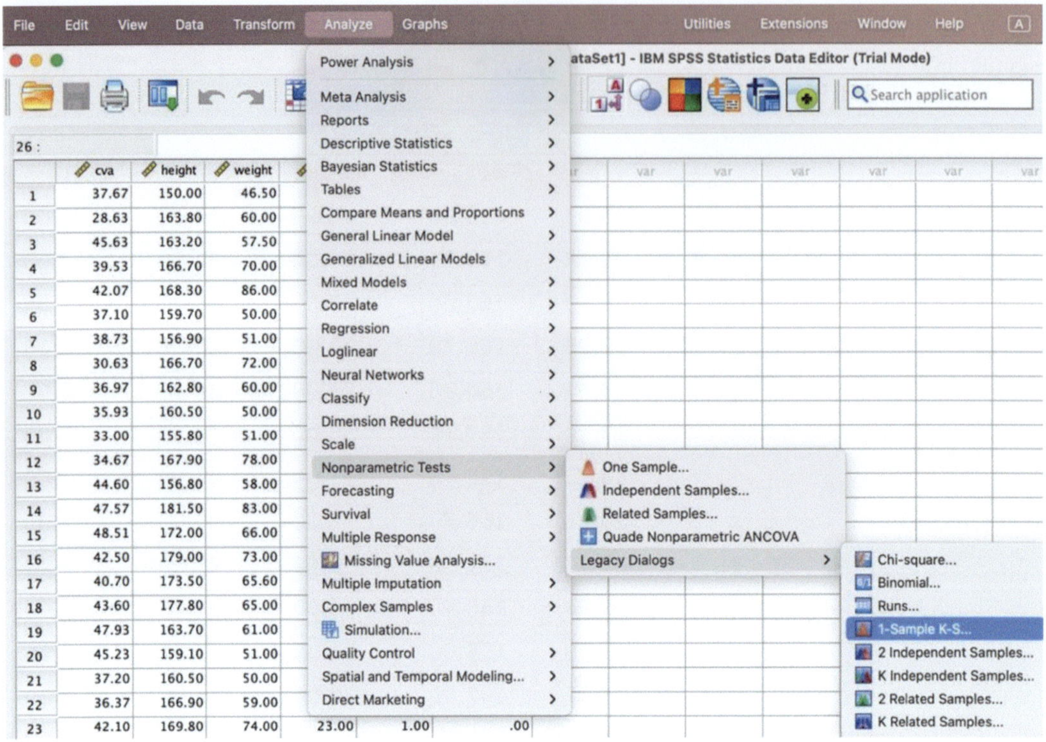

Fig. 15.2 Path to the one-sample Kolmogorov–Smirnov test in SPSS

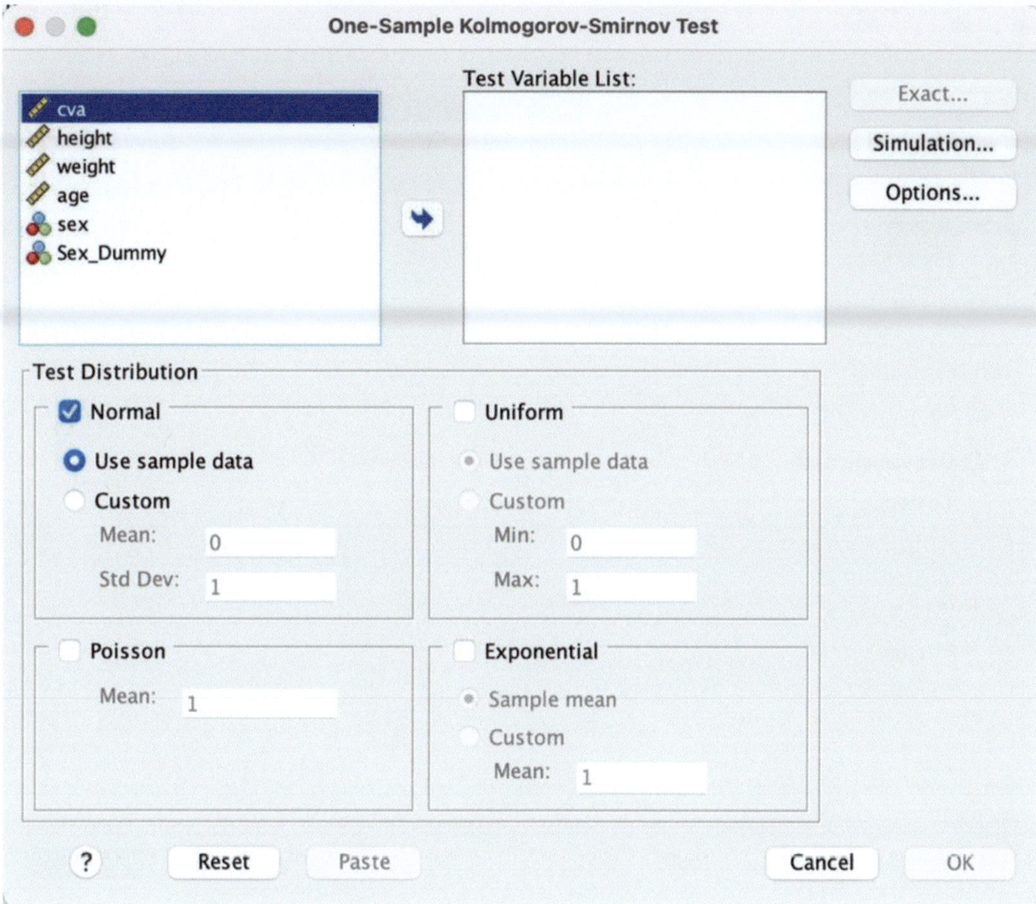

Fig. 15.3 One-sample Kolmogorov–Smirnov test dialog box in SPSS

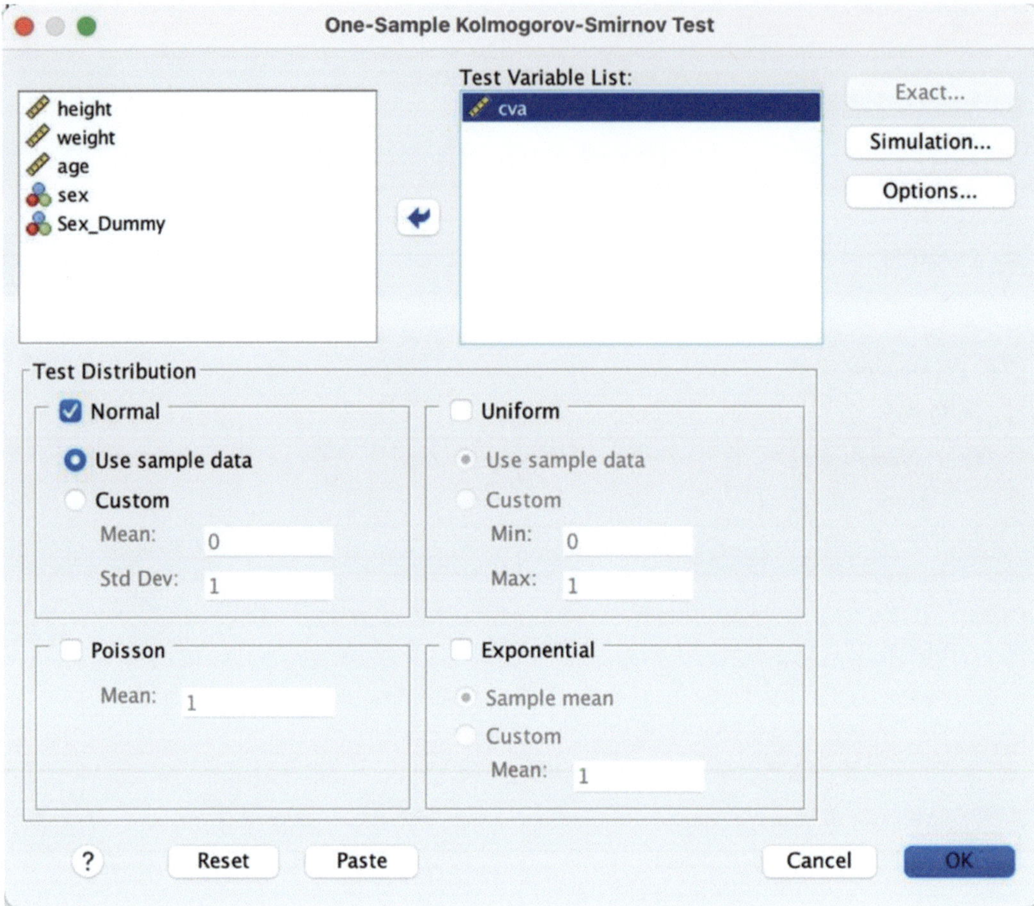

Fig. 15.4 Variable assigned to the test variable list for one-sample K-S test in SPSS

Fig. 15.5 Output window displaying results of the one-sample Kolmogorov–Smirnov test in SPSS

One-Sample Kolmogorov-Smirnov Test

			cva
N			48
Normal Parameters[a,b]	Mean		40.6531
	Std. Deviation		6.25455
Most Extreme Differences	Absolute		.110
	Positive		.063
	Negative		-.110
Test Statistic			.110
Asymp. Sig. (2-tailed)[c]			.190
Monte Carlo Sig. (2-tailed)[d]	Sig.		.144
	99% Confidence Interval	Lower Bound	.135
		Upper Bound	.153

a. Test distribution is Normal.

b. Calculated from data.

c. Lilliefors Significance Correction.

d. Lilliefors' method based on 10000 Monte Carlo samples with starting seed 299883525.

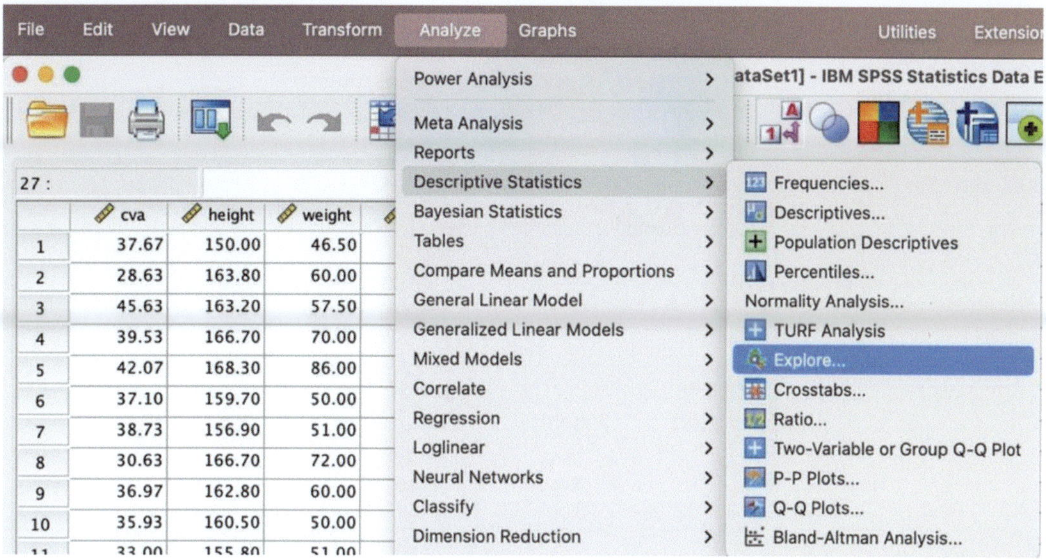

Fig. 15.6 Path to access the Shapiro–Wilk test via Analyze

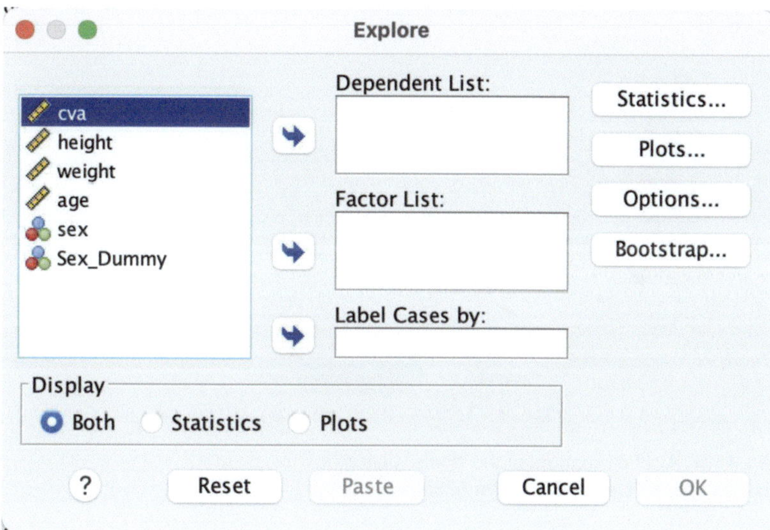

Fig. 15.7 Explore dialog window displayed after selecting Explore

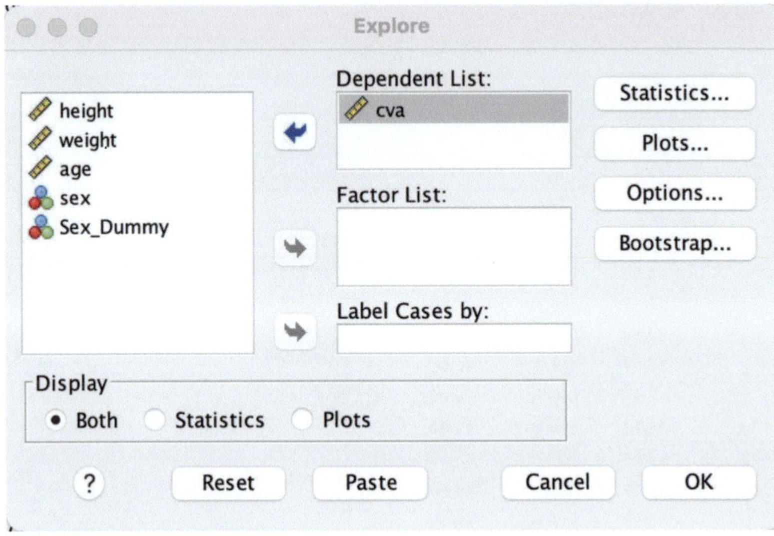

Fig. 15.8 Variables moved to the dependent list for Shapiro–Wilk normality test in the Explore dialog

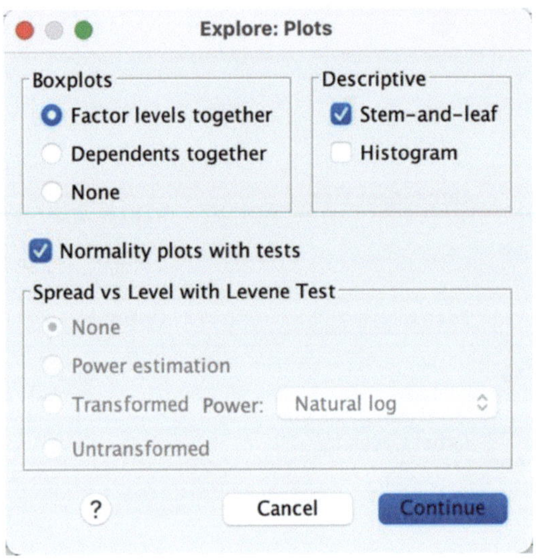

Fig. 15.9 Available options in the “Plots” dialog box for the Shapiro–Wilk normality test in SPSS

Fig. 15.10 SPSS output window showing results of the tests of normality

Tests of Normality

	Kolmogorov–Smirnov[a]			Shapiro–Wilk		
	Statistic	df	Sig.	Statistic	df	Sig.
cva	.110	48	.190	.971	48	.271

a. Lilliefors Significance Correction

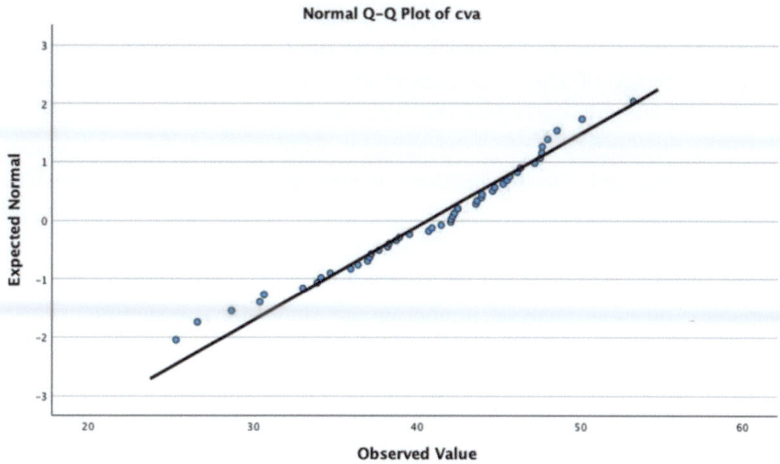

Fig. 15.11 Normal Q–Q plot displaying the distribution of data compared to a theoretical normal distribution

15.2 When Outliers Are Present

Parametric methods based on the assumption of normal distribution are highly sensitive even to a small number of outliers. Consider a simple example. Suppose we have five values: 3, 7, 9, 10, and 11. In nonparametric tests, the median is typically used, whereas parametric methods use the mean. For these five values, the median is 9 and the mean is 8. Now imagine that one of the values is either mismeasured or misrecorded. Suppose the value 11 is mistakenly entered as 61, and this error goes unnoticed. In this case, the median remains unchanged, but the mean becomes 18—more than double its original value. Statistical techniques used in nonparametric methods are less affected by such errors compared to methods based on the assumption of a normal distribution.

15.3 Characteristics of Nonparametric Statistical Methods

Nonparametric statistical methods have the following characteristics:

1. These methods are generally used under relaxed or minimal distributional assumptions compared to parametric methods.
2. Most nonparametric procedures do not rely on actual quantitative observations but rather on their relative evaluation. In other words, they can be applied even when only ordinal or ranked data are available.
3. The computational procedures involved in inference are much simpler than those of parametric methods. Since ranks are usually represented as integers such as 1, 2, 3, and so on, the calculations are easier than those based on raw data.
4. They are generally easier to understand.

Nonparametric tests should be used in the following situations:

1. When the dependent variable does not meet the assumptions of normality or homogeneity of variance.
2. When the dependent variable is measured at the nominal or ordinal level.
3. When the sample size is too small (typically six or fewer) to assess the underlying distribution.

15.4 Considerations When Selecting Statistical Methods

In statistical analysis, tests are commonly categorized based on the number of groups or samples being studied: single-sample tests, two-sample tests, and tests involving three or more samples. Therefore, the number of samples directly influences the choice of statistical method. It is also crucial to determine whether the data involve repeated measures, whether the samples were paired or matched during selection, or whether they are independent.

When the number of variables under analysis is one, a univariate approach is used; with two variables, bivariate analysis is appropriate; and with three or more variables, multivariate analysis should be employed. As such, choosing the appropriate statistical method requires consideration of these factors. In addition, it is essential to evaluate whether the assumptions underlying each statistical method are satisfied.

For example, in an independent samples *t*-test, the following assumptions must be met: the distributions of the two populations should be normal, the two groups must be independent, and the population variances should be equal. While parametric tests have multiple assumptions, some are essential and must be met, whereas others are less strict and may tolerate slight violations. It is often difficult for nonspecialists to judge whether these assumptions have been violated, especially when advanced statistical methods are involved. Therefore, consulting a statistics expert is highly recommended when applying complex analyses.

Statistical methods frequently used in the fields of cosmetic dermatology and plastic surgery research are summarized in Table 15.1.

Table 15.1 Summary of statistical methods

Statistical method	Test type	Purpose of use	Level of measurement	
			Independent variable	Dependent variable
Independent *t*-test	P[a]	To test the mean differences between two independent groups	Nominal scale	Interval/Ratio scale
Paired *t*-test	P	To compare means from two related groups or pre–post measurements in the same group	Nominal scale	Interval/Ratio scale
Median test	NP	To compare medians across two or more independent groups	Nominal scale	Ordinal scale
Mann–Whitney *U* test[b]	NP	To test differences in ranks between two independent groups	Nominal scale	Ordinal scale
Wilcoxon signed-rank test	NP	To test differences in ranks between two related groups	Nominal scale	Ordinal scale
Analysis of variance (ANOVA)[c]	P	To test mean differences across three or more independent groups	Nominal scale	Interval/Ratio scale
Kruskal–Wallis test	NP	To compare rank differences among three or more independent groups	Nominal scale	Ordinal scale
Friedman test	NP	To test rank differences across three or more related groups	Nominal scale	Ordinal scale
Chi-square test	NP	To test associations between categorical variables, or goodness of fit	Nominal scale	Nominal scale
Pearson correlation	P	To test the correlation between two continuous variables	Interval/Ratio scale	Interval/Ratio scale
Spearman's rho	NP	To test the correlation between two ranked variables	Ordinal scale	Ordinal scale
Multiple regression analysis	P	To predict a continuous dependent variable from multiple independent variables	Interval/Ratio scale	Interval/Ratio scale

[a] *P* parametric test, *NP* nonparametric test
[b] Also known as the Wilcoxon rank-sum test
[c] When there is only one independent variable, it is referred to as one-way ANOVA. When there are two or more independent variables, it is referred to as multiway ANOVA. If the independent variables are related (e.g., repeated measures), repeated-measures ANOVA is used

15.5 Statistical Analysis Using Software

Although the statistical methods discussed above can technically be calculated by hand, the process is often tedious and time-consuming. With the widespread availability of personal computers, most statistical analyses are now conducted efficiently using statistical software packages. Entering raw data into a computer is a relatively straightforward process with minimal guidance from statistical experts. However, interpreting the results properly still requires the involvement of professionals.

The following are examples of commonly used commercial statistical software programs for computer-based data analysis:

1. SAS/STAT—*SAS/STAT User's Guide*, Version 6, 4th edition, SAS Institute, Inc., Cary, NC (1990)
2. SPSS—*Statistical Package for the Social Sciences*, 444 North Michigan Avenue, Chicago, IL 60611 (1995)—also known as PASW (*Predictive Analytics Software*)

Besides, Minitab is also a widely used statistical software package. These statistical packages are available for both Windows and Macintosh operating systems. In most cases, data stored in one program can be imported into another, as they support interoperability. Furthermore, most statistical software programs are highly compatible with Microsoft Excel, allowing users to import data directly from Excel spreadsheets. For users familiar with Excel, this means they can conveniently enter data in Excel, import it into the statistical software, and proceed with the analysis.

If one does not have access to commercial statistical software and only needs to compute basic statistics with a small dataset, online tools can be an effective alternative. By visiting search engines such as http://www.google.com and entering keywords like "statistical computation website" or "free statistics," one can find websites that offer free statistical analysis tools or trial-based statistical software. After navigating to one of these sites, users can input data and perform analyses through a series of guided steps directly online.

Commercial statistical packages such as SAS and SPSS require a paid license due to copyright restrictions. However, a widely used and freely available statistical software called R can be downloaded from the internet. R is an open-source program that is free to use, user-friendly, and offers powerful graphics capabilities, making it a popular choice among researchers. Because it is open-source, R has a vast and growing ecosystem of community-contributed packages tailored to various fields of study. A commonly used format for importing data into R is the CSV (comma-separated values) format, which separates variables with commas and is compatible with most other statistical software, including Excel, SPSS, and SAS. For users familiar with Excel, data can be entered in Excel and saved as a .csv file, which can then be easily imported into R for analysis. Installing RStudio, an integrated development environment (IDE) for R, further simplifies the user experience by allowing graphical data import without the need to type command-line code. To install R, visit http://www.r-project.org, click on Download, then select CRAN, choose a CRAN mirror (e.g., Korea), click base, and then Download R x.x.x for Windows. For RStudio, visit http://rstudio.com and download the free desktop version.

A summary of commonly used commercial statistical packages is provided in Table 15.2.

Figure 15.12 is a flowchart that can serve as a reference when conducting statistical analysis. Table 15.3 provides a summary to assist in selecting appropriate statistical methods.

Table 15.2 Commonly used statistical software packages

InStat
Medcalc
Minitab
R (Open-source software available for free download at http://www.r-project.org)
SAS(Statistical Analysis System)
SPlus
SPSS(Statistical Package for the Social Sciences)
STATA
Statistical Navigator
StatXact
StatView
StatsDirect
StatSoft
STATISTICA
SysStat
S-Link(ISP) (Korean statistical software available for free at http://www.s-link.co.kr)
dBSTAT (Korean statistical software package)

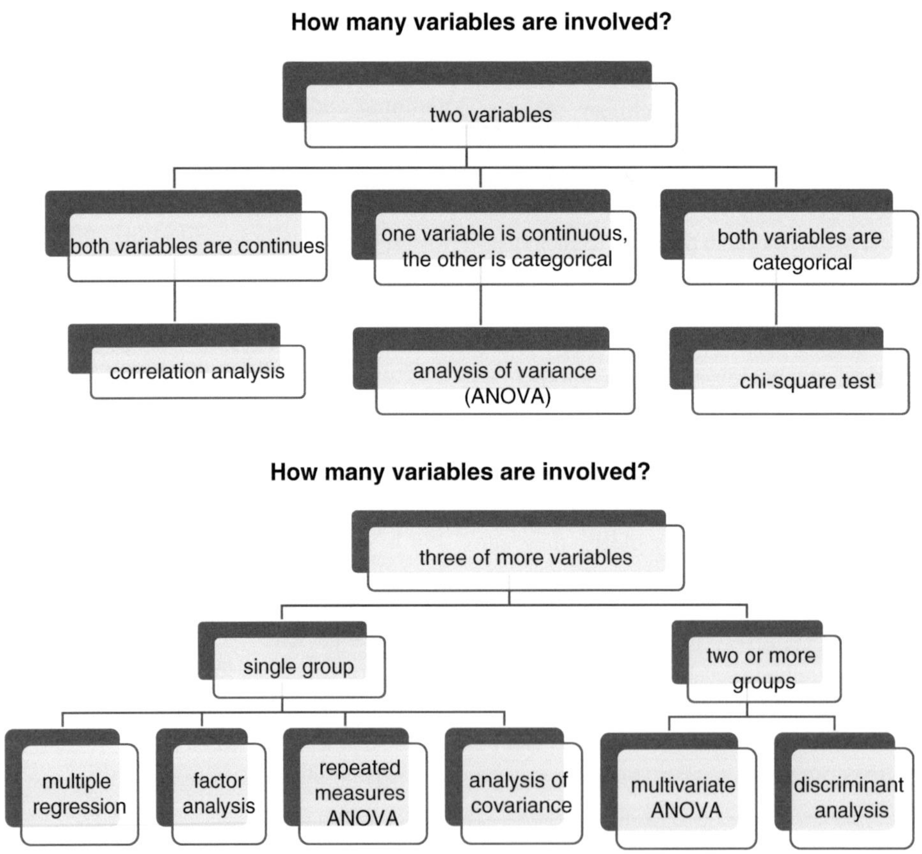

Fig. 15.12 Statistical methods by number of variables and groups

Table 15.3 Summary of statistical methods

	Number of samples					
		2 samples		3 or more samples		
Measurement scale	1 sample	Independent	Dependent (correlated)	Independent	Dependent (correlated)	Correlation
Nominal (nonparametric statistics)	Chi-square test	Chi-square test	McNemar test	Chi-square test	Cochran's Q test	Spearman's rank correlation
Ordinal (nonparametric statistics)		Mann–Whitney *U* test	Wilcoxon signed-rank test	Kruskal–Wallis one-way ANOVA	Friedman two-way ANOVA	
Interval or ratio (parametric statistics)—Normality (one-sample Kolmogorov–Smirnov test, Shapiro–Wilk test); homogeneity of variance (Levene's test, Bartlett's test)	Paired *t*-test(pre–post)	Independent *t*-test (use Welch's *t*-test if unequal variances)	Paired *t*-test	One-way ANOVA → Post hoc tests (see Table 12.7)	Repeated-measures ANOVA (requires sphericity) → Post hoc tests	Pearson's correlation (When independent variables are present, multiple regression, logistic regression, and discriminant analysis)
		Two-way ANOVA, two-way repeated-measures ANOVA, Multifactorial analysis				

Meta-Analysis

16

Meta-analysis is a form of systematic review used to quantitatively integrate findings from multiple studies. Researchers identify all relevant research—published articles, theses, and unpublished studies—pertinent to a specific topic and apply statistical procedures to synthesize the results and present a collective conclusion. A systematic review is a structured process of integrating all available evidence with a clearly defined research objective. It uses a predetermined methodology for selecting studies (primary studies), setting inclusion and exclusion criteria, collecting data, and analyzing the results in an objective and reproducible manner. Systematic reviews are essential in evidence-based medicine (EBM), which combines the best available external evidence with clinical expertise to inform clinical decision-making. As a core component of EBM, systematic reviews guide treatment by summarizing the current state of research. To support this effort, clinicians and research methodology experts have formed an international network known as the Cochrane Collaboration, which continuously publishes up-to-date systematic reviews.

Systematic reviews help refine and summarize vast amounts of medical information, prevent redundant research efforts, and expedite the translation of findings into clinical practice. Furthermore, by aggregating data across multiple studies, they improve generalizability to broader patient populations and provide more robust conclusions about the effectiveness of specific interventions than single studies alone.

The databases and search tools commonly used in evidence-based medical decision-making are summarized in Tables 16.1 and 16.2.

Meta-analysis is a type of systematic review that presents results in numerical form. Its primary goal is to synthesize the findings of individual studies to determine the overall effectiveness of a treatment or intervention. Researchers often consider meta-analysis as a method to statistically integrate and summarize the outcomes of diverse, independently conducted prior studies on a specific topic. Although methods for statistical integration of research findings have a long history, the development of a formal theoretical framework has become more active since the 1970s. As the prefix "meta" implies—meaning "after"—meta-analysis refers to an "analysis of analyses," aiming to integrate accumulated research findings on a specific field or topic. By aggregating the results of multiple studies, meta-analysis enables the derivation of generalizable conclusions.

The key characteristics of meta-analysis are as follows:

1. Quantitative Approach: Meta-analysis adopts a quantitatively oriented approach.
2. Comprehensive Inclusion: It considers all relevant studies conducted within the target research domain.

K.-H. Yi, *Statistical Research Methods for Dermatologists and Plastic Surgeons*,
https://doi.org/10.1007/978-981-95-5668-7_16

Table 16.1 Databases and search tools used in evidence-based medicine

Feature	Evidence matters	Google Scholar	PubMed	Cochrane
Evidence-based focus	Yes	–	–	Yes
Update frequency	Daily	Daily	Daily	Every ≥2 years; new reviews quarterly
Structured clinical questions	Yes	–	–	–
Integrated real-time synthesis	Yes	–	–	–
Search result classification	By patient, age, sex, country, disease stage, study design, and study quality	Ranked by relevance	Chronologically	–
Standardized article summaries	Yes	–	–	–
Multilingual availability	Yes	–	–	–

http://www.evidencematters.com/emweb/

Table 16.2 Databases providing meta-analysis resources

Database	Web address
MEDLINE	http://www.ncbi.nlm.nih.gov/entrez/query.fcgi?db=PubMed
Cochrane library	http://www.thecochranelibrary.com/view/0/index.html
Evidence-based medicine reviews	http://www.ovid.com/site/catalog/DataBase/904.jsp

3. Systematic Generalization: It aims to comprehensively synthesize research outcomes to derive a general and structured conclusion about the research question.
4. Reproducibility and Objectivity: Meta-analysis is conducted systematically and can be replicated by other researchers. This reduces the subjective bias of the researcher conducting the synthesis and allows for re-evaluation by subsequent investigators.

Despite its widespread application across various academic fields, meta-analysis faces several limitations:

1. Validity Issues: Combining studies with different populations, experimental designs, and measurement scales may raise concerns about the validity of the synthesis.
2. Value-Based Concerns: It may indiscriminately integrate findings from both high-quality and low-quality studies without appropriate distinction.
3. File Drawer Problem: Studies that remain unpublished or are left in "file drawers" may be excluded from the analysis, potentially omitting significant findings due to the reliance on published literature alone.

Another major concern in meta-analysis is that the included studies may not adequately represent the entire population of completed studies on a given topic, which is generally referred to as publication bias. While commonly labeled as publication bias, a closer examination reveals that it encompasses several types of bias: language bias, in which only studies published in English are selectively included; availability bias, where researchers include studies that are more readily accessible; familiarity bias, in which studies from the researcher's own field are preferentially selected; outcome-reporting bias, in which only statistically significant results are reported; and cost bias, which refers to the inclusion of studies that are free or low-cost to access. Because of these various potential sources of bias, it is essential to assess for publication bias at the final stage of a meta-analysis [1].

Despite such criticisms and limitations, meta-analysis offers several advantages.

First, it enables a more systematic synthesis or overview of previous studies.

Second, by integrating multiple individual studies on the same topic, meta-analysis effectively increases the overall sample size of the study population, thereby enhancing statistical power and narrowing confidence intervals, which leads to improved precision in estimating treatment effects.

In the results of a meta-analysis, the *effect size* (ES or *d*) is often reported. The effect size is defined as the difference between the means of two groups (e.g., experimental and control groups) divided by the standard deviation of the control group (or the pooled standard deviation of both groups). The advantage of using effect size is that it provides a standardized statistical index that enables comparison across studies, even if different measurement scales have been used. The formula for calculating effect size is as follows:

$$Effect\ size\left(ES\right)=\frac{Mean\ of\ experimental\ group - Mean\ of\ control\ group}{Standard\ deviation\ of\ control\ group}$$

Through the effect size, it is possible to assess the magnitude of the difference between groups or the effectiveness of an intervention. An effect size of 0 indicates no treatment effect. According to Cohen's [2] criteria, an effect size of 0.8 or above is considered large, around 0.5 is considered moderate, and 0.2 or below is considered small. While the statistical significance of a research result informs us about the probability of the observed outcome occurring by chance, it does not provide meaningful information about the magnitude of the effect. Therefore, it is necessary to report the effect size in addition to statistical significance when presenting research findings.

Meta-analysis is typically conducted through the following five steps:

1. Formulating research questions.
2. Defining the target population and setting inclusion and exclusion criteria.
3. Conducting a literature search and selecting relevant studies, including the classification of study characteristics.
4. Assessing study quality and extracting data, including the calculation of effect sizes.
5. Performing statistical analysis and presenting the results.

Statistical methods commonly used in meta-analysis include:

1. The sign test.
2. Combination of p-values.
3. Combination of estimates of effect sizes.

In a study by Park and Shin [3], a meta-analysis was conducted to evaluate the effectiveness of fall prevention exercise programs on improving muscle strength in older adults in Korea. The overall effect size of the fall prevention programs collected from the included studies was 0.8, and the 95% confidence interval for the overall effect size ranged from 0.72 to 0.93, indicating a large effect.

A trial version of the meta-analysis software used in the study can be downloaded free of charge at http://www.meta-analysis.com/.

Examples of Meta-Analyses in the Fields of Cosmetic Dermatology and Plastic Surgery

1. de Araujo CM, Schroder AGD, de Araujo BMM, et al. Impact of orthodontic-surgical treatment on quality of life: a meta-analysis. *Eur J Orthod.* 2020;42(3):281–289.

2. Dreher R, Blaya C, Tenório JL, Saltz R, Ely PB, Ferrão YA. Quality of Life and Aesthetic Plastic Surgery: A Systematic Review and Meta-analysis.*Plast Reconstr Surg Glob Open.* 2016 Sep 15;4(9):e862.
3. Gallo L, Kim P, Churchill IF, et al. Measuring the Impact of Surgical and Non-surgical Facial Cosmetic Interventions Using FACE-Q Aesthetic Module Scales: A Systematic Review and Meta-Analysis. *Plast Surg (Oakv).* Published online January 23, 2024.
4. Jia Z, Lu H, Yang X, et al. Adverse Events of Botulinum Toxin Type A in Facial Rejuvenation: A Systematic Review and Meta-Analysis. *Aesthetic Plast Surg.* 2016;40(5):769–777.
5. Kucukguven A, Galandarova A, Bitik O. A Systematic Review and Meta-Analysis of Early Relapse After Facelift. *Aesthetic Plast Surg.* 2023;47(1):144–155.
6. Oliver JD, Eells AC, Saba ES, et al. Alloplastic Facial Implants: A Systematic Review and Meta-Analysis on Outcomes and Uses in Aesthetic and Reconstructive Plastic Surgery. *Aesthetic Plast Surg.* 2019;43(3):625–636.
7. Pour Mohammad A, Gholizadeh Mesgarha M, Seirafianpour F, et al. A systematic review and meta-analysis of efficacy, safety, and satisfaction rates of laser combination treatments vs laser monotherapy in skin rejuvenation resurfacing. *Lasers Med Sci.* 2023;38(1):228. Published 2023 Sep 30.
8. Rahman E, Rao P, Philipp-Dormston W, et al. Intradermal Botulinum Toxin A on Skin Quality and Facial Rejuvenation: A Systematic Review and Meta-analysis. *Plast Reconstr Surg Glob Open.* 2024;12(8):e6084. Published 2024 Aug 23.
9. Santos S, Almeida I, Oliveiros B, Castelo-Branco M. The Role of the Amygdala in Facial Trustworthiness Processing: A Systematic Review and Meta-Analyses of fMRI Studies. *PLoS One.* 2016;11(11):e0167276. Published 2016 Nov 29.
10. Seirafianpour F, Pour Mohammad A, Moradi Y, et al. Systematic review and meta-analysis of randomized clinical trials comparing efficacy, safety, and satisfaction between ablative and non-ablative lasers in facial and hand rejuvenation/resurfacing. *Lasers Med Sci.* 2022;37(4):2111–2122.

Bibliography

1. Jin ZC, Zhou XH, He J. Statistical methods for dealing with publication bias in meta-analysis. Stat Med. 2015;34(2):343–360. https://doi.org/10.1002/sim.6342.
2. Cohen J. Statistical power analysis for the behavioral sciences. 2nd ed. Hillsdale (NJ): Lawrence Erlbaum Associates; 1988.
3. Park S, Shin I. Effects of Fall Prevention Exercise Programs on Muscle Strength in Korean Older Adults: A Meta-Analysis. Journal of Korean Academy of Physical Therapy Science. 2011;18(3):38–48.
4. Song H. Meta-Analysis Method. Jayu Academy; 1992.
5. Oh S. Theory and Practice of Meta-Analysis. Konkuk University Press; 2009.
6. Borenstein M, Hedges LV, Higgins JPT, et al. Introduction to Meta-Analysis. UK, John Wiley & Sons, Ltd, 2009.
7. Glase GV. Integrating findings: the meta analysis of research. Review of Research in Education. 1977;5:351–379.

Rasch Analysis

17

Rasch analysis was developed in 1953 by the Danish mathematician Georg Rasch. Most of the assessment tools used in the field of cosmetic dermatology and aesthetic medicine are scored using ordinal scales, and total scores are typically calculated. For example, to assess the level of difficulty experienced during the recovery period after a cosmetic skin procedure, the items shown in Table 17.1 might be included in a questionnaire.

If a patient is able to independently perform all three tasks-cleansing the face, applying sunscreen, and attending follow-up appointments, then the total score would be 9 points. However, if the patient experiences substantial difficulty with all of these activities, the total score would be 3 points. For this total score to be meaningful, three conditions must be met. First, the items must measure a unidimensional concept. Second, each item must be arranged in order of increasing difficulty. That is, all items comprising the assessment tool should be sequenced from easier to more difficult, allowing the tool to consistently measure how much of a particular trait (e.g., recovery-related functional capacity) is reflected in each respondent. The difficulty of each item should apply equally to all individuals. Therefore, if the scale is well constructed, "cleansing the face" should consistently be easier than "applying sunscreen," and "applying sunscreen" should be easier than "attending follow-up appointments" across all patients. Third, the scale should be able to measure changes that occur both within an individual and between individuals. A tool developed using ordinal scales has limitations in sensitivity and precision. For instance, a patient may experience meaningful improvement in their ability to attend follow-up appointments, but such progress might not be enough to be recognized as a higher functional level under the original scoring system. For example, if a patient initially scored as "requiring assistance" for attending appointments and, after two weeks of recovery and supportive care, improved but still did not reach full independence, the score would remain the same. Therefore, to capture such

Table 17.1 Degree of difficulty in performing daily activities during recovery after facial cosmetic procedures

	Very difficult to perform independently (1 point)	Slightly difficult to perform independently (2 points)	Able to perform independently (3 points)
Washing the face	○	○	○
Applying sunscreen	○	○	○
Visiting a clinic for follow-up	○	○	○

K.-H. Yi, *Statistical Research Methods for Dermatologists and Plastic Surgeons*, https://doi.org/10.1007/978-981-95-5668-7_17

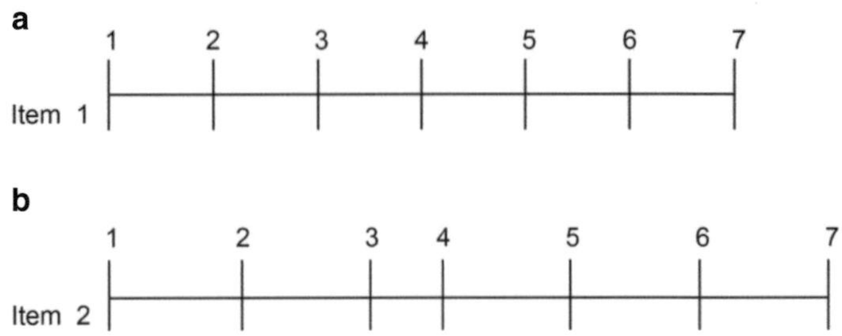

Fig. 17.1 Ordinal nature of raw scores (**a**: equal intervals, **b**: unequal intervals)

incremental changes, the scale should ideally be constructed using equal-interval levels.

One effective way to address this issue is by applying Rasch analysis to convert ordinal scales into interval scales. The Xerosis Severity Scale (XSS) is a widely used tool in dermatology to assess the severity of skin dryness (xerosis), particularly in patients undergoing treatments that compromise the skin barrier, such as chemical peels, laser resurfacing, or retinoid therapy. The XSS consists of multiple items designed to evaluate observable characteristics such as scaling, roughness, redness, and fissures across different body sites. Each item on the XSS is rated on an ordinal scale, typically from 0 (no xerosis) to 6 (severe xerosis). A higher score indicates more pronounced symptoms of skin dryness.

The total score, obtained by summing across all items, is often used as a representative measure of the patient's overall skin condition or treatment response. However, summing raw scores across ordinal items in this way is statistically problematic. While the numerical difference between a score of 3 and 4 may appear equal to that between 4 and 5, we cannot assume that these differences reflect equivalent changes in the actual severity of xerosis. Because ordinal scales like the XSS do not have equal intervals between score levels, adding, subtracting, or multiplying raw scores is not logically appropriate (see Fig. 17.1).

Thus, the degree of skin dryness indicated by a score of 5 on one item is not necessarily equivalent to a score of 5 on another. Consequently, any conclusions or inferences derived from the total raw score may be misleading.

In order to produce meaningful and interpretable results, it is necessary to transform ordinal scores into interval-level data. This transformation is achieved through Rasch modeling, which converts ordinal scores into logit scores. Logit scores represent measurements on an interval scale, where the distance between each score level is uniform across all items. This allows for valid arithmetic operations and supports more accurate and objective interpretation of results. When using measurement tools based on ordinal scales, such as the XSS, researchers and clinicians must remain cautious of the limitations inherent in raw score interpretation.

17.1 Rasch Model

Figure 17.2 illustrates the items within the skin maintenance domain, arranged in order of functional level (i.e., item difficulty). Items representing lower levels of ability (easier tasks) are located at the bottom of the vertical line, while more difficult items are positioned at the top. When conducting Rasch analysis using computer software such as Rasch Unidimensional Measurement Models (RUMM2030) or WINSTEPS, the relative difficulty of each item can be determined and visually mapped onto a single continuum. Rasch analysis examines how each individual responds to each item and estimates their ability level. It also evaluates whether the data conform to a unidimensional model appropriate for assessing skin maintenance capabilities. Based on these response patterns, Rasch analysis provides a continuous scale on which each individual's ability can be placed-ranging from low to high levels of skin maintenance proficiency.

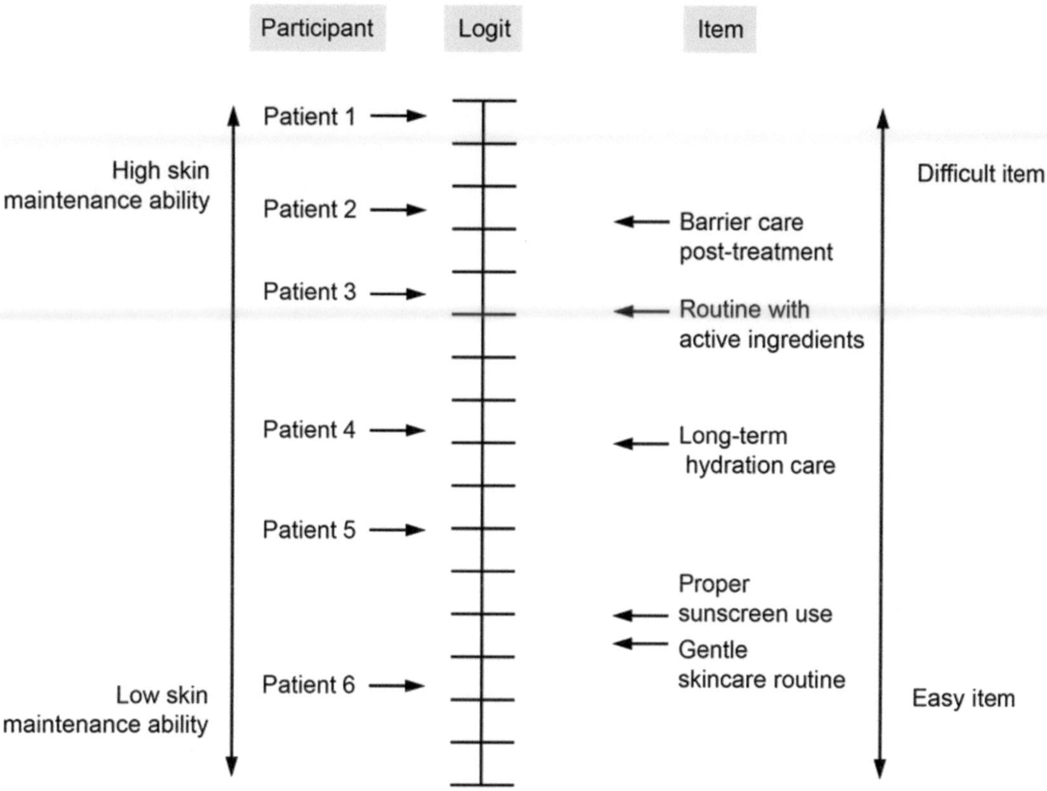

Fig. 17.2 Example output of Rasch analysis: locations of skin maintenance items and patient abilities (hypothetical data)

Figure 17.2 presents the Rasch analysis results for five representative items in the skin maintenance domain. Two key features are depicted: on the right, the items are ordered by increasing difficulty, and on the left, individuals are positioned based on their ability levels. The more difficult an item is, the higher its logit score. Individuals capable of performing more challenging tasks are plotted higher along the vertical line, indicating superior skin maintenance ability and greater independence in managing post-treatment care. In contrast, individuals with lower levels of ability are positioned toward the bottom of the continuum, as they are only able to perform the easier items, which are associated with lower logit scores. For example, in Fig. 17.2, Individual 5 can only complete the items gentle skincare routine and proper sunscreen use, while Individuals 1 and 2 demonstrate the ability to perform all five tasks, including more advanced routines such as barrier care post-treatment and routine with active ingredients.

When a measurement instrument is designed to assess a single functional construct, such as skin maintenance ability, it must satisfy three fundamental measurement principles. First, the total score must reflect the underlying functional level that each item is intended to measure. Second, the items must be arranged in order of increasing difficulty, based on the level of skill or independence required. Third, the hierarchy of item difficulty must remain invariant across individuals. That is, the relative difficulty order should not differ from one individual to another. For example, if the items barrier care post-treatment, routine with active ingredients, long-term hydration care, proper sunscreen use, and gentle skincare routine are ordered from most to least difficult for one person, this order must remain consistent for all individuals. The difficulty sequence should not vary such that another person finds long-term hydration care harder than barrier care post-treatment or considers proper sunscreen use to be the most difficult.

Rasch analysis ensures that the item difficulties and individual ability levels are estimated through a mathematical process known as maximum likelihood estimation. This estimation not only indicates where each individual falls along the ability continuum, but also expresses the difficulty level of each item on an interval scale. Moreover, the Rasch model provides information about item fit-that is, how well each item conforms to the assumptions of a cumulative scale. Through this process, items that do not align well with the overall scale can be identified and potentially removed.

17.2 Measurement Criteria

To determine whether a given dataset is suitable for Rasch modeling, several measurement criteria are employed. The first of these is item difficulty, which refers to the location of each item along a hierarchical scale, expressed in units of logits (log-odds units). In Rasch measurement, odds refer to the probability of successfully completing (or passing) an item divided by the probability of failing it. Taking the natural logarithm (base e, where $e = 2.7183$) of this odds ratio yields the log-odds, or logit score. The logit thus expresses the odds of success versus failure in responding to a test item. For example, an odds ratio of 1:1 results in a logit score of 0, since $\ln(1) = 0$.

The logit scale is centered at 0, with values extending in both positive and negative directions. Items are arranged along this scale according to their difficulty level: more difficult items are associated with higher logits, while easier items have lower logits. Likewise, individuals with higher skin maintenance ability are more likely to pass more difficult items. Importantly, item difficulty is not limited to a simple rank order; it also allows us to quantify the magnitude of difference between items. Ideally, the items are spaced at equal intervals along a continuous scale, forming an interval-level measurement. For instance, a difference of 0.693 logits implies that the odds of success on a particular item are twice as high as those for another item, since $e^{0.693} \approx 2.0$. This log-odds scale possesses two important statistical properties: linearity and equal interval spacing, which together provide an additive structure suitable for quantitative interpretation. As shown in Table 17.2 and Fig. 17.2, the five items within the skin maintenance domain—namely barrier care post-treatment, routine with active ingredients, long-term hydration care, proper sunscreen use, and gentle skincare routine—are appropriately ordered along the logit scale, ranging from −0.43 to +0.52 logits. The most difficult item is barrier care post-treatment, while the easiest is gentle skincare routine.

Item fit refers to the degree to which each item conforms to a unidimensional model—a model based on the assumption that all items measure a single underlying ability or trait. Person fit, on the other hand, reflects how well an individual's pattern of responses aligns with the assumptions of the unidimensional model. In a well-structured assessment, individuals with higher skin care ability would be expected to succeed on more difficult items (e.g., barrier care post-treatment), while those with lower ability would tend to succeed only on easier tasks (e.g., gentle skincare routine). Accordingly, individuals with high ability should be located toward the upper end of the logit scale, whereas those with low ability should appear near the lower end.

Rasch analysis builds a probabilistic model that predicts the likelihood of a person succeeding on each item based on their estimated ability and the item's difficulty. If an item or person displays response patterns that deviate significantly

Table 17.2 Results of Rasch analysis for skin maintenance items (hypothetical data)

Item	Logit
Barrier care post-treatment	0.52
Routine with active ingredients	0.31
Long-term hydration care	0.00
Proper sunscreen use	−0.41
Gentle skincare routine	−0.43

from these predictions, it is considered a misfit. For instance, suppose Rasch analysis is applied to a 30-item assessment that combines items related to post-treatment care protocols and daily skincare adherence. If many items appear misfitting, this may indicate that individuals with high ability are not consistently passing the more difficult items, or that easier items are unexpectedly being failed. This suggests the two item clusters may not reflect a single construct and should be analyzed separately.

Fit statistics are calculated for each item to evaluate how well it aligns with the hierarchical structure. The most commonly used index is the Mean Square Residual (MNSQ), which measures the discrepancy between observed scores and scores expected by the model. An MNSQ of 1.0 indicates a perfect fit—i.e., observed performance matches the model's expectations. Larger MNSQ values signify greater deviation, suggesting that item difficulty was not applied consistently across individuals. Although misfitting items or persons may be statistically excluded, it is more appropriate to view fit statistics as diagnostic tools. In the case of item misfit, poor wording or ambiguity may be the issue; in such cases, rephrasing or reconstructing the item is recommended. If a person shows misfit, a closer examination of their characteristics is warranted. For example, in aesthetic dermatology studies, patients undergoing ablative laser treatment versus those treated with nonablative modalities may exhibit different skin recovery patterns even when responding to the same items. If such heterogeneous groups are combined, their differing recovery trajectories might distort fit statistics. Therefore, identifying and understanding sources of misfit is essential for maintaining the validity of the measurement instrument.

Item Response Theory (IRT) provides a framework that addresses the limitations inherent in Classical Test Theory (CTT). While IRT includes several models, such as the one-parameter model (1PL), two-parameter model (2PL), and three-parameter model (3PL), the Rasch model corresponds to the one-parameter model, focusing solely on item difficulty. When the Rasch model is applied, it offers several advantages over CTT. For instance, it enables the identification of items with either excessively high or low discriminative power using infit (information-weighted fit statistic) and outfit (outlier-sensitive fit statistic), which are unaffected by the distribution of respondent ability. The model also provides measures of item reliability and person reliability, independent of one another. Additionally, Rasch analysis supports the validation of item ordering, response category structure, and the fit of each item and respondent to the underlying latent construct being measured. By examining person fit statistics, we can assess whether respondents answered in a consistent and interpretable manner. Similarly, category fit statistics help determine whether respondents used rating categories in the way that researchers intended. When items or respondents are flagged as misfitting, removing them from the analysis and re-estimating the model typically improves overall measurement quality (Hong 1999).

Before applying the Rasch model, unidimensionality must be established. This is typically done through factor analysis, which identifies whether items cluster around a single latent trait. If the number of items is small and inter-factor correlations are high, the dataset may still be treated as unidimensional and thus suitable for Rasch modeling. When choosing between more complex models, such as the Partial Credit Model (PCM), and simpler alternatives like the Rating Scale Model (RSM), it is often reasonable to use the RSM if both models yield similar reliability indices. In RSM, the expected value of both infit and outfit MNSQ (mean square residual) is 1.0, indicating a perfect model-data fit. In standardized multiple-choice assessments, an infit MNSQ value below 0.7 or above 1.3 is typically considered misfitting. For instance, an infit MNSQ of 1.3 suggests that the observed responses deviate by 30% from what the Rasch model predicts. Outfit, which can be adversely affected by one or two extreme responses, and infit, which was developed to compensate for this limitation, should both be examined.

Infit indicates how well an item measures individuals whose ability is close to the item's difficulty level. Outfit indicates how well an item measures individuals whose ability is much higher or lower than the item's difficulty level. For example, when assessing a barrier care post-treatment item, infit would indicate how well the item measures individuals whose skin maintenance ability closely matches the difficulty of the task. Outfit, on the other hand, reflects how well the item performs when administered to individuals whose ability is either far below (e.g., only able to perform gentle skincare routine) or far above (e.g., beyond the scope of standard routines) the expected level. Additionally, the ZSTD (standardized mean square residual) converts MNSQ to a standardized metric with a mean of 0 and standard deviation of 1; values of 2.0 or greater are typically regarded as problematic. In survey-based research or instruments using Likert-type scales, a misfitting item is generally defined as one with an MNSQ below 0.6 or above 1.4 and a Z-value beyond ±2.0. According to the Winsteps software, values between 0.5 and 1.5 are considered to support productive measurement. Similarly, a misfitting person is typically flagged when the person's infit MNSQ lies outside the range of acceptable variation ($Z < -2$ or $Z > +2$), indicating inconsistency or unexpected response behavior.

Person reliability refers to the extent to which individuals can consistently distinguish between items based on their relative difficulty. A person reliability index below 0.8 may indicate that the responses were inconsistent or lacked discernment. Item reliability, on the other hand, reflects how well the items distinguish among individuals with varying levels of the underlying trait—such as skin maintenance ability. Like Cronbach's alpha, a value above 0.8 is generally considered acceptable. Item separation refers to how well the items are distributed across different ability levels based on participants' responses. The separation index serves as a relative metric to compare the spread of item difficulty, particularly when item reliability is similar across the scale. Ideally, Rasch analysis should yield a spread of items that represent at least low, medium, and high difficulty levels. Statistically, item distribution is related to measurement error and overall reliability: higher reliability implies that item or person scores more accurately reflect their true values.

The many-faceted Rasch model is an extension of the one-parameter model based on Item Response Theory, and it provides a framework for quantifying item difficulty, person ability, and rater leniency on the same linear scale. Analysis using the many-faceted Rasch model not only statistically recalibrates raw scores to provide fairer evaluation results but also supplies data that allow for a detailed examination of the validity and reliability of each facet. This model presents fit statistics and standard errors for rater variables, respondent variables, and item variables, thereby enabling verification of the internal validity and reliability of each variable.

Linacre (1993) extended the basic Rasch model-within Item Response Theory-that estimates a person's task performance probabilistically based only on person ability and item difficulty, by incorporating rater severity into the original equation. In doing so, he developed the many-faceted Rasch model, which allows for the estimation of person ability parameters while accounting for the rater's level of stringency. Whereas the rating scale model (Andrich 1978) and the partial credit model (Masters 1982), which are applicable to polytomous response formats, are concerned only with person ability and item difficulty, the many-faceted Rasch model further includes the rater (judge, rater, grader) as an additional facet of interest. The key feature of this model is the inclusion of a parameter representing judge severity. To apply the many-faceted Rasch model, the FACETS program (Linacre, 1988) was developed. This program provides information on item fit statistics, differences in rater severity, and enables the estimation of each individual respondent's ability.

The issue of inter-rater reliability can be explained through the reliability for separation provided by the FACETS program. This separation reliability indicates the degree to which differences among raters can be distinguished, and it provides a chi-square (χ^2) test result, allowing for verification of statistical significance. A high rater separation reliability suggests meaningful differences in severity between evaluators, while (1—separation reliability) can be interpreted as the degree of agreement among raters. Rater fit indices are also provided in FACETS. In general, a fit index between 0.6 and 1.5 is considered to indicate valid and trustworthy scoring. A fit index above 1.5 suggests that a rater may have been overly lenient or severe, whereas a value below 0.6 may indicate that the rater gave nearly identical ratings across all subjects.

In the MFRM, higher positive logit values correspond to higher person ability, more lenient raters, and more difficult items. Conversely, lower logits represent lower ability, stricter raters, or easier items. To determine whether the items effectively distinguish between individuals of different ability levels (person separation index), whether raters effectively distinguish between items of varying difficulty levels (item separation index), and whether raters effectively distinguish between individuals of different ability levels (rater separation index), the reliability of the separation statistic is examined. The reliability of separation indices is conceptually similar to reliability coefficients in Classical Test Theory, as they represent the proportion of observed score variance that can be attributed to true variance. A high separation reliability score for items implies that there are systematic differences in item difficulty, while a high rater separation score indicates systematic differences in rater severity.

17.3 Examples of Rasch Analysis Applications

Preparing the Data File

The following data were collected from 206 patients who underwent cosmetic skin procedures affecting the skin barrier, such as chemical peels, laser resurfacing, or topical retinoid treatment. Their skin recovery was assessed using the Xerosis Severity Scale (XSS), a clinical tool designed to evaluate post-treatment xerosis. The XSS consists of 88 items divided into five domains: barrier care post-treatment (17 items), routine with active ingredients (20 items), long-term hydration care (14 items), proper sunscreen use (13 items), and gentle skincare routine (24 items). Each item is scored on a 4-point ordinal scale: 0 = no signs, 1 = mild (less than 10% of area affected), 2 = moderate (10% to less than 100%), 3 = severe (fully present or widespread involvement).

Example of a Data File

```
001 33322323332233333200223021100З
0000000999999999999999 ...omitted... 0
002 33333333332333333332333333312
3332333223333333231023 ................ 9
003 33333333333333333333333333333
3333333233333333321113 ................ 0
004 33311333333233333323333331333
1332220032232222000000 ................ 0

        :
        :omitted
        :

204 33111103310003300100110000000
0000000000000000000000 ................ 0
205 33333333332333333333333333333
3333333232322339922213З ................ 2
206 33133333310001200111210000000
0000000000000000000000 ................ 0
```

*Responses in the data file should be recorded using the values "0," "1," "2," and "3." Any other numeric entry is treated as a missing value. Both the data file and the control file must be saved as text files in ANSI format. If the files are saved in Unicode format, the Rasch analysis software may not read the data correctly. When exporting a text file from Excel, it is recommended to save it as a.csv file. If using a text editor such as UltraEdit, the file should be saved as a plain text file in ANSI/ASCII format using the "Save As" function

Creating the Control File

The following is an example of a control file created for Rasch analysis using the data file "XSS2025.txt".

```
TITLE = "Skin Recovery Function
Measure 2025" ← Title displayed in
the analysis output
CODES = 0123 ← Valid numeric codes
used in the data
NI = 88 ← Number of items
NAME1 = 1 ← Column number where the
person label begins
NAMELEN = 3 ← Length of the person
label in the output
ITEM1 = 5 ← First item starts in
column 5 of the data file
DATA = C:\XSS2025.txt ← Name and
location of the data file
&END ← End of basic control settings

1 RED; erythema visibly reduced ← The
name of item 1 to be analyzed
2 RED; skin coolness maintained ← The
name of item 2 to be analyzed
3 RED; stinging or burning sensation
resolved
4 RED; post-inflammatory redness
improved
...
84 ADH; consistently uses moisturizer
as directed
85 ADH; applies sunscreen every
morning
86 ADH; follows evening cleansing
protocol
87 ADH; keeps all scheduled follow-up
visits
88 ADH; independently manages daily
skincare ← The name of item 88 to be
analyzed
END NAMES ← End of item name list
```

A more detailed control file may be constructed as follows:

```
&INST
TITLE = "XSS Extended 2025"
PERSON = Person ; persons are ...
ITEM = Item ; items are ...
ITEM1 = 5 ; column of response to first
item
NI = 13 ; number of items
NAME1 = 1 ; column of first character
of person label
NAMELEN = 4 ; length of person label
XWIDE = 1 ; number of columns per item
response
CODES = 0123 ; valid response codes
UIMEAN = 50 ; item mean for local
origin
USCALE = 10 ; user-defined scaling for
logits
UDECIM = 2 ; number of decimal places
to report
PDFILE = *
7
12
14
22
26
33
36
37
41
49
53
54
58
71
72
80
81
```

```
89
94
104
106
107
141
144
150
151
161
168
217
242
259
263
*
DIF = *
$S1W1 ; start in person label column 2
with a width of 1 ? Clinic location
$S2W1 ; start in person label column 3
with a width of 1 Gender
$S3W1 ; start in person label column 4
with a width of 1? Age group: 1 =
under 40s, 2 = 50s, 3 = 60s, 4 = 70s,
5 = 80s
$S4W1 ; start in person label column 5
with a width of 1 ? Number of
treatment sessions
*
;IDFILE-*
;3
;7
;*
&END

1
2
3
4
5
6
7
8
9
10
11
12
13
END LABELS

12424433444344334
12524444444334334
12424423222323223
12404434332223233
12414443342323333
11514434444443333
12414432443333333
12514433343342223
11424434443433333
41502242432223223
... (omitted) ...
41414432232243322
42403322322222222
42324422442233222
42314431241123113
42414421121122112
42424422422222222
42414431312223323
42424421441122222
42423321232232222
```

Example of Output Tables

Table Ordered by Item Difficulty

Table 17.3 presents the items ordered by difficulty level. In this table, entry number refers to the item number, measure indicates the item's

Table 17.3 Winsteps output: items ordered by difficulty

TABLE 13.1 XSS 2025 ZOU295WS.TXT Jan 16 16:332012
INPUT: 206 PERSON 88 ITEM REPORTED: 206 PERSON 88 ITEM 4 CATS WINSTEPS 3.71.0.1

PERSON: REAL SEP.: 10.93 REL.: 0.99 ... ITEM: REAL SEP.: 17.52 REL.: 1.00
ITEM STATISTICS: MEASURE ORDER

Entry	Total	Total		Model	Infit		Outfit		PT-Measure		Exact	Match
Number	Score	Count	Measure	S.E.	MNSQ	ZSTD	MNSQ	ZSTD	CORR.	EXP.	OBS%	EXP%
82[a]	32	203	4.88	0.19	1.03	0.2	0.64	−0.5	0.45	0.45	91.1	90.1
83	35	203	4.78	0.18	1.11	0.5	1.07	0.3	0.46	0.47	93.1	90.1
80	50	203	4.35	0.16	0.35	−4.3	0.10	−2.5	0.62	0.53	92.6	85.7
88	64	203	3.98	0.15	0.78	−1.2	0.26	−1.7	0.59	0.58	87.2	85.1
81	67	203	3.95	0.15	0.71	−1.6	0.36	−1.3	0.61	0.59	88.7	84.5
⋮												
8	562	204	−3.71	0.15	1.00	0.1	9.90	8.7	0.48	0.52	85.3	85.0
22	568	206	−3.75	0.15	0.70	−1.7	0.26	−1.6	0.55	0.51	86.4	84.6
10	573	205	−3.94	0.16	0.99	0.0	9.46	5.6	0.45	0.48	87.8	85.9
1	582	206	−4.11	0.17	0.90	−0.4	1.08	0.3	0.45	0.45	87.9	87.2
21	588	206	−4.30	0.18	0.94	−0.2	0.24	−1.07	0.44	0.42	90.3	88.8
MEAN	325.8	203.3	0.00	0.13	0.98	−0.3	1.59	−0.2			79.9	78.5
S.D.	160.8	1.9	2.41	0.02	0.35	1.9	2.28	2.4			5.5	4.1

[a]This table shows the item numbers from the Xerosis severity scale(XSS)

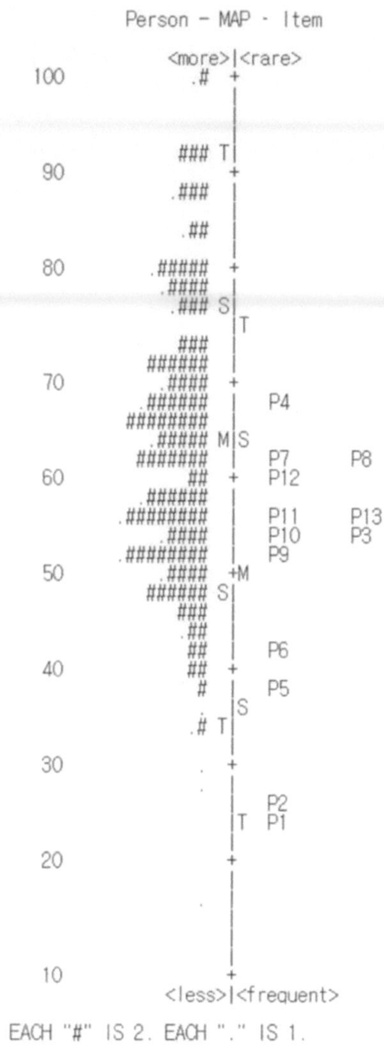

Fig. 17.3 Person-item map displaying the distribution of 238 participants and 13 items from a Rasch analysis output. *Person-item map displaying the distribution of 238 participants and 13 items

estimated difficulty, infit MNSQ represents the infit mean square statistic, and outfit MNSQ represents the outfit mean square statistic

The figure below is an example of output generated using a different dataset (Figs. 17.3 and 17.4).

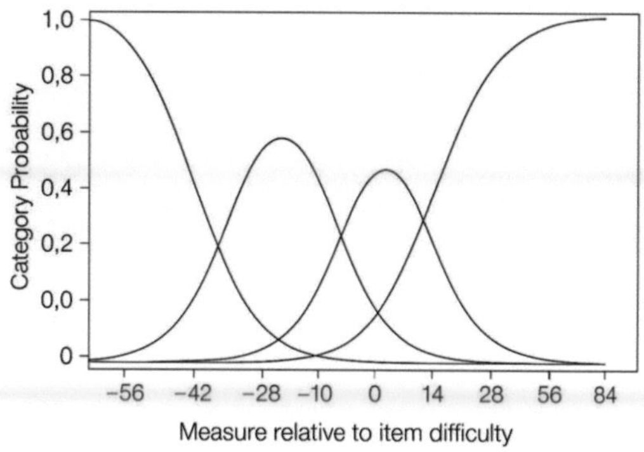

Fig. 17.4 Category probability curves showing the relationship between measure relative to item difficulty (X-axis) and category probability (Y-axis)

Bibliography

Andrich D. A rating formulation for ordered response categories. Psychometrika. 1978;43:561–573. https://doi.org/10.1007/BF02293814.

He Z, Lo Martire R, Lu C, et al. Rasch Analysis of the Dermatology Life Quality Index Reveals Limited Application to Chinese Patients with Skin Disease. *Acta Derm Venereol.* 2018;98(1):59–64.

Hong, S. H. Scale development and validation using item response theory and factor analysis. *Proceedings of the 3rd Workshop of the Korean Society of Clinical Psychology.* 1999.

Linacre JM. Facets Rasch analysis computer program. Chicago (IL): MESA Press; 1988.

Linacre JM. Generalizability theory and many-facet Rasch measurement. Paper presented at: Annual Meeting of the American Educational Research Association (AERA); 1993 Apr 12–16; Atlanta, GA. (ERIC Document No. ED364573).

Liu Y, Li T, An J, et al. Rasch analysis holds no brief for the use of the Dermatology Life Quality Index (DLQI) in Chinese neurodermatitis patients. *Health Qual Life Outcomes.* 2016;14:17.

Masters GN. A Rasch model for partial credit scoring. Psychometrika. 1982;47:149–174. https://doi.org/10.1007/BF02296272.

Rencz F, Mitev AZ, Szabó Á, et al. A Rasch model analysis of two interpretations of 'not relevant' responses on the Dermatology Life Quality Index (DLQI). *Qual Life Res.* 2021;30(8):2375–2386.

Sanclemente G, Mora-Gaviria C, Aguirre-Acevedo DC. Rasch Analysis of the Dermatology Life Quality Index. *Actas Dermosifiliogr.* 2025;116(4):349–356.

18 Methods of Evaluating Reliability

18.1 Standard Error of Measurement and Minimal Detectable Change

Each observed value is composed of the true score and measurement error. Measurement error can arise from the process of measurement itself or from factors such as carelessness, fatigue, or imprecision. When using measurement instruments or outcome measures, various sources of error can be introduced. While some sources of error, such as unclear instructions or ambiguous scoring criteria, can often be addressed during the tool's development or design phase, observed values will inevitably contain uncontrollable measurement error. Reliability should not be understood as a binary concept (i.e., present or absent), but rather as a continuum. Thus, it is more appropriate to describe reliability as "low" or "high" depending on where it falls along this continuum.

Reliability can be divided into two types: relative reliability and absolute reliability. Relative reliability includes inter-rater reliability, intra-rater reliability, and internal consistency. Absolute reliability is represented by the Standard Error of Measurement (SEM) and is expressed using the same units as the original measurement scale.

Table 18.1 summarizes these aspects of reliability.

The Standard Error of Measurement (SEM) is a method of assessing response stability as an indicator of reliability. SEM estimates the standard error of a series of repeatedly measured scores. There are multiple formulas for calculating SEM; one common approach is as follows:

Table 18.1 Summary of reliability in measurement

Type	Definition	Meaning	Statistical indicators
Relative reliability (inter–/intra-rater)	Agreement between raters or over two time points	Reflects the degree of random error present in the items of an assessment tool	Bland–Altman method, % agreement, kappa coefficient, weighted kappa, intra-class correlation coefficient
Absolute reliability	Reliability expressed in the original measurement unit	Indicates the degree of change that exceeds measurement error	Minimal detectable change at 90% or 95% confidence level
Internal consistency	Consistency of measurements taken at the same point in time	Degree of homogeneity among items within the instrument	Cronbach's alpha coefficient

K.-H. Yi, *Statistical Research Methods for Dermatologists and Plastic Surgeons*,
https://doi.org/10.1007/978-981-95-5668-7_18

$$\text{SEM} = \text{standard deviation of the values at the first time point} \times \sqrt{1 - \text{ICC}}$$

ICC: Intraclass Correlation Coefficient

Interpretation of SEM implies that there is a 68% probability that the true value lies within ±1 SEM around the observed value.

Various formulas used to calculate SEM are presented in Table 18.2.

SEM is also used to calculate the Minimal Detectable Change (MDC). MDC refers to the smallest score change that can be interpreted as a true change in the individual, rather than a fluctuation due to measurement error. The MDC is commonly reported at 90% or 95% confidence levels. To estimate the MDC, measurements must be taken at two different time points, and these time points should be close enough that the subject's actual performance is assumed to remain unchanged. This ensures that any detected change reflects measurement error alone and not real clinical change.

The Minimal Detectable Change (MDC) is a statistically estimated value representing the smallest amount of change that can be detected by a measurement instrument when a real and meaningful change in the individual has occurred. It reflects the minimal score change that can be interpreted as a true change, rather than one attributable to measurement error.

The MDC is often calculated at a 95% confidence level using the following formula:

$$\text{MDC}_{95} = 1.96 \times \text{SEM} \times \sqrt{2}$$

For example, in the FACE-Q Aesthetic Module, the reported MDC_{95}(individual-level smallest detectable change) ranged from 9.34 to 32.91 points, while the MDC_{95}(group-level smallest detectable change) ranged from 0.95 to 3.23 points. It is important to note that the MDC may vary across score ranges, depending on the total score obtained by the subject.

Additionally, the Minimally Clinically Important Difference (MCID) refers to the smallest change in score that is perceived as important by either the patient or the clinician.

18.2 Pearson Correlation Coefficient and Intraclass Correlation Coefficient

There are several methods for assessing reliability, including test–retest reliability, inter-rater reliability, parallel-forms reliability, the Pearson product-moment correlation coefficient, the Spearman rank correlation coefficient, and internal consistency.

These correlation coefficients reflect either the covariance or the rank-order relationships within the data. A high correlation coefficient is often interpreted as an indicator of high reliability. However, there are several limitations to this

Table 18.2 Methods for calculating the standard error of measurement (SEM)

Method	Design	Outcome	Formula
Method 1	Measurement at two time points, assuming equal variances across both	Standard deviation (SD), Pearson correlation coefficient (r)	$s\sqrt{1-r}$
Method 2A	Measurement at two time points	Relative reliability is estimated using one-way ANOVA, with within-subject mean squares	$\sqrt{\text{MSW}}$
Method 2B	Measurement at two time points with a randomized block design	Relative reliability is estimated using one-way ANOVA, with mean square error from the ANOVA table	$\sqrt{\text{MSE}}$
Method 3	Measurement at two time points	Standard deviation (SD) of the difference scores is estimated	$\text{SD}/\sqrt{2}$

approach. First, a correlation coefficient does not represent agreement. Second, the Pearson correlation coefficient only captures the linear relationship between two variables and cannot represent multivariate relationships. Third, the Pearson correlation includes variance caused by error, and therefore cannot be considered a pure estimate of reliability. In other words, it does not reflect a true reliability coefficient that accounts for measurement error.

In fact, instead of interpreting the raw correlation coefficient (*r*), it is often more meaningful to use the coefficient of determination (r^2). For example, if $r = 0.66$, then $r^2 = 0.43$, which indicates that 43% of the variance in one measurement can be explained by the variance in the second measurement.

As noted earlier, the Pearson correlation reflects the degree to which two sets of scores vary together, not how closely they agree. Despite its frequent use in reliability studies, its interpretation must be approached with caution. The following section describes how to calculate reliability (*r*) using the Pearson correlation coefficient in SPSS (Fig. 18.1).

In SPSS, click on Analyze → Correlate → Bivariate (Fig. 18.2).

Move the variables for Rater 1 and Rater 2 into the Variables box (Fig. 18.3).

Click OK to run the analysis (Fig. 18.4).

The following output will appear (Fig. 18.5).

When using the Pearson correlation coefficient, if the two groups differ substantially in means or standard deviations, the resulting correlation coefficient (r) merely reflects the degree to which the two sets of scores vary in the same direction. It does not indicate how closely the scores actually agree (see Table 18.3 and Fig. 18.6). To address this limitation, one

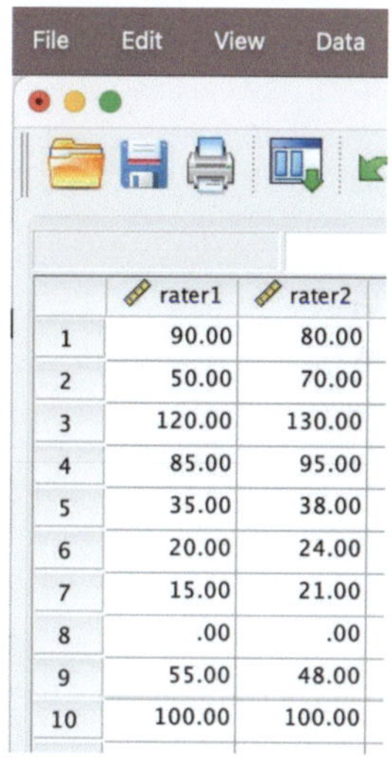

Fig. 18.1 Example dataset used to compute the Pearson Correlation Coefficient in SPSS

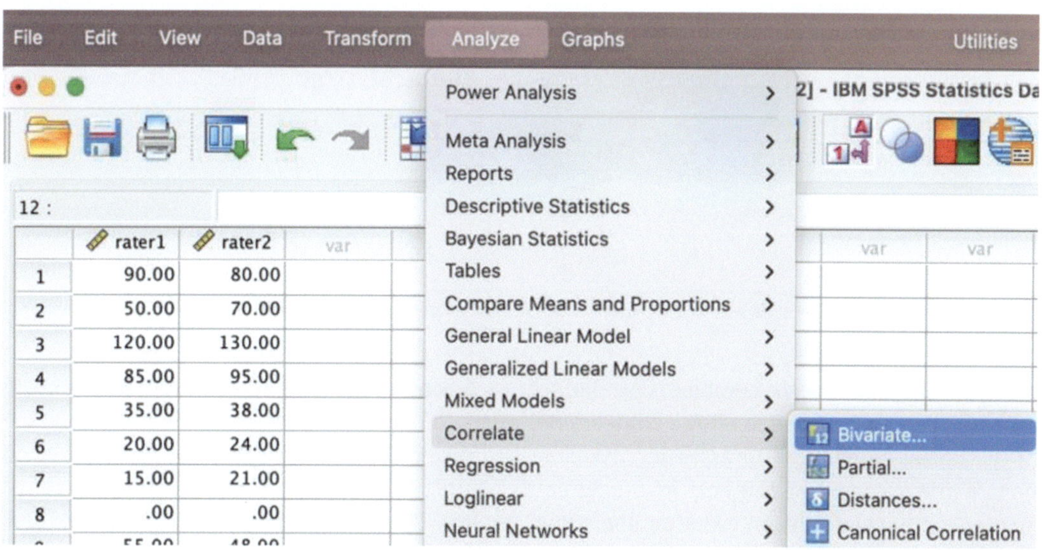

Fig. 18.2 Menu path in SPSS to access Pearson correlation analysis

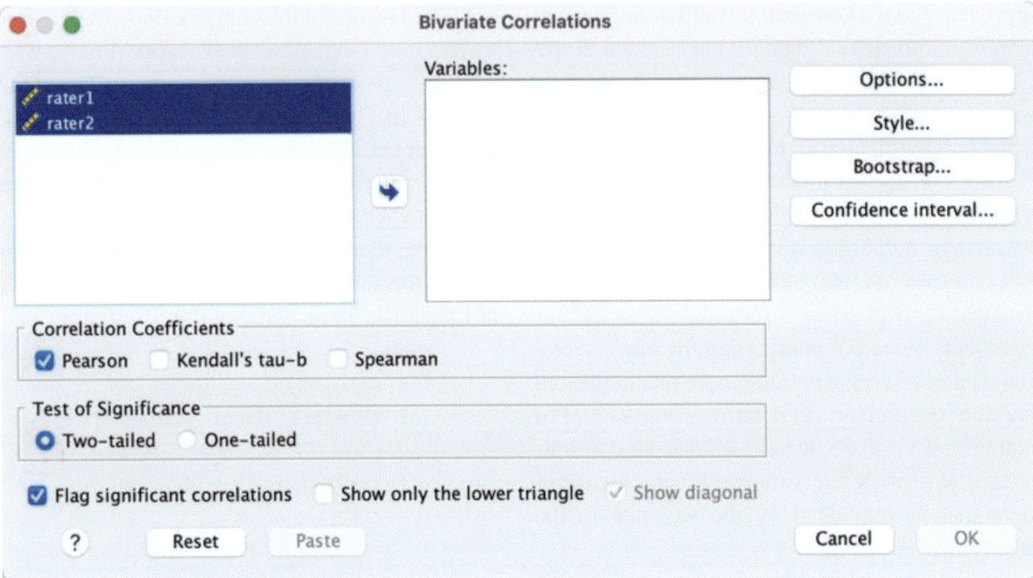

Fig. 18.3 SPSS dialog window for Bivariate Correlations after selecting Analyze → Correlate → Bivariate

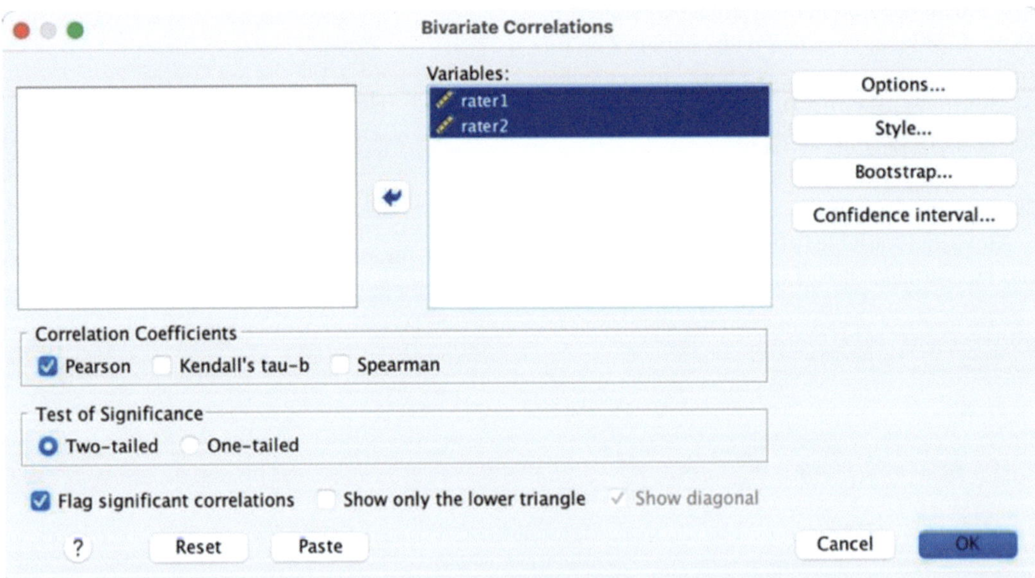

Fig. 18.4 Bivariate Correlations dialog box in SPSS with variables moved to the analysis list

possible approach is to combine correlation analysis with a t-test, which allows comparison of the means in addition to assessing association. While this method can help assess agreement to some extent, it is somewhat cumbersome and not ideal as a single index of reliability.

Even when measurement values appear consistent, there may be cases where a statistically significant difference is observed between the first and second measurements. Conversely, the correlation coefficient (r) may be low, despite no significant difference between the two sets of scores. These situations raise the question of how such results should be interpreted. This leads to the need for a single index that can represent both the consistency and agreement between measure-

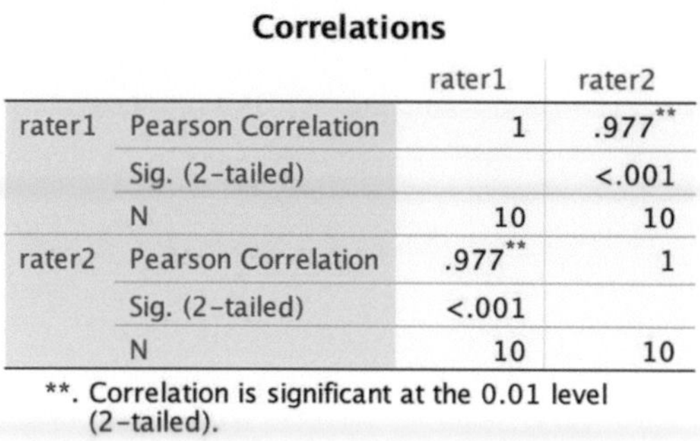

Correlations

		rater1	rater2
rater1	Pearson Correlation	1	.977**
	Sig. (2-tailed)		<.001
	N	10	10
rater2	Pearson Correlation	.977**	1
	Sig. (2-tailed)	<.001	
	N	10	10

**. Correlation is significant at the 0.01 level (2-tailed).

Fig. 18.5 SPSS output table displaying Pearson correlation coefficients, significance levels (2-tailed), and sample size (N)

Table 18.3 Example of two sets of measurements by two raters

	Data A		Data B	
Participant	Rater 1	Rater 2	Rater 1	Rater 2
1	10	10	10	20
2	20	20	20	40
3	30	30	30	60
4	40	40	40	80
5	50	50	50	100
6	60	60	60	120
7	70	70	70	140
8	80	80	80	160
9	90	90	90	180
10	100	100	100	200
	$r = 1$		$r = 1$	

The correlation coefficient (r) for both datasets is 1.00.

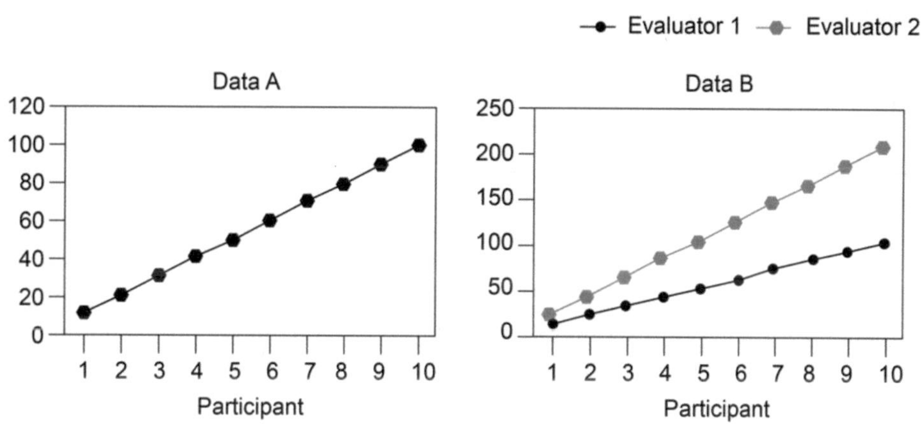

Fig. 18.6 A visual comparison demonstrating that two evaluators can yield the same correlation coefficient while differing in the level of agreement

ments. One solution to this problem is the use of the Intraclass Correlation Coefficient (ICC). The ICC is commonly used to assess reliability, and its calculation is typically based on values derived from analysis of variance (ANOVA).

A visual representation of this concept is shown in Fig. 18.6.

Figure 18.6 and Table 18.4 demonstrate that even when the correlation coefficient is the same, the level of agreement between raters, as reflected by the intraclass correlation coefficient (ICC), can differ.

Table 18.4 Variance components and intraclass correlation coefficients

	Mean square	Intraclass correlation coefficient
Data A		
Subjects	1833	1.00
Raters	0	
Subjects by raters	0	
Data B		
Subjects	4125	0.49
Raters	15,125	
Subjects by raters	458	

From a statistical perspective, the ICC offers several advantages. First, it provides a single index to represent the level of agreement among two or more raters. Second, it is clinically useful, as it does not require all raters to assess every subject. Third, although the ICC was originally developed for use with interval or ratio-level data, it can also be applied to ordinal scales as long as the assumption of equal intervals between values is reasonable.

There are six types of Intraclass Correlation Coefficients (ICCs) commonly used: ICC(1,1), ICC(1,k), ICC(2,1), ICC(2,k), ICC(3,1), and ICC(3,k) (Shrout & Fleiss, 1976). The two numbers inside the parentheses represent different aspects of the model. The first number indicates the type of model used. The second number (k) represents the unit of analysis, indicating whether the ICC is based on a single measurement (1) or the mean of k measurements.

For example, in ICC(1,k), k refers to the number of measurements averaged. The initial "1" indicates that a one-way analysis of variance (ANOVA) model was used. ICC(1,1) and ICC(1,k) are appropriate when raters are considered randomly selected from a larger population, and each subject is not rated by all raters. This implies that the raters assessing each subject are randomly assigned. Clinically, ICC(1,1) and ICC(1,k) are rarely used, as they have limited applicability in typical clinical contexts. For purposes of generalizability in clinical settings, ICC(2,1) is often the most appropriate model. Models such as ICC(2,k) and ICC(3,k) are based on a two-way ANOVA design. ICC(2,k) assumes that the raters are randomly selected, and thus the results can be generalized to the larger population of raters.

In contrast, ICC(3,k) assumes that the raters are fixed, meaning that the analysis only applies to the specific raters involved in the study and cannot be generalized beyond them. The "1" in the second position of any ICC model (e.g., ICC(2,1)) indicates that the calculation is based on a single measurement, not an average. Among these, ICC(2,1) is the most commonly used in clinical and applied research, because it reflects the level of reliability expected when different raters use the same assessment tool. Each type of ICC is calculated using a different formula, depending on the underlying model.

```
bms = between target mean square
wms = within target mean square
jms = mean square for judges (raters)
k = number of judges
bms = ss/df for targets
msw = ((ems×edf) + (jms×jdf)) / (edf+jdf)
wms = msw
jms = ss/df for judges (raters)

ICC(1,1) = (bms-wms) / (bms+(k-1)×wms)
ICC(2,1) = (bms-ems) / ((bms)+((k-
1)×ems) + ((k×(jms-ems))/n))
ICC(3,1) = (bms-ems) / (bms+((k-1)×ems))
ICC(1,k) = (bms-wms) / bms
ICC(2,k) = (bms-ems) /
(bms)+((jms-ems)/n))
ICC(3,k) = (bms-ems) / bms
```

The Intraclass Correlation Coefficient (ICC) ranges from 0 to +1. In general, ICC values are interpreted as follows. < 0.50: Poor reliability, 0.50–0.74: Moderate reliability, 0.75–0.90: Good reliability, and >0.90: Excellent reliability. These thresholds, however, should be considered as guidelines rather than absolute standards. The interpretation of ICC values should always be made in the context of the specific study.

When the same dataset is analyzed using ICC(1,1), ICC(2,1), and ICC(3,1), the ICC(1,1) value tends to be lower than ICC(2,1) or ICC(3,1). In most cases, ICC(2,1) is also lower than ICC(3,1). ICC can also be used to assess intra-rater reliability in repeated measures designs. In this case, ICC(1,k) is often used, where k refers not to the number of raters but to the number of measurement occasions (time points).

ICC(2,1) is commonly calculated using a two-way random effects model. The formula is provided below.

$$\mathrm{ICC}(2,1) = \frac{\mathrm{BMS} - \mathrm{EMS}}{\mathrm{BMS} + (k-1)\mathrm{EMS} + k(\mathrm{JMS} - \mathrm{EMS})/n}$$

k = number of raters or investigators
n = number of subjects
BMS= between subjects mean squared
JMS = between judges (raters) mean squared (within subjects)
EMS = error or residual mean squared

Table 18.5 Data for intraclass correlation coefficient (ICC) calculation

Subject	Rater 1	Rater 2	Rater 3	Rater 4
A	2	4	3	3
B	5	7	5	6
C	1	3	1	2
D	7	9	9	8
E	2	4	6	1
F	6	8	8	4

ANOVA summary table

ANOVA

	Sum of squares	df	Mean square	F	p-value
Between subjects	122.500	5	24.500		
Within subjects between items	17.500	3	5.833	4.730	0.016
Residual	18.500	15	1.233		
Total	36.000	18	2.000		
Total	158.500	23	6.891		

Grand mean = 4.7500

Table 18.5 presents hypothetical data in which four raters independently assessed six subjects. For example, for subject A, Rater 1 assigned a score of 2, Rater 2 a 4, Rater 3 a 3, and Rater 4 also a 3. The researcher is interested in determining the degree of agreement among the four raters. To evaluate this, an analysis of variance (ANOVA) can be conducted. The results of the ANOVA are presented below.

Using the results of the ANOVA summary table, the Intraclass Correlation Coefficient (ICC) can be calculated by applying the appropriate formula. In this section, we will use SPSS to calculate the ICC based on the hypothetical dataset presented earlier. To begin, open SPSS and navigate to: Analyze → Scale → Reliability Analysis. Select the variables to be analyzed and move them into the Items box. Then, click on the Statistics button in the upper right corner. In the dialog box, check the Intraclass correlation coefficient in the lower left section. To compute ICC(2,1), select the following options: Model: Two-way random effects (Assumes that both subjects and raters are randomly sampled from larger populations) and Type: Absolute agreement. To compute ICC(3,1), select: Model: Two-way mixed effects (Assumes that subjects are randomly sampled but raters are fixed) and Type: Consistency. Click Continue, then OK to run the analysis.

In the output window, refer to either the single-measures ICC or the average-measures ICC, depending on the purpose of your analysis. Use the single-measures ICC when the unit of analysis is an individual rating. Use the average-measures ICC when the reliability is based on the mean of multiple ratings per subject. In most cases, the single-measures ICC is reported, as it represents the reliability of a single observation from a single rater. The following section demonstrates how to calculate ICC(3,1) using SPSS based on the same hypothetical dataset (Figs. 18.7, 18.8, 18.9, 18.10, 18.11, 18.12, and 18.13).

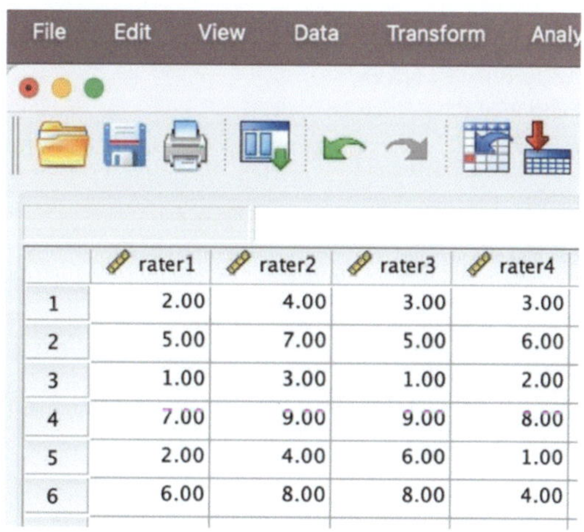

Fig. 18.7 Example SPSS dataset for calculating the Intraclass Correlation Coefficient (ICC)

In this example, the ICC(3,1), assuming that the reliability is based on a single measurement, is 0.825 (Fig. 18.14). If the goal is to assess reliability based on the average of multiple ratings per subject, the ICC(3,k) yields a value of 0.950. However, interpretation should not rely solely on the ICC point estimate. It is essential to also con-

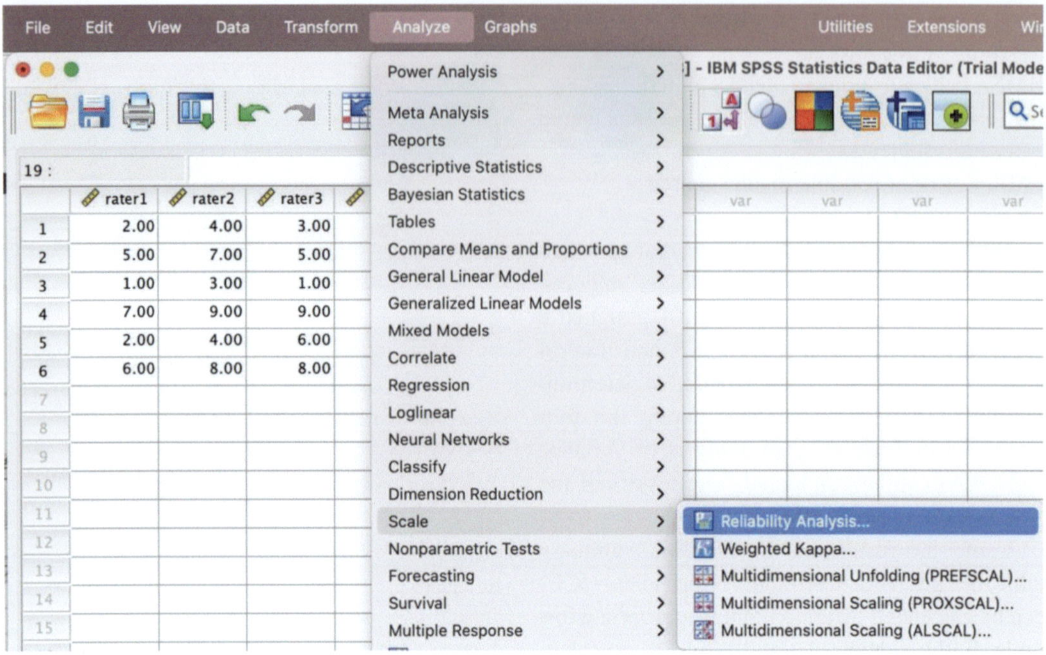

Fig. 18.8 SPSS menu path to access Reliability Analysis for calculating the Intraclass Correlation Coefficient (ICC)

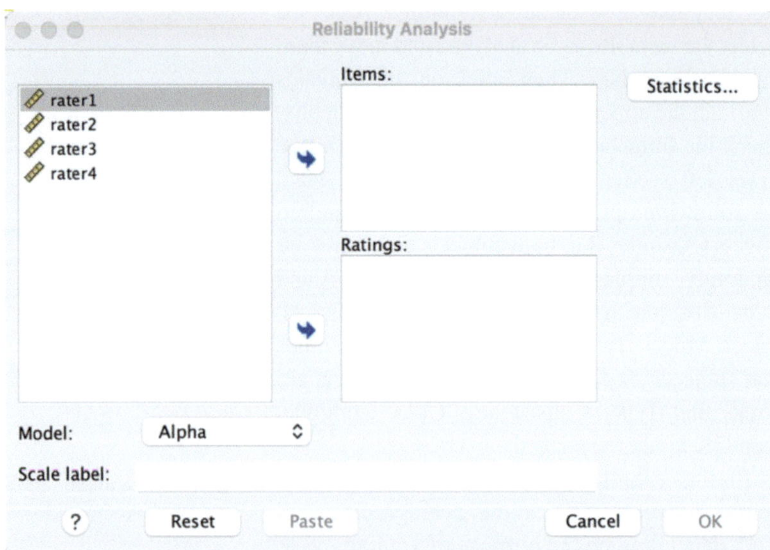

Fig. 18.9 Reliability Analysis dialog box in SPSS used for calculating the Intraclass Correlation Coefficient (ICC)

sider the 95% confidence interval (CI). In this case, the CI for ICC(3,k) is 0.820 to 0.992, suggesting that rater reliability should be described as falling between "good" and "excellent", rather than definitively concluding that it is excellent.

Let us review the steps for selecting the appropriate ICC model in reliability studies. When evaluating test–retest or intra-rater reliability, proceed as follows. First, choose a two-way mixed effects model. Second, decide whether to use ICC(3,1) (for a single measurement) or ICC(3,k) (for the mean of multiple measurements). Third, in SPSS, under Reliability Analysis, select Consistency rather than Absolute

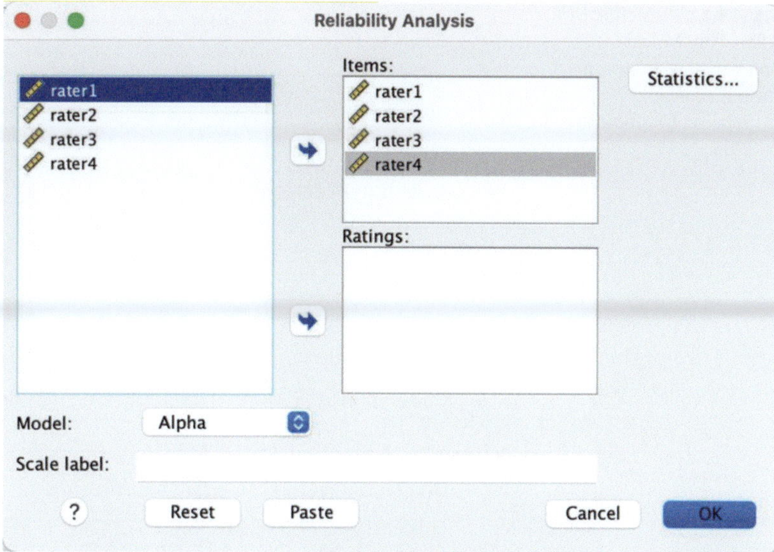

Fig. 18.10 Variables moved to the "Items" box in the Reliability Analysis dialog

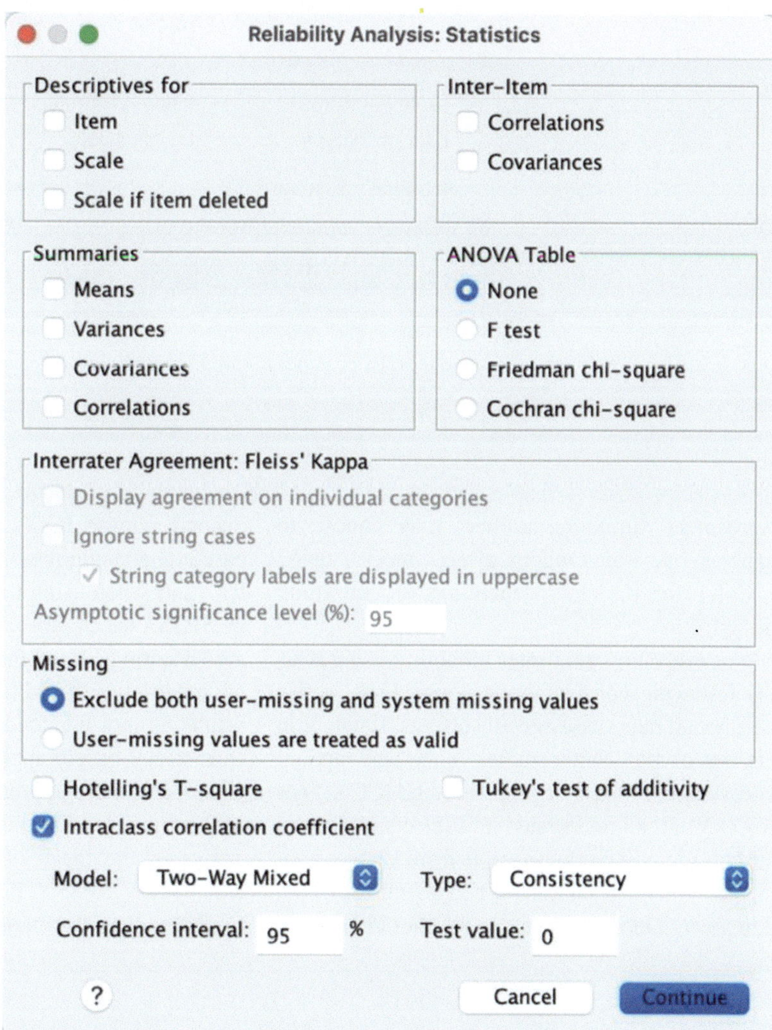

Fig. 18.11 Available options after clicking the "Statistics" button in the Reliability Analysis dialog in SPSS

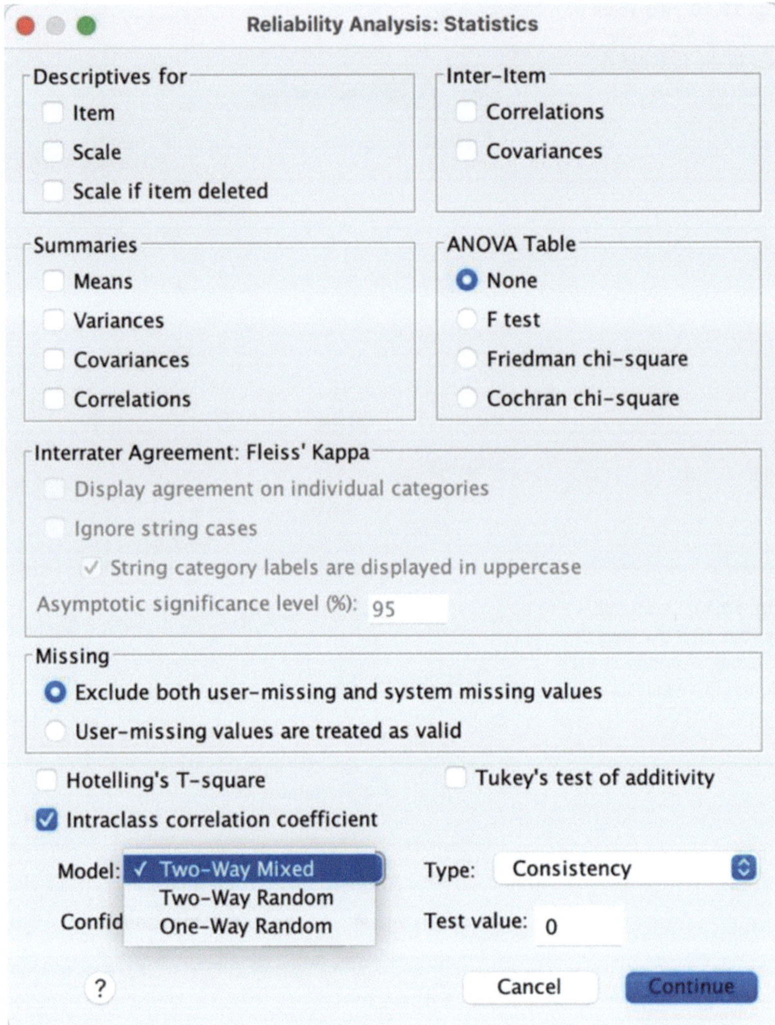

Fig. 18.12 Selection of "Two-Way Mixed" under the Model option for Intraclass Correlation Coefficient in SPSS

Agreement. Some researchers may choose to apply a one-way random effects model, using ICC(1,1) or ICC(1,k) depending on the study design.

For evaluating inter-rater reliability using ICC, the following considerations apply. First, verify whether all raters assessed all subjects. If not, or in the case of multicenter studies, a one-way random effects model should be selected (e.g., ICC(1,1) or ICC(1,k)). If all raters rated all subjects, and raters are considered a random sample from a larger population (and the results are to be generalized), then a two-way random effects model should be used. Second, choose ICC(2,1) when the reliability is based on a single measurement from one rater, or ICC(2,k) when using the mean of k raters. Third, in SPSS, select Absolute Agreement under the model settings. If, on the other hand, the raters are not randomly selected (i.e., they are fixed), and the results are not intended to be generalized, then a consistency-based approach using ICC(3,1) or ICC(3,k) is more appropriate. Use ICC(3,1) when analyzing individual ratings. Use ICC(3,k) when analyzing the mean of multiple ratings. In this case, under SPSS's Reliability Analysis, select Consistency as the model type.

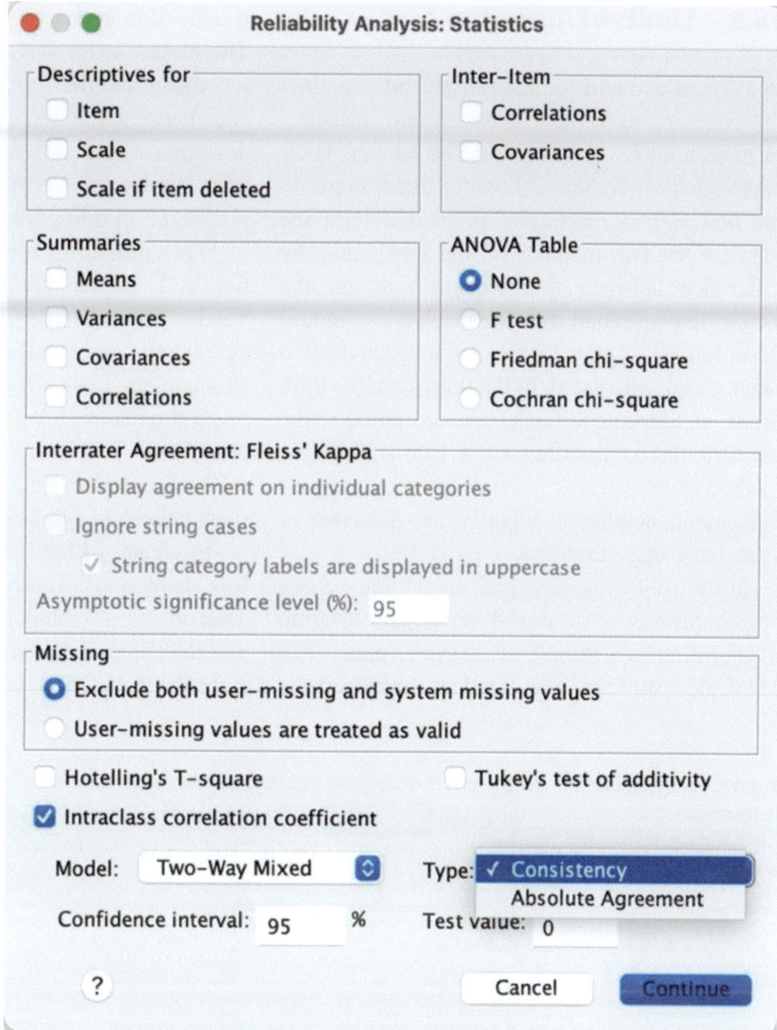

Fig. 18.13 Selection of "Consistency" under the Type option for Intraclass Correlation Coefficient in SPSS

Intraclass Correlation Coefficient

	Intraclass Correlation[b]	95% Confidence Interval		F Test with True Value 0			
		Lower Bound	Upper Bound	Value	df1	df2	Sig
Single Measures	.825[a]	.532	.969	19.865	5	15	<.001
Average Measures	.950[c]	.820	.992	19.865	5	15	<.001

Two-way mixed effects model where people effects are random and measures effects are fixed.

a. The estimator is the same, whether the interaction effect is present or not.

b. Type C intraclass correlation coefficients using a consistency definition. The between-measure variance is excluded from the denominator variance.

c. This estimate is computed assuming the interaction effect is absent, because it is not estimable otherwise.

Fig. 18.14 Output window displaying Intraclass Correlation Coefficient (ICC) results in SPSS

18.3 Limits of Agreement

In 1986, Bland and Altman introduced a method for assessing agreement between two measurement techniques, published in *The Lancet*. Their approach involves the following three steps. In the first step, a scatterplot is created with the mean of the two methods on the x-axis and the difference between the two methods on the y-axis. In the second step, the mean and standard deviation (SD) of the differences between the two methods are calculated. In the third step, the 95% limits of agreement (LoA) are computed using the formula: mean difference ± 1.96 × SD. This method allows for a visual interpretation of agreement, helping to identify the presence of systematic bias or outliers.

In the following example, maximum oxygen consumption was measured before and after an intervention in a sample of 30 participants. The MedCalc software was used to perform the Bland–Altman analysis (Figs. 18.15 and 18.16). The pretest mean was 46.4 ml/kg/min, the posttest mean was 48.0 ml/kg/min, the mean difference between the two was −1.7, and the standard deviation of the differences was 6.5. Thus, the 95% limits of agreement are calculated as −1.7 ± 12.74 ml/kg/min (Fig. 18.17).

When measuring maximum oxygen consumption in 27 participants before and after an intervention, the Bland–Altman 95% limits of agreement can be calculated using SPSS. In this example, the pretest mean is 46.4 ml/kg/min, the posttest mean is 48.0 ml/kg/min, the mean difference is −1.7, and the standard deviation of the differences is 6.5. Thus, the 95% limits of agreement are calculated as −1.7 ± 12.74 ml/kg/min.

To create a Bland–Altman plot in SPSS, follow these steps. To create new variables, go to Transform → Compute Variable. For the first variable, name it Difference, and set the Numeric Expression as Difference = pretest—posttest and

Fig. 18.15 Example dataset loaded in MedCalc for statistical analysis

	pretest	posttest
1	31	27
2	33	35
3	42	47
4	40	44
5	63	63
6	28	31
7	43	54
8	44	54
9	68	68
10	47	58
11	47	48
12	40	43
13	43	45
14	47	52
15	58	48
16	61	61
17	45	52
18	43	44
19	58	48
20	40	44
21	48	47
22	42	52
23	61	45
24	48	43
25	43	52
26	50	52
27	39	40

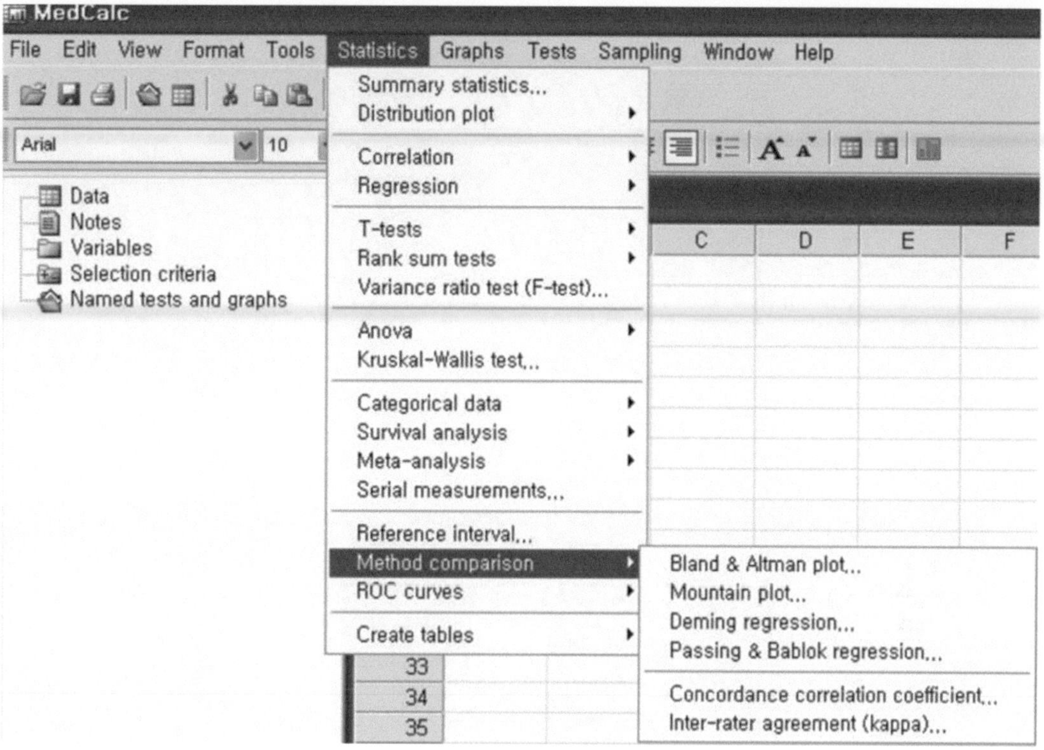

Fig. 18.16 Navigation path to generate Bland & Altman plot in MedCalc

Fig. 18.17 Output of Bland & Altman plot displaying mean difference and limits of agreement

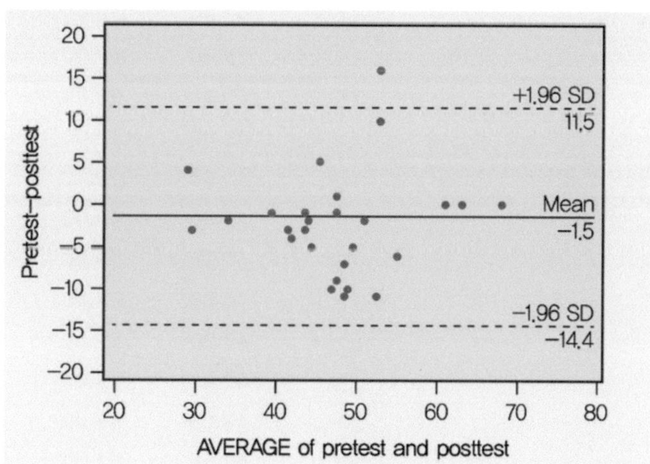

Average = (pretest + posttest) / 2. Click OK. These two new variables—Difference and Average—will now appear in your data file (Fig. 18.18).

Next, go to Analyze → Descriptive Statistics → Descriptives. Select the Difference variable and click OK to obtain its mean and standard deviation. Now, go to Graphs → Scatter/Dot, and select Simple Scatter (Figs. 18.19 and 18.20). For the y-axis, use the Difference variable. For the x-axis, use the Average variable (Fig. 18.21). Then click OK. Double-click on the chart to open the Chart Editor (Fig. 18.22). Go to Edit → Select y-Axis → Properties, and set the Minimum to −20 and the Maximum to

Fig. 18.18 Example dataset for creating a Bland–Altman plot in SPSS

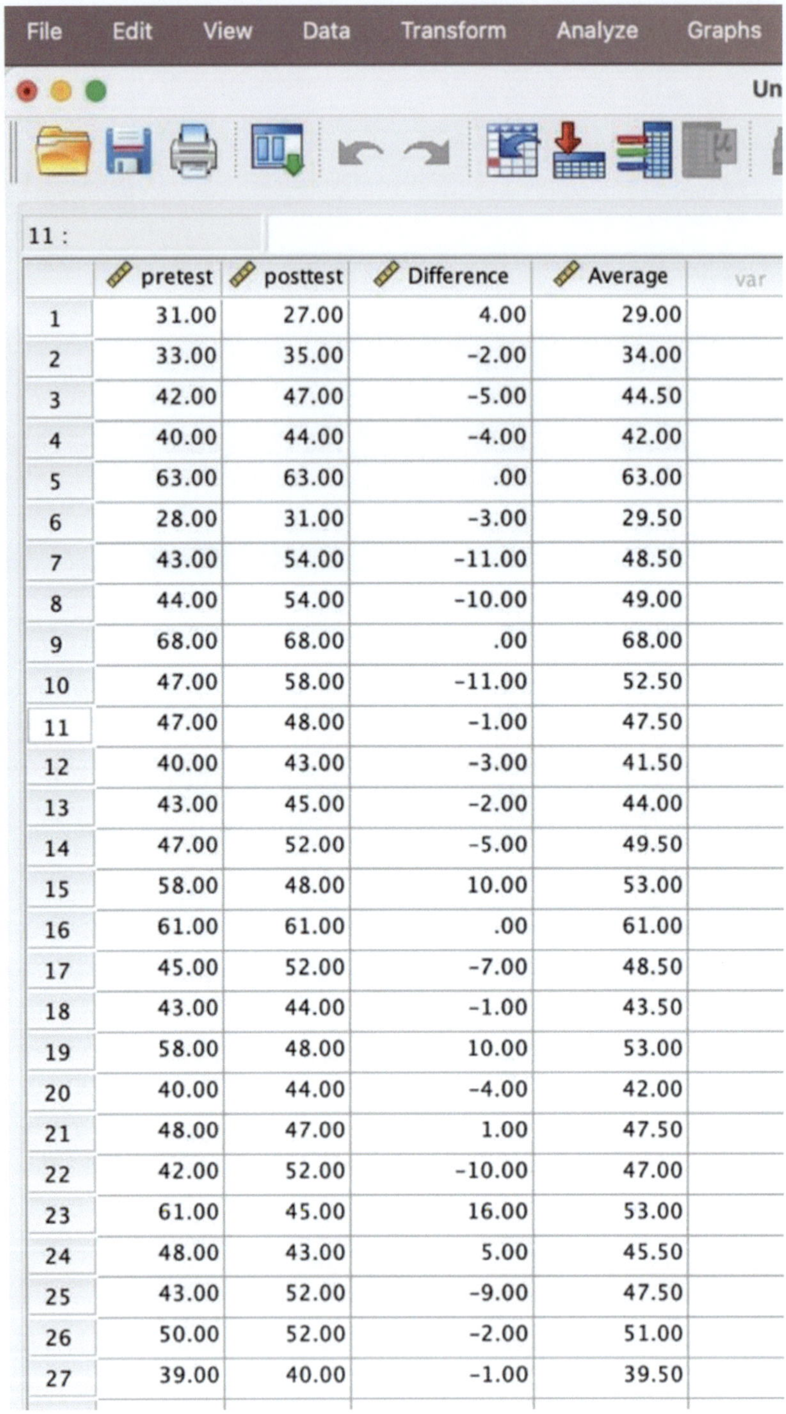

	pretest	posttest	Difference	Average	var
1	31.00	27.00	4.00	29.00	
2	33.00	35.00	-2.00	34.00	
3	42.00	47.00	-5.00	44.50	
4	40.00	44.00	-4.00	42.00	
5	63.00	63.00	.00	63.00	
6	28.00	31.00	-3.00	29.50	
7	43.00	54.00	-11.00	48.50	
8	44.00	54.00	-10.00	49.00	
9	68.00	68.00	.00	68.00	
10	47.00	58.00	-11.00	52.50	
11	47.00	48.00	-1.00	47.50	
12	40.00	43.00	-3.00	41.50	
13	43.00	45.00	-2.00	44.00	
14	47.00	52.00	-5.00	49.50	
15	58.00	48.00	10.00	53.00	
16	61.00	61.00	.00	61.00	
17	45.00	52.00	-7.00	48.50	
18	43.00	44.00	-1.00	43.50	
19	58.00	48.00	10.00	53.00	
20	40.00	44.00	-4.00	42.00	
21	48.00	47.00	1.00	47.50	
22	42.00	52.00	-10.00	47.00	
23	61.00	45.00	16.00	53.00	
24	48.00	43.00	5.00	45.50	
25	43.00	52.00	-9.00	47.50	
26	50.00	52.00	-2.00	51.00	
27	39.00	40.00	-1.00	39.50	

20 (Figs. 18.23 and 18.24). To add reference lines, go to Options → Y Reference Line (Fig. 18.25). Add a reference line at the mean difference: −1.7 (Fig. 18.26). Add reference lines for the limits of agreement, upper limit: 11.04 and lower limit: −14.44. These steps will result in a Bland–Altman plot with three horizontal reference lines (Fig. 18.27).

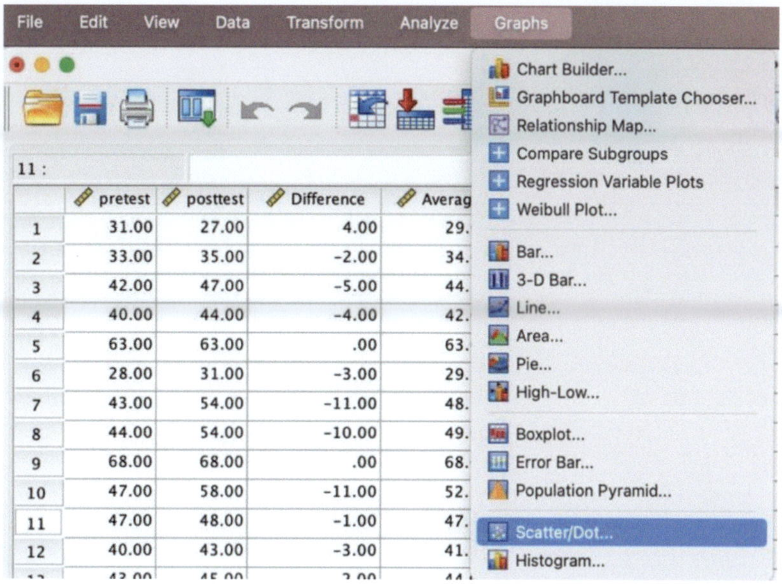

Fig. 18.19 Navigation path to Descriptive Statistics → Descriptives in SPSS

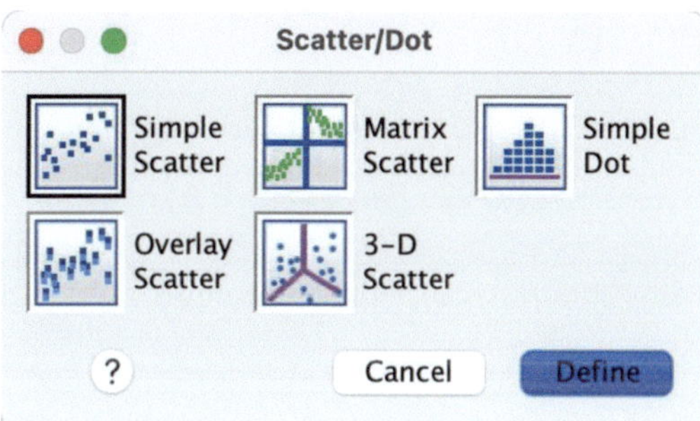

Fig. 18.20 Scatter/Dot dialog window with selectable plot types

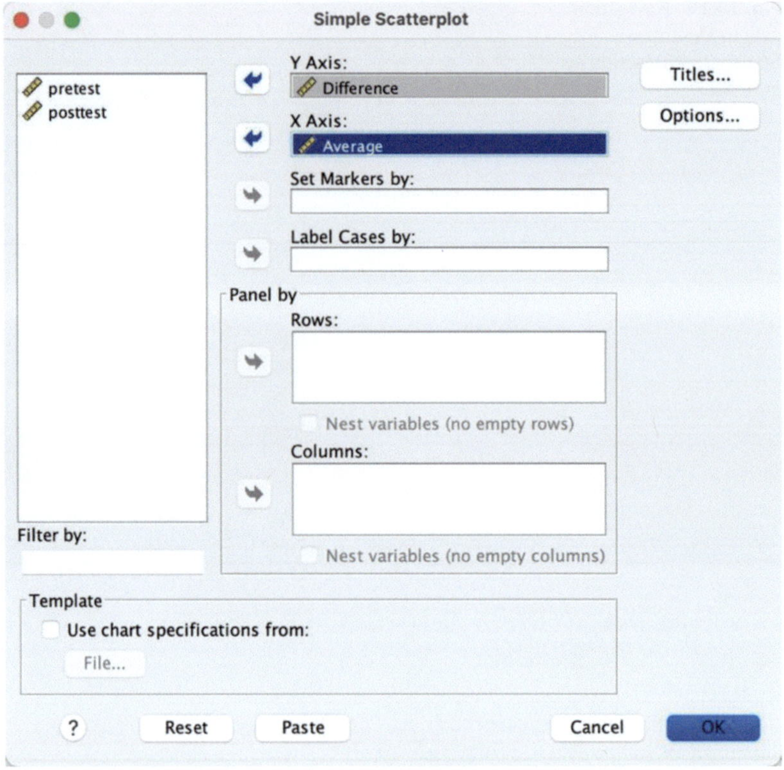

Fig. 18.21 SPSS interface showing the Simple Scatterplot option with selected variables assigned to the x-axis and y-axis

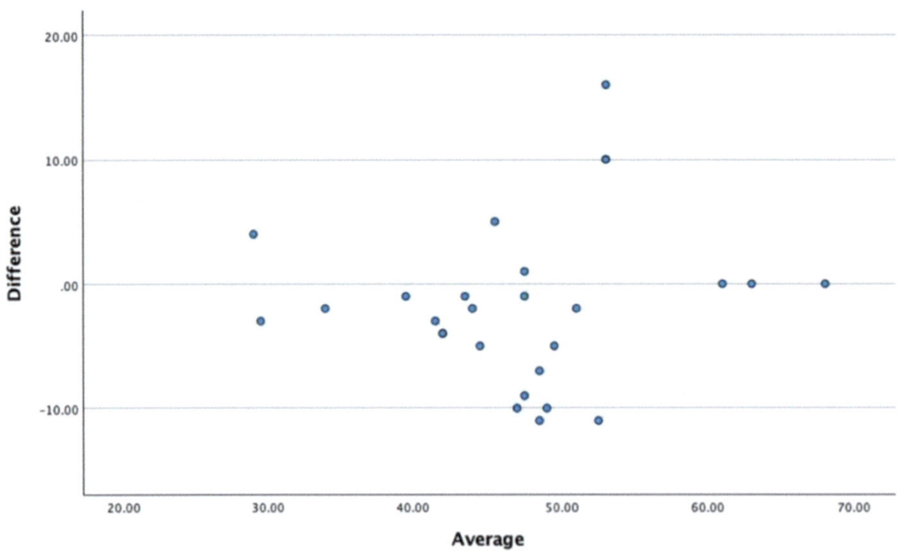

Fig. 18.22 Output scatterplot displaying the relationship between the selected variables

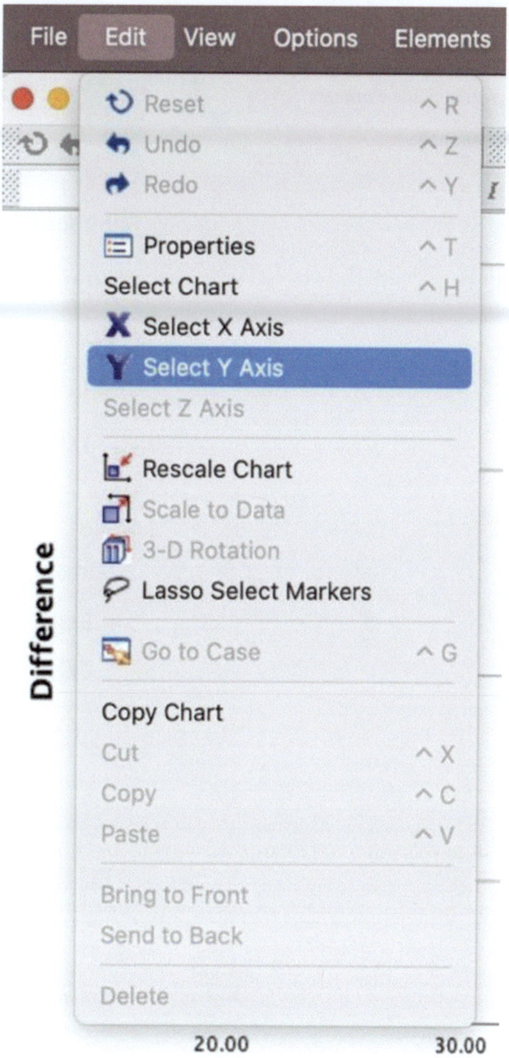

Fig. 18.23 Path to select and edit the y-axis in the Chart Editor of an SPSS scatterplot

Descriptive statistics					
	N	Minimum	Maximum	Mean	Std. deviation
Pretest	27	28.00	68.00	46.3704	9.77103
Posttest	27	27.00	68.00	48.0370	9.04468
Difference	27	−11.00	16.00	−1.6667	6.53394
Average	27	29.00	68.00	47.2037	8.82987
Valid N (listwise)	27				

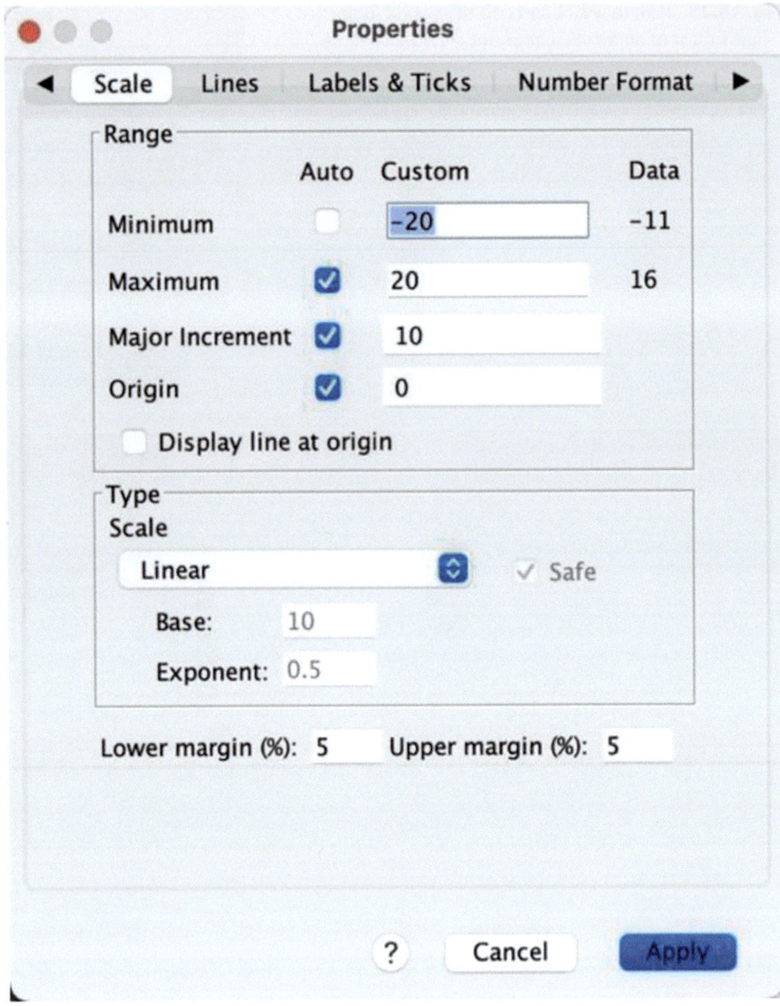

Fig. 18.24 Chart Editor's Properties window highlighting customizable elements

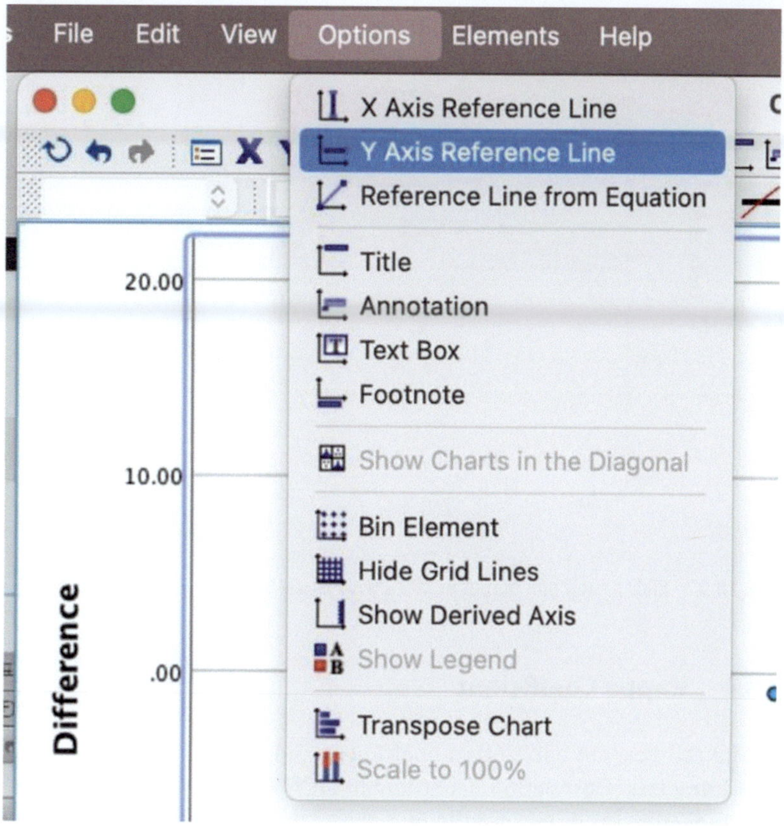

Fig. 18.25 Path to a y-axis reference line using the Chart Editor in SPSS

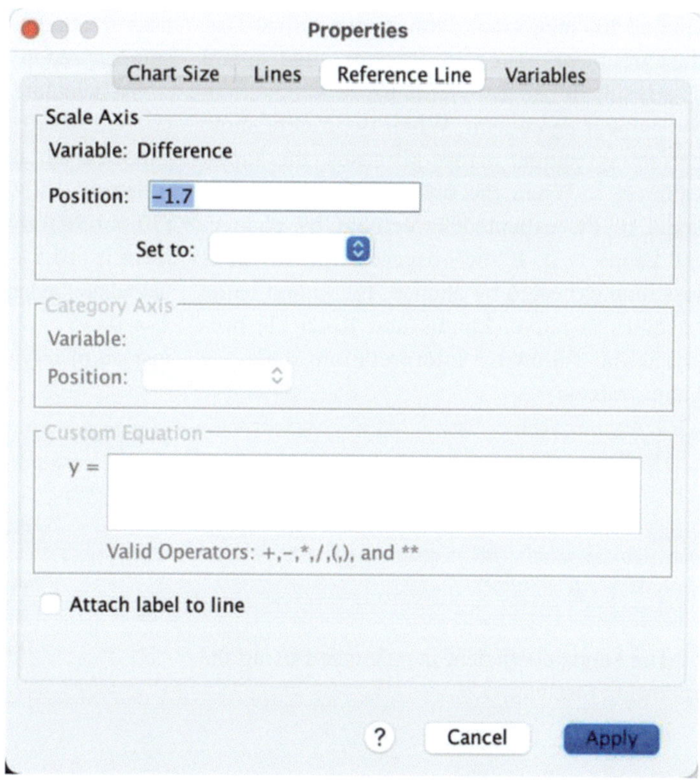

Fig. 18.26 Entering a reference line value of −1.7 under "Reference Line Position" in the SPSS Chart Editor

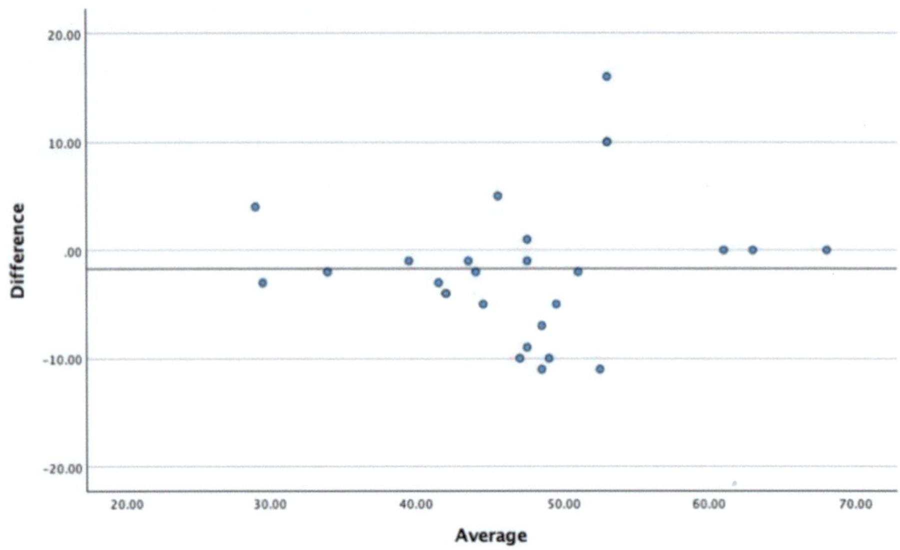

Fig. 18.27 Final scatter plot output in SPSS with y-axis and reference line added

18.4 Kappa Coefficient

While the Pearson correlation coefficient and the Intraclass Correlation Coefficient (ICC) are typically used for continuous data, the kappa coefficient, developed by Cohen, is applied to categorical data. Kappa adjusts for the agreement that could occur by chance, and as a result, it usually yields lower values than the percent agreement. When two raters show perfect agreement across all cases, the kappa value is 1. When the observed agreement is equal to the expected agreement by chance, the kappa is 0. If the observed agreement is less than expected by chance, the kappa value becomes negative. Landis and Koch [1] proposed the following interpretation scale for kappa values:

```
<.20 = poor
 .21 ≤ k ≤ .40 = fair
 .41 ≤ k ≤ .60 = moderate
 .61 ≤ k ≤ .80 = substantial
 k >.80 = good
```

The kappa coefficient is calculated using the following formula:

$$k = \frac{(\text{observed proportion} - \text{expected proportion})}{(1 - \text{expected proportion})}$$

Suppose that two dermatologists independently assess the presence or absence of post-inflammatory hyperpigmentation (PIH) following laser treatment in 100 patients. Their ratings are summarized in Table 18.6.

To calculate the overall observed agreement, (20 + 55)/100= 0.75. However, to calculate the expected agreement by chance, we proceed as follows: (35 × 30)/100=10.5 and (70 × 65)/100=45.5. Thus, the expected agreement is (10.5 + 45.5)/100 = 0.555. Now, we can calculate the kappa coefficient using the formula: k = (0.75 − 0.555)/(1 − 0.555) = 0.43. Thus, instead of relying on the original agreement rate

Table 18.6 Results between two observers on the presence of post-inflammatory hyperpigmentation (PIH) in 100 patients

	Observer 2			
Observer 1		Present	Absent	Total
	Present	20	15	35
	Absent	10	55	65
	Total	30	70	100

of 0.75, we are able to calculate an agreement coefficient that excludes chance agreement.

The minimum assumptions for the use of kappa statistics are as follows. First, the subjects being evaluated must be independent of one another. Second, the raters must evaluate the subjects independently, without influencing each other. Third, the response categories (classification labels) must be mutually exclusive and independent.

$$\text{Agreement rate} \quad = (36/53) \times 100 = 67\%$$

$$\text{Disgreement rate} \quad = (17/53) \times 100 = 33\%$$

$$\text{Agreement due to chance} \quad = 67\% - 33\% = 34\%$$

$$\text{Percent Agreement} \quad = 67\%$$

$$\text{Kappa} = \frac{\text{Observed agreement rate} - \text{Agreement due to chance}}{1 - \text{Agreement due to chance}} = \frac{0.67 - 0.34}{1 - 0.34} = 0.51$$

To compute the kappa value using SPSS based on the data presented in Table 18.7, follow the steps below: When entering data into SPSS, each row represents a combination of ratings from the two raters along with the corresponding frequency. For example, the first row represents the number of times both Rater 1 and Rater 2 gave a rating of 1 and the frequency is 4. The second row represents the number of times Rater 2 rated as 1, while Rater 1 rated as 2, with a frequency of 2. Each remaining row can be interpreted in the same way.

After entering the data, you must define the structure of the dataset in SPSS (Fig. 18.28). Click on Data → Weight Cases (Fig. 18.29).

The following dialog box will appear. Select "Weight cases by" and move the frequency variable into the box labeled Frequency Variable (Fig. 18.30).

Click OK to apply the weights and return to the data view. Next, go to the Analyze menu and select Descriptive Statistics → Crosstabs (Fig. 18.31).

Move Rater 2 to the TargetList box and Rater 1 to the Columns box. Click on the Statistics button (Fig. 18.32).

In the window that appears, check the box next to Kappa (Fig. 18.33). Then click Continue and finally click OK.

The output window will display the Crosstabulation table along with Cohen's kappa statistic (Fig. 18.34).

In the Symmetric Measures table of the SPSS output, the Measure of Agreement: Kappa is reported as 0.508. When rounded, this value becomes k = 0.51, which is consistent with the result obtained through manual calculation.

Table 18.7 Example of two raters using a 4-point scale

	Rater 1				
Rater 2	Grades	1	2	3	4
	1	4	2	2	0
	2	3	20	4	0
	3	1	3	9	1
	4	0	0	1	3

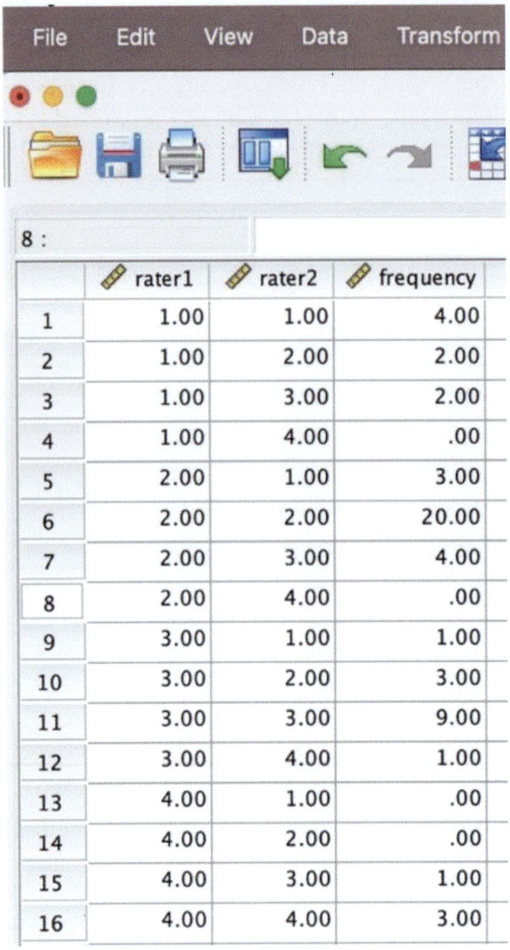

	rater1	rater2	frequency
1	1.00	1.00	4.00
2	1.00	2.00	2.00
3	1.00	3.00	2.00
4	1.00	4.00	.00
5	2.00	1.00	3.00
6	2.00	2.00	20.00
7	2.00	3.00	4.00
8	2.00	4.00	.00
9	3.00	1.00	1.00
10	3.00	2.00	3.00
11	3.00	3.00	9.00
12	3.00	4.00	1.00
13	4.00	1.00	.00
14	4.00	2.00	.00
15	4.00	3.00	1.00
16	4.00	4.00	3.00

Fig. 18.28 Example dataset for calculating Cohen's kappa coefficient in SPSS

If a statistical software package is not available, the kappa coefficient (including unweighted kappa) can also be calculated online.

1. http://vassarstats.net/
   → Click on Clinical Research Calculators.
2. http://www.graphpad.com/quickcalcs/Kappa1.cfm

Examples of Reliability Studies

1. Cohen JL, Thomas J, Paradkar D, et al. An interrater and intrarater reliability study of 3 photographic scales for the classification of perioral aesthetic features. *Dermatol Surg.* 2014;40(6):663–670.
2. Faure-Brac M, Antezack A, Melloul S, Hadj Saïd M, Raskin A, Monnet-Corti V. Smile Aesthetic Evaluation on Videographs: An Intra-Rater and Inter-Rater Agreement Study. *Dentistry Journal.* 2022;10(5):87.
3. Kantor J. Reliability and Photographic Equivalency of the Scar Cosmesis Assessment and Rating (SCAR) Scale, an Outcome Measure for Postoperative Scars. *JAMA Dermatol.* 2017;153(1):55–60.
4. Lorenc ZP, Smith S, Bass LS, Bank D, Weiss R, Canfield D, D'Alessandro BM, Cramer LM. Validating the Reliability and Clinical Relevance of an Infraorbital Hollow Photonumeric Scale. *Aesthetic Surgery Journal Open Forum.* 2023;5.
5. Topsakal O, Akbaş Mİ, Smith BS, Perez MF, Guden EC, Celikoyar MM. Evaluating the agreement and reliability of a web-based facial analysis tool for rhinoplasty. *Int J Comput Assist Radiol Surg.* 2021;16 (1):1381–1391.

As an example, we will demonstrate how to analyze interrater agreement using Cohen's kappa in SPSS.

In this scenario, two board-certified dermatologists independently assessed the severity of post-laser erythema on the right cheek in 20 patients using a 4-point Erythema Severity Scale (0 = none, 1 = mild, 2 = moderate, 3 = severe). Because the scale represents categorical, noncontinuous data, Pearson correlation is not an appropriate statistic to evaluate agreement. In SPSS, navigate to Analyze → Descriptive Statistics → Crosstabs (Figs. 18.35 and 18.36). Place the two raters' scores in the row and column variables (Fig. 18.37). Click Statistics, then check the box for Kappa (Fig. 18.38). Click Continue, then OK to generate the results.

The results are presented in Fig. 18.39.

Example of Cohen's kappa is presented in Table 18.8.

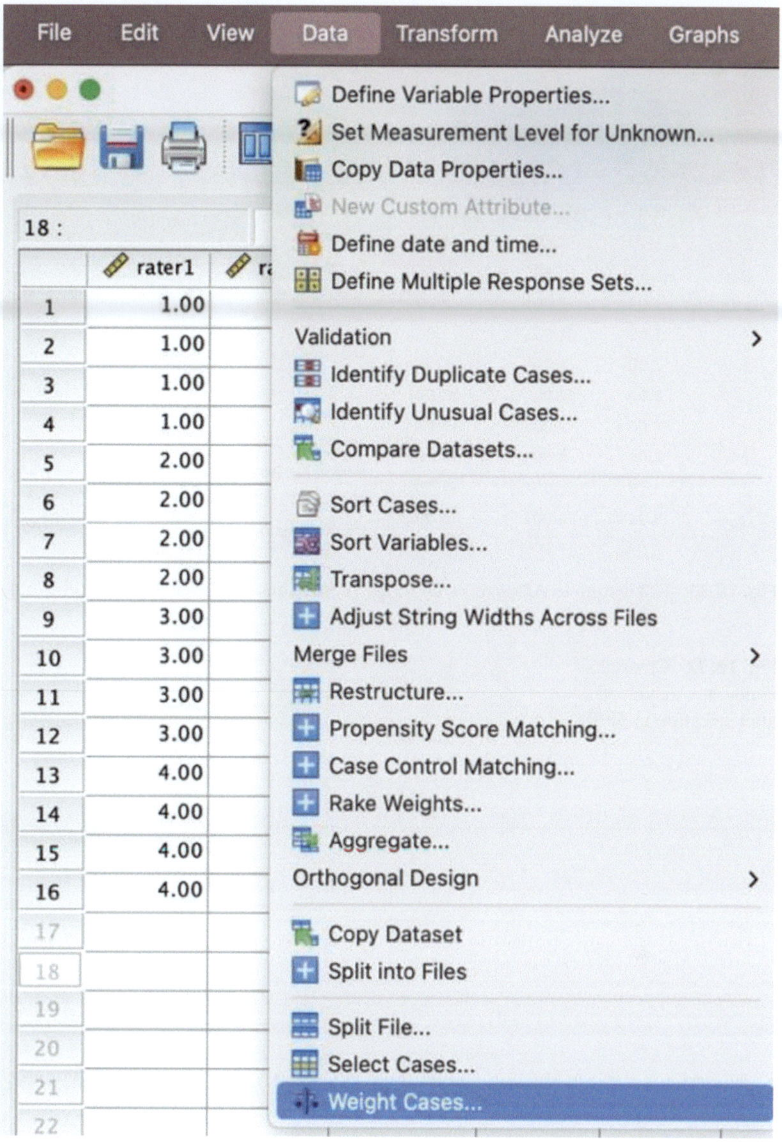

Fig. 18.29 Accessing the "Weight Cases" Function in SPSS via Data Menu

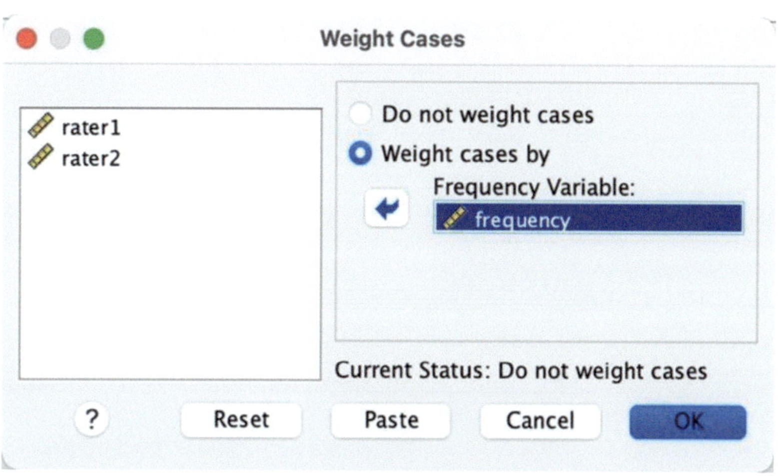

Fig. 18.30 Specifying the frequency variable in the "Weight Cases by" dialog box

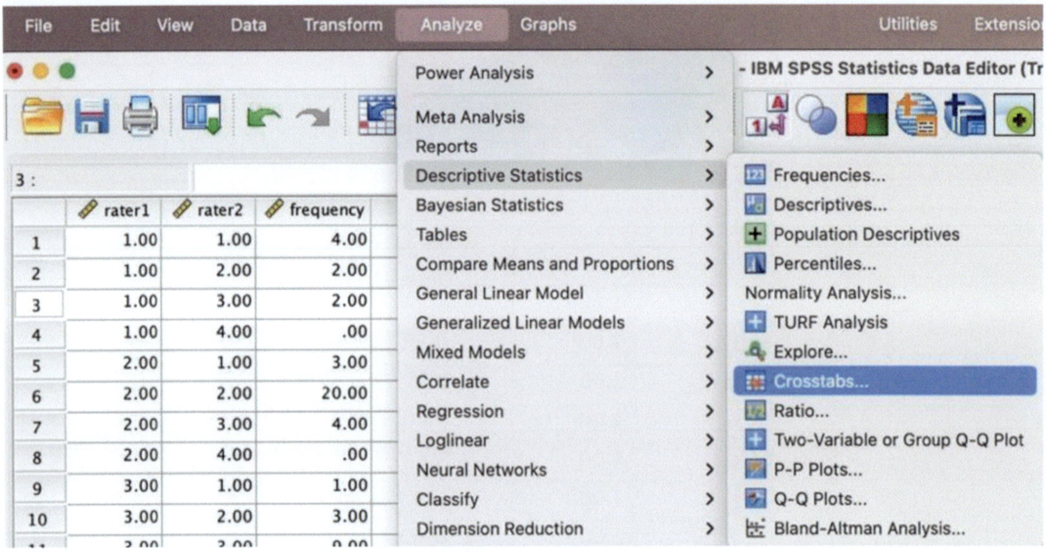

	rater1	rater2	frequency
1	1.00	1.00	4.00
2	1.00	2.00	2.00
3	1.00	3.00	2.00
4	1.00	4.00	.00
5	2.00	1.00	3.00
6	2.00	2.00	20.00
7	2.00	3.00	4.00
8	2.00	4.00	.00
9	3.00	1.00	1.00
10	3.00	2.00	3.00

Fig. 18.31 Navigating to Analyze → Descriptive Statistics → Crosstabs in SPSS

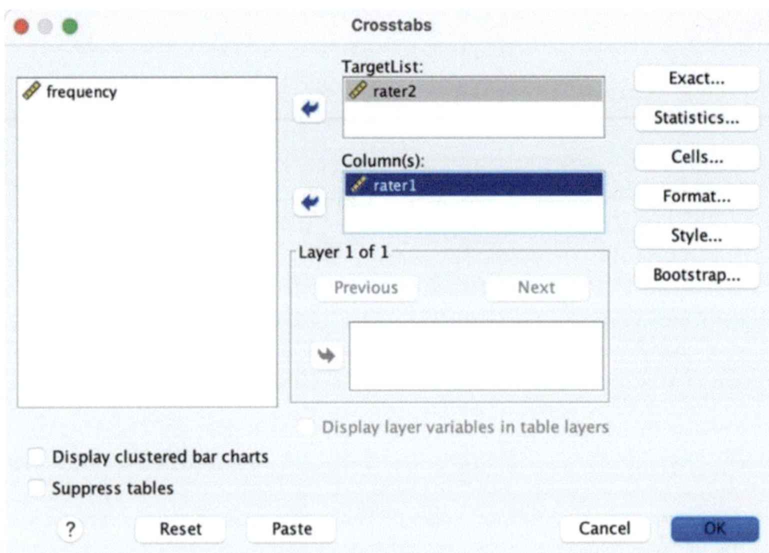

Fig. 18.32 Crosstabs dialog box displayed after selection in SPSS

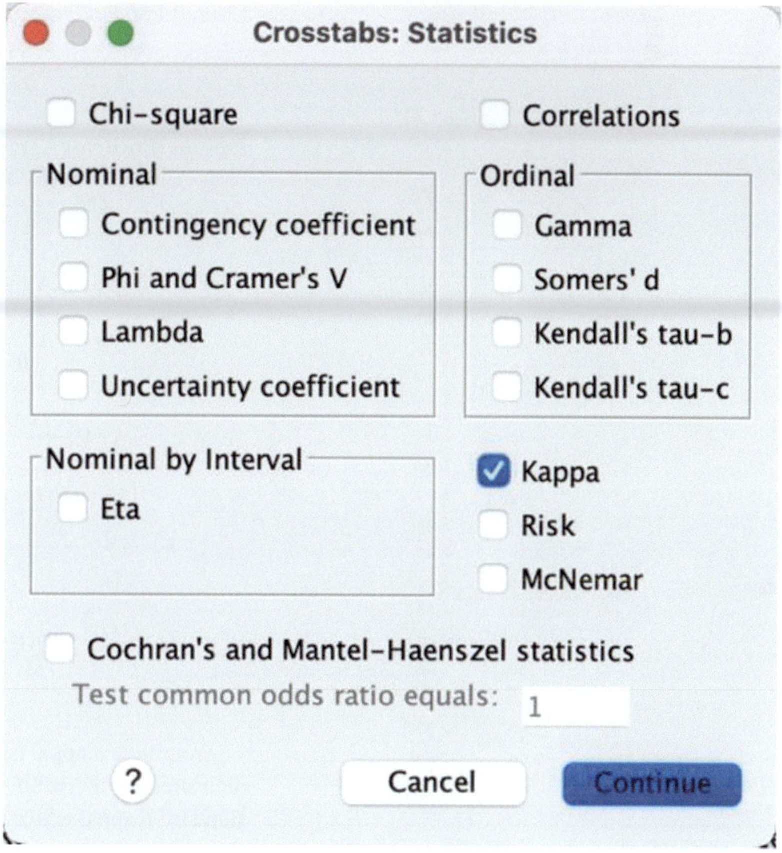

Fig. 18.33 Statistics options available in the Crosstabs dialog box in SPSS

rater2 * rater1 Crosstabulation

Count

		rater1				
		1.00	2.00	3.00	4.00	Total
rater2	1.00	4	3	1	0	8
	2.00	2	20	3	0	25
	3.00	2	4	9	1	16
	4.00	0	0	1	3	4
Total		8	27	14	4	53

Symmetric Measures

		Value	Asymptotic Standard Error[a]	Approximate T[b]	Approximate Significance
Measure of Agreement	Kappa	.508	.097	5.654	<.001
N of Valid Cases		53			

a. Not assuming the null hypothesis.

b. Using the asymptotic standard error assuming the null hypothesis.

Fig. 18.34 Output of Cohen's kappa coefficient calculation in SPSS

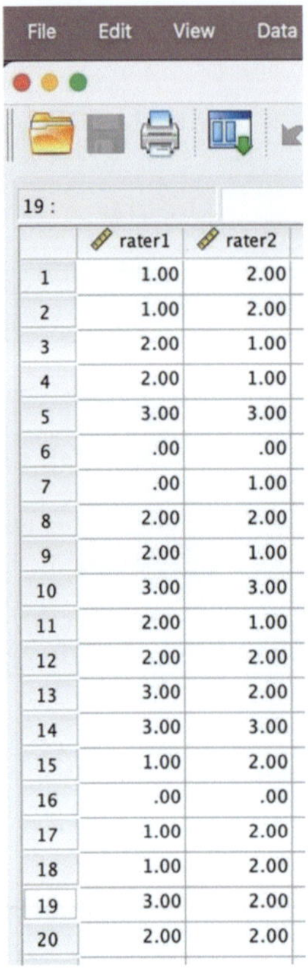

	rater1	rater2
1	1.00	2.00
2	1.00	2.00
3	2.00	1.00
4	2.00	1.00
5	3.00	3.00
6	.00	.00
7	.00	1.00
8	2.00	2.00
9	2.00	1.00
10	3.00	3.00
11	2.00	1.00
12	2.00	2.00
13	3.00	2.00
14	3.00	3.00
15	1.00	2.00
16	.00	.00
17	1.00	2.00
18	1.00	2.00
19	3.00	2.00
20	2.00	2.00

Fig. 18.35 Example dataset for interrater agreement using Cohen's kappa in SPSS

Overall Percentage Agreement

$$T\% = \frac{A+D}{N} \times 100.$$

Present (Positive) Agreement Percentage

$$O\% = \frac{A}{A+B+C} \times 100$$

Absent (Negative) Agreement Percentage

$$NO\% = \frac{D}{B+C+D} \times 100$$

$$K = \frac{(A+D) - \left(\left(\frac{(A+B)(A+C)}{N}\right) + \left(\frac{(C+D)(B+D)}{N}\right)\right)}{(N) - \left(\left(\frac{(A+B)(A+C)}{N}\right) + \left(\frac{(C+D)(B+D)}{N}\right)\right)} = 0.59$$

Weighted Kappa is used when the data are measured on an ordinal scale, as opposed to the standard Kappa, which is appropriate for nominal data. For example, let us assume that two board-certified dermatologists evaluated the severity of

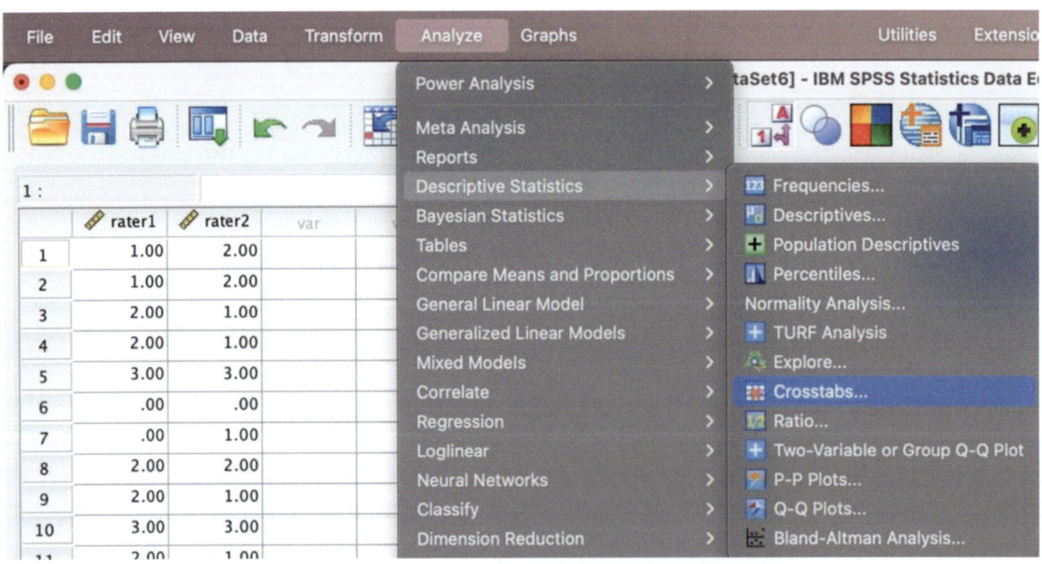

Fig. 18.36 Navigation path to perform interrater agreement using Cohen's kappa in SPSS

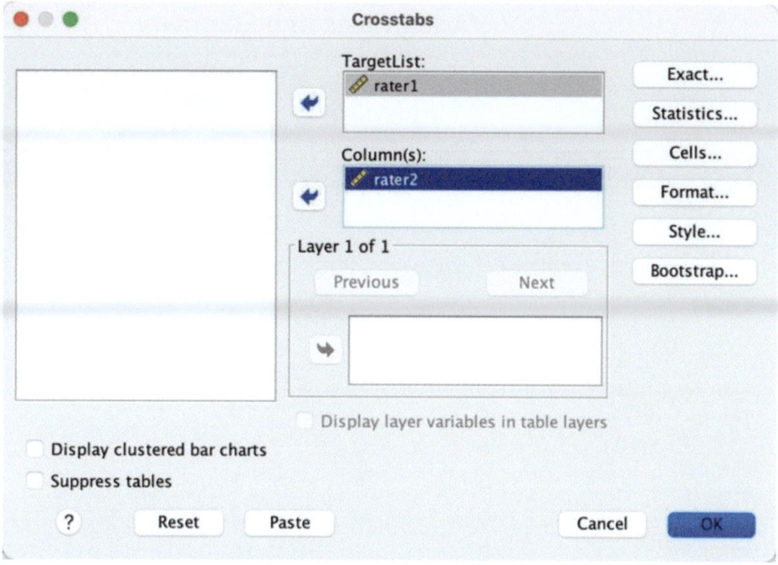

Fig. 18.37 Variables assigned to the appropriate row and column fields in the Crosstabs dialog box

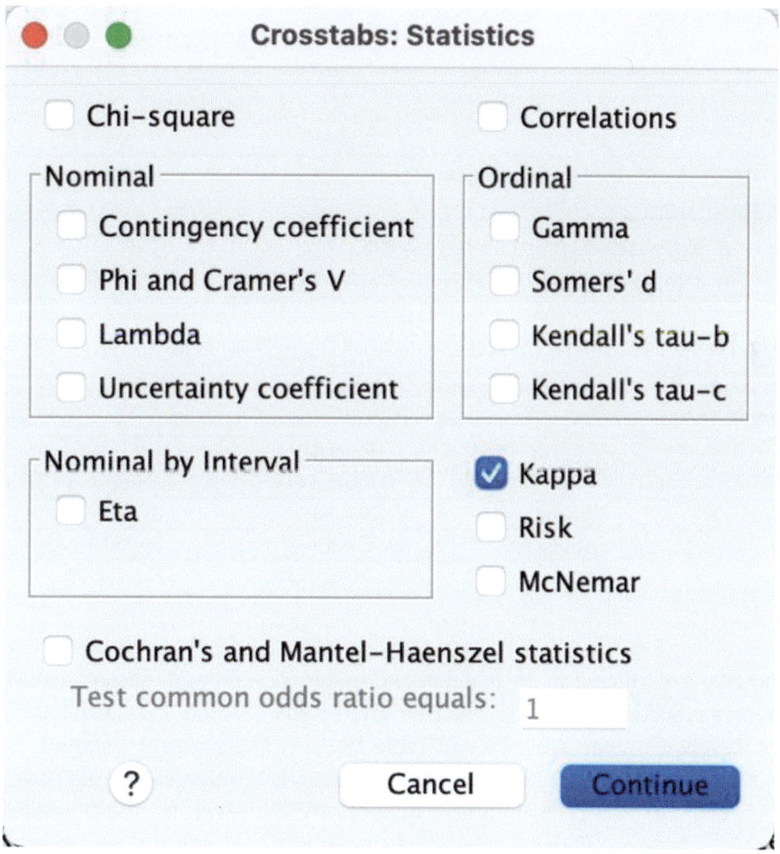

Fig. 18.38 Selection of the Kappa option under the Statistics menu in the Crosstabs dialog box

Case Processing Summary

	Cases					
	Valid		Missing		Total	
	N	Percent	N	Percent	N	Percent
rater1 * rater2	20	100.0%	0	0.0%	20	100.0%

rater1 * rater2 Crosstabulation

Count

		rater2				
		.00	1.00	2.00	3.00	Total
rater1	.00	2	1	0	0	3
	1.00	0	0	5	0	5
	2.00	0	4	3	0	7
	3.00	0	0	2	3	5
Total		2	5	10	3	20

Symmetric Measures

		Value	Asymptotic Standard Error[a]	Approximate T[b]	Approximate Significance
Measure of Agreement	Kappa	.155	.172	1.175	.240
N of Valid Cases		20			

a. Not assuming the null hypothesis.

b. Using the asymptotic standard error assuming the null hypothesis.

Fig. 18.39 Output screen displaying the result of kappa interrater agreement analysis in SPSS

Table 18.8 Frequencies of agreement and disagreement between two raters for a single event

		Rater 1		
		Present (+)	Absent (−)	Total
Rater 2	Present (+)	A = 30	B = 15	A + B = 45
	Absent (−)	C = 5	D = 50	C + D = 55
	Total	A + C = 35	B + D = 65	N = 100

post-laser erythema in 16 patients and assigned scores reflecting increasing severity. The results of their assessments are shown in Table 18.9.

Among the 16 patients, exact agreement between the two dermatologists was observed only in 5 cases (Patients 1, 3, 4, 11, and 14). Therefore, the exact agreement rate is relatively low. However, in some cases, although the ratings were not identical, they were very close, such as Patients 2 and 6. In contrast, some cases showed substantial disagreement, such as Patients 9 and 15. In situations like these, where near-agreement should still be acknowledged, weighted scoring is applied—higher weights are given to near-agreement, and lower weights to greater discrepancies. This is why the method is referred to as Weighted Kappa (or Generalized Kappa). To compute Weighted Kappa in SPSS version 25, follow these steps. In the menu bar, click on Extensions. In the Extension Hub win-

Table 18.9 Post-laser erythema severity scores rated by two dermatologists

	Patient															
Rater	1	2	3	4	5	6	7	8	9	10	11	12	13	14	15	16
A	9	14	29	17	34	17	38	29	4	29	25	4	16	25	25	45
B	9	13	29	17	22	14	45	10	29	4	25	34	9	25	8	50

Table 18.10 Hypothetical dataset

	Rater 1				
Rater 2		**Independent**	**Needs assistance**	**Dependent**	**Total**
	Independent	25	5	7	37
	Needs assistance	6	24	4	34
	Dependent	11	1	17	29
	Total	42	30	28	100

dow, type "kappa" in the search field. Click Apply in the lower-left panel. On the right-hand side, check both boxes labeled Import Extension (Top and Bottom). Click OK, agree to the terms of use, and then click Finish. After installation, go to Analyze → Scale → Weighted Kappa (or Fleiss' Kappa) in the menu. The submenus will now display options for both Fleiss Kappa and Weighted Kappa.

Table 18.10 presents a hypothetical dataset in which two board-certified dermatologists independently assessed the functional recovery level of 100 patients following laser-based aesthetic procedures.

When analyzed using the StatsDirect software, the results yielded kappa = 0.49 and weighted kappa = 0.41.

General agreement over all categories(2 raters)

```
    Cohen's kappa(unweighted)
    Observed agreement = 66%
    Expected agreement = 33.86%
    Kappa = 0.485939 (se = 0.070742)
    95% confidence interval = 0.347287
to 0.624591
    z (for k = 0) = 6.869153
    p < 0.0001

    Cohen's kappa (weighted by
1-abs(i-j)/(1-k))
    ratings weighted by:
      1         0.5        0
      0.5.       1         0.5
     0         0.5        1
    Observed agreement = 74%
    Expected agreement = 55.66%
    Kappa = 0.413622 (se = 0.079267)
    95% confidence interval for kappa =
0.258262 to 0.568982
    z (for kw = 0) = 5.218118
    p < 0.0001
```

In cases where there are three or more raters (multirater), it is necessary to use statistical software packages such as STATA or StatsDirect to compute interrater agreement using kappa statistics. Furthermore, when the data are measured on an ordinal scale and the goal is to evaluate agreement among three or more raters, the appropriate measure is Kendall's coefficient of concordance.

Bibliography

1. Landis JR, Koch GG: The measurement of observer agreement for categorical data. *Biometrics.* 1977;33:159-174.
2. Gallo L, Rae C, Kim PJ, et al. Establishing test-retest reliability and the smallest detectable change of FACE-Q Aesthetic Module scales. *J Plast Reconstr Aesthet Surg*. 2024;95:231–238

19 Reporting Research Results

The final stage of a research study is the reporting of its results. Through this process, researchers are able to share new information and contribute to the expansion of the scientific knowledge base. To disseminate their work, researchers may present their findings at academic forums under various names, such as conferences, seminars, symposia, or scientific meetings. Among these, the following three methods are the most commonly used:

1. Submission to scientific journals
2. Poster presentations
3. Oral reports

When submitting a study for publication in a journal, the research becomes part of a permanent scientific record, allowing a wide audience to access and refer to the findings. In contrast, poster presentations and oral reports are typically shared with a smaller audience, such as during professional meetings or academic conferences. This chapter outlines the process of preparing manuscripts for each of these methods of scientific communication.

1. Original research and review articles on topics relevant to the safe and effective practice of aesthetic surgery including anatomical studies, outcomes of clinical techniques, and patient safety.

19.1 Submission to Scientific Journals

Selection of an Appropriate Journal

Before writing the final version of a manuscript, the researcher must decide which journal to submit the paper to. Many journals clearly state the scope and nature of the articles they accept, often in the publisher's notes or the instructions to authors section. For instance, *Aesthetic Surgery Journal* (ASJ) specifies: "Original research and review articles on topics relevant to the safe and effective practice of aesthetic surgery including anatomical studies, outcomes of clinical techniques, and patient safety."

Understanding the mission and focus of a journal helps the author determine whether their study aligns with the journal's aims, thereby avoiding inappropriate journal selection. Authors should also consider the intended readership of the journal. The research findings should reach an audience that can meaningfully interpret and apply the information. For example, if the study focuses on interventions following cosmetic procedures, such as laser therapy or filler injection, it should be submitted to a journal that is widely read by dermatologists, aesthetic physicians, or plastic surgeons.

While there are general conventions for manuscript preparation, each journal has its own for-

K.-H. Yi, *Statistical Research Methods for Dermatologists and Plastic Surgeons*,
https://doi.org/10.1007/978-981-95-5668-7_19

matting and submission guidelines. These may include specifications for table formatting, figures, graphs, and illustrations. Failure to follow such guidelines may result in rejection or the manuscript being returned for revision prior to review.

19.2 Structure and Content

A research report is generally organized into the following sections: Introduction, Methods, Results, Discussion, and Conclusion. The Introduction and Methods sections reiterate the objectives outlined in the research proposal, but they must also explain the theoretical framework and the specific procedures used for data collection. Although the content in these sections may be similar to the proposal, the author must revise and adapt it to meet the submission guidelines of the target journal.

Introduction

The introduction section, much like in the research proposal, presents the background and purpose of the study. After reading the first or second paragraph, the reader should clearly understand what problem is being addressed and why it is important. The literature review provides the theoretical foundation supporting the rationale for the study and offers the context needed to understand how the research question is framed and why it is relevant. This section should also explain how the research question will be answered in a way that is clear and logical to the reader. The introduction must clearly state the research objective, outline the key variables, and conclude with a statement of the hypothesis.

Methods

This section begins with a description of the study participants, including the sample size, the recruitment process, and the group assignment method, if applicable. General characteristics of the participants, such as age, sex, or other relevant demographics, should be summarized using means, ranges, or appropriate descriptive statistics. Many scientific journals require explicit mention of whether participants provided informed consent and whether the study was approved by an Institutional Review Board (IRB) or equivalent ethics committee.

Next, the section should describe the instruments used and the data collection procedures, preferably in chronological order. If the measurement or intervention procedures are standardized and well established, a brief description is sufficient. Each variable should be clearly operationally defined.

Figures, diagrams, and tables can be useful tools for presenting complex procedures in a clear and concise manner. The Methods section concludes with a description of all procedures used to analyze the data, including the statistical tests employed. If any specialized or novel statistical methods are used, relevant references should be provided.

Results

The Results section should present only the findings of the study. If the study was designed to test a single, focused hypothesis, the results can be stated in clear and concise sentences. Statistical outcomes should be accompanied by interpretations that help explain or support the findings. While it is important to report test statistics, degrees of freedom, and p-values, these numbers should be presented within the context of meaningful statements. For instance, instead of writing: "A statistically significant difference in melanin index was observed between the treatment and control groups ($t = -3.13$, $p < 0.01$)," it is more informative to state: "Patients who received fractional laser treatment showed a significantly greater reduction in melanin index compared to the control group ($t = -3.13$, $p < 0.01$)." Readers typically prefer to interpret data more easily through the use of tables and figures. These visual aids help summarize findings in a format that is both accessible and efficient.

There are two key principles in organizing the results. First, avoid redundant reporting between the text and tables or figures. The narrative should be understandable even without referring to the table, and likewise, the table should make sense on its own, independent of the text. Second, the discussion or interpretation of the results should not be included in this section. Any explanation or contextualization of the findings belongs in the Discussion section.

Discussion

The Discussion section forms the core of the research report, as it reflects the author's interpretation of the findings. It is the only section where the author may express their own perspective and critical insights. In this section, the author should explain the clinical and theoretical significance of the results, identify the limitations of the study, and propose implications for future research and practice. New findings should be compared with those of previous studies, and the author should offer logical explanations to account for the observed outcomes. It is essential to address both statistically significant and nonsignificant results, providing a balanced interpretation. Authors are also encouraged to discuss the clinical applicability of their findings.

Any potential confounding variables—whether anticipated before the study or recognized during data collection or analysis—should be acknowledged. Understanding and explaining the possible impact of these extraneous factors can help readers interpret the results more accurately and critically.

Conclusion

The Conclusion should briefly restate the main purpose of the study and highlight the key findings.

Abstract

Most journals require a structured or unstructured abstract at the beginning of the manuscript. Authors usually prepare the abstract after completing the full manuscript. For Korean language submissions, an English abstract is typically required; for English-language articles, the abstract is presented under the title "Abstract" or "Summary." The abstract should summarize the objective, sample size, methods, major results, and conclusions. Since most journals impose a word limit—typically 200 to 300 words—it is important to adhere strictly to the journal's submission guidelines. The abstract often determines whether readers will proceed to read the full article, and therefore, it must be written clearly and succinctly. Additionally, a well-written abstract improves the discoverability of the paper in electronic databases and search engines.

Abstract

Lateral Eyebrow Lifting and Eye-Opening Point Injection With Botulinum Neurotoxin: Anatomical Perspective

Yi, Kyu-Ho & Kim, Soo-Bin & Park, Hyun-Jin & Kim, Hee-Jin.

Background: The orbicularis oculi muscle plays a critical role in eye-opening and closure. Identifying precise injection sites for botulinum neurotoxin can improve both functional and esthetic outcomes, particularly for conditions like blepharospasm or ptosis. Materials and methods: Three fresh cadavers were dissected, separating soft tissues from bones to observe the muscle layers. A 29-year-old Korean female was administered a botulinum neurotoxin injection. Before the injection, ultrasound was used to identify the lateral superior part of the orbicularis oculi muscle. The injection point, at the edge of the superolateral orbital rim, received a 1-unit intradermal injection of letibotulinum neurotoxin. Changes in eye-opening were observed 4 weeks postinjection. Results: Dissection revealed intermingling of the frontalis and orbicularis oculi muscles, with the orbicularis oculi muscle exclusively present at the edge of the superolateral orbital rim. This point was targeted for the injection, resulting in improved eye-opening and eyebrow elevation. The patient reported a GAIS score of 2, indicating noticeable improvement. Discussion: Targeting the edge of the superolateral orbital rim for botulinum neurotoxin injections effectively reduces involuntary muscle contractions, facilitating easier eye-opening and eyebrow lifting. The anatomic specificity of this site minimizes risks to surrounding muscles. These findings suggest potential clinical applications for enhancing eyelid function and esthetic outcomes. Further research with larger samples and long-term studies is recommended to validate these results and explore additional benefits.

Tables and Graphs

Tables and graphs are frequently used in the Results section of scientific papers to facilitate visual explanation and improve the clarity of statistical findings. The narrative portion of a manuscript typically conveys general knowledge and overarching interpretations, while tables and figures present the detailed data.

Tables

A standard table consists of five elements: the title, column headings (horizontal content), row headings (vertical content), the body (data cells organized according to column and row headings), and footnotes. Most scientific journals allow horizontal lines only below the column headings and at the bottom of the table. Other grid lines are generally omitted. Tables are most effective when used to present relationships between independent and dependent variables, whether in the form of raw data or summary statistics. The title of the table should clearly reflect these relationships. Column headings should be arranged from left to right in logical order—for example, based on temporal sequence. When reporting pre- and post-treatment data (as is common in cosmetic dermatology studies), pre-treatment values should be listed first. Footnotes may be used to indicate statistical significance

Table 19.1 Comparison of skin hydration levels before and after a hyaluronic acid mask application (Unit: arbitrary units)

Time point	Skin hydration (Mean ± SD)	df	F	*p*
Before application	7.9 ± 4.5	2	1.52	0.23
5 minutes after application	9.3 ± 5.8			
25 minutes after application	6.9 ± 3.6			

(e.g., *p*-values), define abbreviations, or cite references. Each journal has its own formatting rules for footnotes. The *American Medical Association (AMA)*, for instance, recommends the following standard footnote symbols: *, †, ‡, §, ||, ¶, #. Table 19.1 is an example modeled after a table format actually published in a scientific journal. The title should appear above the table.

Graphs

Graphs are used to visually communicate research findings. When explaining trends, relationships, or comparisons, graphs are often more effective and concise than lengthy textual descriptions. Graphs can be constructed in various formats. For frequency data, bar charts and line graphs are commonly used. A line graph typically connects the frequency points of a bar chart in a continuous line (Fig. 19.2). Pie charts are used to show proportional distributions of a particular characteristic within a sample. Bar charts are most appropriate when comparing discrete variables between groups, such as control vs. treatment, or pre- vs. post-treatment values in separate samples.

When designing graphs, authors should pay careful attention to the scales of measurement used. Since graphs are meant to convey meaningful trends or differences, the chosen scale must be rational and proportionate. For example, Fig. 19.1 presents the skin surface roughness depth before and after treatment. Prior to treatment, both the control and experimental groups showed the same mean roughness depth of 0.27 mm. After treatment, the control group had a mean of 0.30 mm, while the experimental group improved to 0.33 mm. Compared to Fig. 19.1a, b appears to exaggerate the treatment effect. This is because

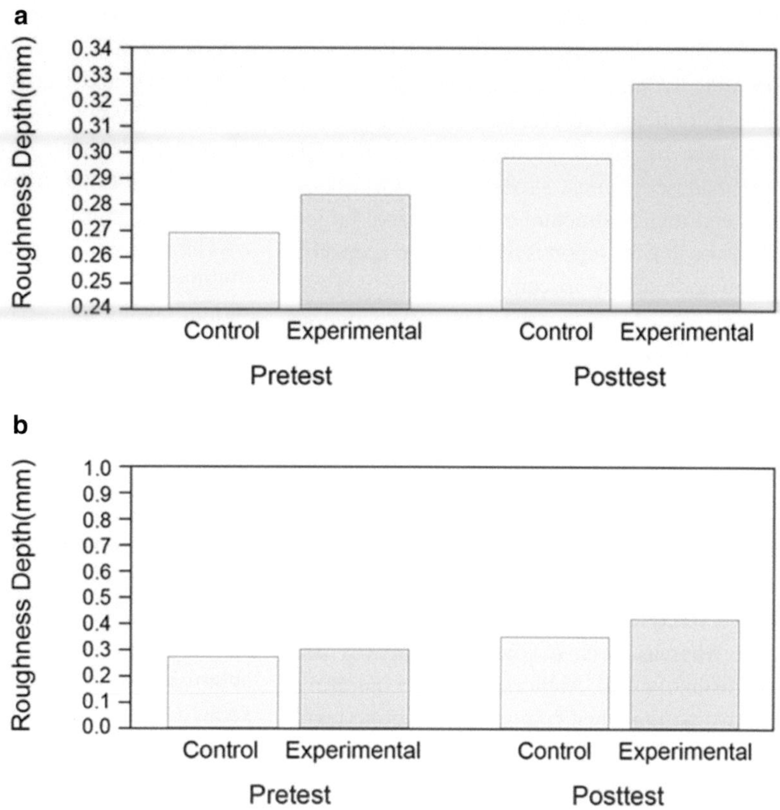

Fig. 19.1 Two graphs depicting the same roughness depth data using different Y-axis scales

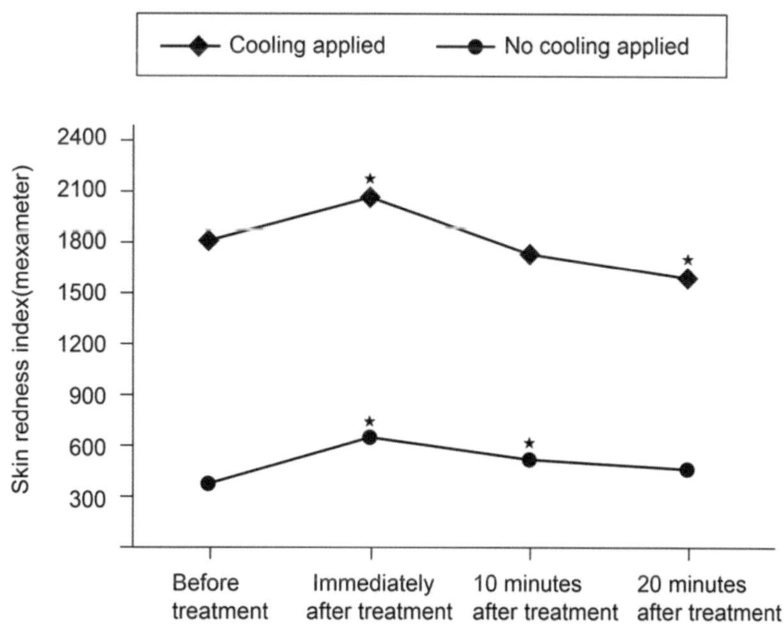

Fig. 19.2 Comparison of repeated measures of skin redness index before and after cooling treatment. *Significantly different from pre-cooling skin redness index, $p < 0.05$

the Y-axis scale in Fig. 19.1a starts at 0.24 mm, whereas the clinically relevant full range of roughness values may extend from 0.0 to 1.0 mm. As a result, Fig. 19.1a visually overstates the clinical improvement. The caption for a figure should be placed below the graph (Fig. 19.2).

19.3 Writing Style

Scientific writing should be well-organized and clear, prioritizing the accurate communication of facts over literary or rhetorical expression. The final manuscript must strongly reflect the objectives and logical structure of the research project. To ensure that the report is readable and accessible, the author's ability to convey meaning precisely through written language is essential. Although scientific writing may not come easily, it is a critical skill for communicating research findings, and authors are encouraged to study writing techniques through relevant guides and reference materials.

Active Versus Passive Voice

Active voice tends to be stronger and more specific, whereas passive voice can make writing feel distant or dull. Authors should be mindful of this distinction when composing scientific texts.

Passive: Improvement in skin hydration was observed following the application of the hyaluronic acid serum.
Active: The application of the hyaluronic acid serum improved skin hydration.

These two versions differ not only in structure but also in emphasis. The passive construction emphasizes the timing of the outcome, while the active construction highlights the agent and its action. In addition, the active version uses fewer words (four fewer in this example).

Passive voice may be appropriate when the subject is unknown or irrelevant, or when the object is the focus of the sentence. However, excessive use of passive constructions may weaken the impact of the content and distract the reader from the main message.

Simplicity of Language

Many authors attempt to avoid repetition by using different words to express the same concept. However, if a particular word clearly conveys a key point, it is often better to repeat it for consistency and clarity. Adverbs and adjectives are generally not useful in scientific writing. For example, describing an outcome as *"very practical"* or *"highly useful"* adds little value and may be unnecessary.

The purpose of a scientific paper is to convey findings, not to write poetry. Therefore, sentences should avoid ornate or complex phrases and instead be written using clear, precise, and straightforward language.

Poster Presentation

A poster presentation is a method of displaying a summary of a research study in a standardized format and size at academic conferences for public viewing. With the growing number of research submissions to conferences, many academic societies now encourage poster presentations.

A poster presentation displays the contents of a research study on a large board, allowing many people to read and view the work in an open and informal setting. Its main advantage is that a large number of interested attendees can study the research at their own walking pace.

A well-constructed poster should clearly and concisely present the key components of the study, including the title, hypothesis, objective, methods, results, discussion, and conclusion. Rather than full sentences, short phrases or key expressions should be used. Unique aspects of the methodology or significant findings are best illustrated through tables, graphs, or images. Standard poster dimensions are typically 85–95 cm in width and 120 cm in height. Posters are often mounted on cork boards or wooden panels to allow for easy pinning and display.

The layout of the content should follow a logical flow of information. The Introduction should be positioned in the top left corner, and the Conclusion in the bottom right corner. An example of a poster layout is shown in Fig. 19.3.

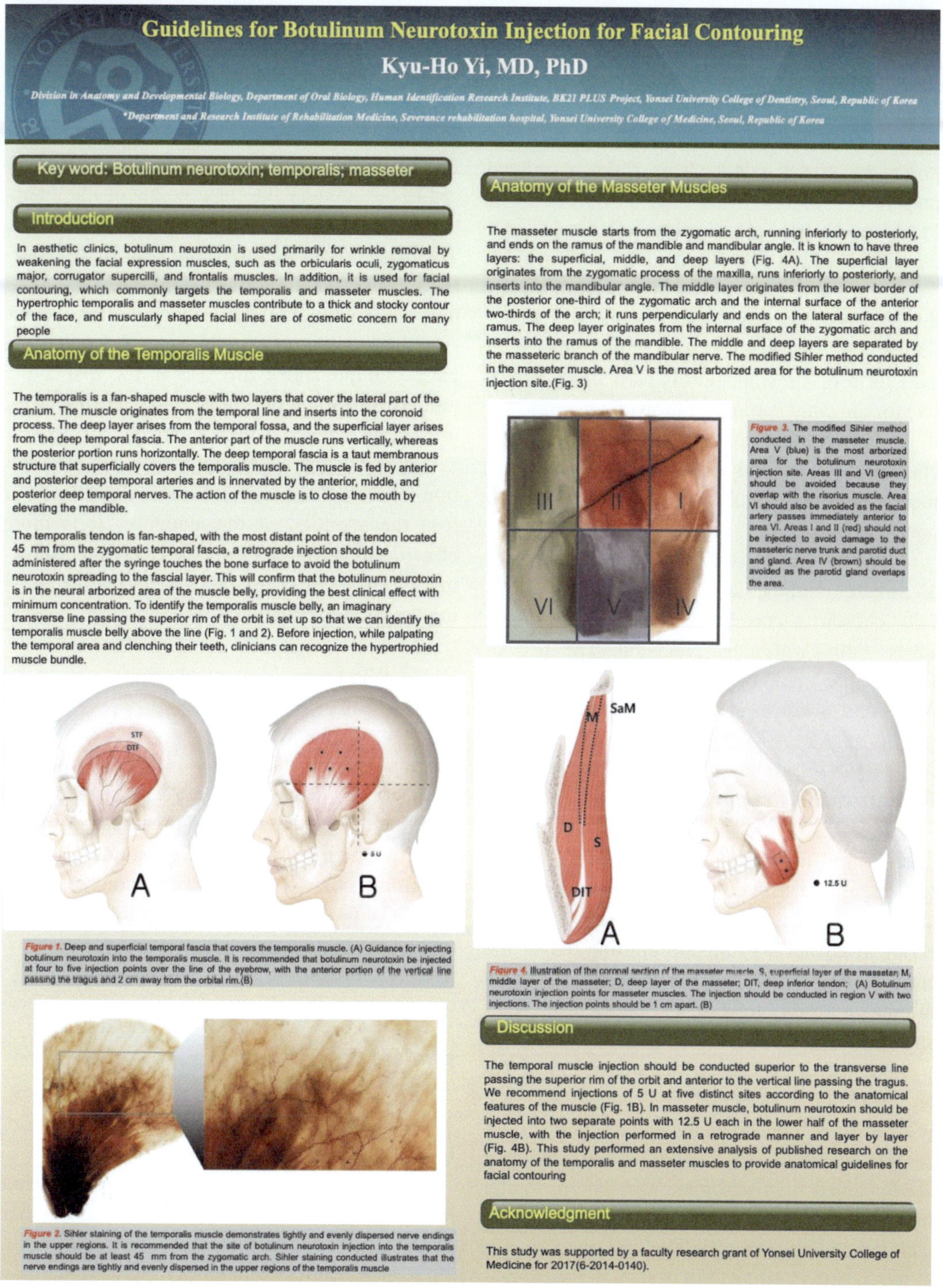

Fig. 19.3 Example format of a poster presentation layout

Platform Presentation

A platform presentation typically involves delivering research findings within a designated time frame, usually between 10 and 30 minutes, supported by visual aids such as slides, overhead projectors (OHPs), Microsoft PowerPoint, or Prezi, a web-based presentation tool that does not require additional software installation.

Oral presentations of research are often conducted at professional forums or symposia, where findings are shared with peers in the same field. This form of dissemination is particularly effective for the rapid communication of new information. For those who find scientific writing challenging, platform presentations may offer a more appealing alternative for research communication.

A typical oral presentation is limited to 10 to 15 minutes, and the language used must be carefully chosen to convey the speaker's key messages with clarity and precision. The use of PowerPoint, Prezi, or OHPs helps reinforce key points and enhances the delivery of the content.

Presentation Preparation

The content of an oral presentation should be well-organized, and due to time constraints, it is advisable for the speaker to prepare a written script in advance. From the drafting stage, the speaker should write with the presentation format in mind, carefully refining key phrases and transitions for emphasis and clarity.

It is also important to practice using visual aids prior to the presentation. A manuscript that is eight pages long, typed in double spacing, typically takes about 10 minutes to deliver when accompanied by visual materials. The presenter must ensure that the entire talk can be delivered within the allotted time.

Visual Presentation

Visual aids are essential for a successful oral presentation. Well-designed PowerPoint slides, Prezi, or OHP transparencies can help highlight key points, maintain the audience's attention, and enhance clarity. However, poorly structured visuals can detract from the presentation and undermine its effectiveness.

The number and type of slides should be chosen to best convey the main points of the manuscript. There are four common types of slides. Text-based slides are used for titles, study objectives, background, protocol summaries, and conclusions. Photographic slides often show equipment setup or procedures involving participants. Graph slides are useful for displaying numerical results, and table slides are ideal for presenting detailed data comparisons.

Overcrowding a slide with too much information results in long, dense text that can distract or lose the attention of the audience. It is more effective to summarize only the key points, allowing the speaker to elaborate verbally while keeping the audience focused.

Rehearsal

Before the actual presentation, it is recommended to practice in front of colleagues or students to ensure that the content of the prepared script and the PowerPoint slides are well-aligned, and to determine how long the presentation will take. Rehearsal provides an opportunity to identify and correct potential issues that may arise during the live presentation.

Effective Presentation Techniques

The following suggestions can help researchers improve their presentation skills:

First, if possible, record yourself practicing the presentation using a video camera. After reviewing your performance, rehearse again while applying the techniques described below.

Second, maintain a relaxed yet upright posture. Avoid standing stiffly. Distribute your body weight evenly across both feet. Shifting your weight to one side may cause a tilt in posture, which can be distracting to the audience.

Third, skilled presenters often move naturally from side to side of the podium or take a few steps toward the audience. This reduces the perceived barrier between the speaker and the listeners, creating a sense of engagement. If no podium is available, standing 1 to 3 meters in front of the audience is ideal. However, avoid either staying rigidly in one spot or moving excessively.

Fourth, adopt natural gestures that do not reveal anxiety. Overly exaggerated movements should also be avoided.

Fifth, avoid looking only at the wall, the floor, the screen, or your notes while speaking. Such behavior can suggest a lack of confidence. Instead, make direct and attentive eye contact with your audience. Identify individuals who appear disengaged and look at them intentionally to re-capture their attention. If the audience is large and you cannot focus on individuals, try to distribute your gaze to different parts of the room. People sitting near the area you're looking at will also feel included. Increasing the distance between you and the audience can help widen your eye contact range.

Sixth, avoid speaking in a monotonous tone, or speaking too fast or too slow, or too loudly or too softly. A monotonous voice is often a sign of anxiety. To maintain a natural and dynamic tone, relax your body and release tension. Gentle upper and lower body movements can help relax muscles and regulate breathing, even if they are not exaggerated. You may also benefit from recording your voice or asking a peer for feedback to better understand your delivery.

Seventh, the average speaking speed for presentations is approximately 125 words per minute. Anxiety often increases speaking speed. While a fast pace is acceptable if your articulation is clear, it's important to adjust the pace in professional settings or when listeners may be taking notes. One common issue with fast speaking is verbal errors. If this occurs, slow down and become more aware of your own speech. Try to listen to the final word of each sentence, pause briefly, and then proceed to the next sentence. Brief pauses during a talk give the audience time to process what you've said. Don't fear moments of silence-they are necessary for comprehension.

Eighth, in most cases, issues with volume can be improved through practice. You need to be aware of how your voice carries. At the beginning of your presentation, ask the audience, "Can those in the back hear me clearly?" Audiences generally respond honestly, as they are eager to hear the presentation.

How to Respond to Questions

First, anticipate potential questions. In most cases, presenters can predict the types of questions they are likely to receive. It is advisable to rehearse answers in advance, especially for difficult or challenging inquiries. If applicable, consider preparing visual aids to support your responses to anticipated questions.

Second, seek clarification if needed. If a question is particularly long, confusing, or includes multiple parts, ask the audience member to rephrase or simplify the question so that you can respond more effectively.

Third, repeat the question. Consider the following: have you ever sat in the back of an auditorium and couldn't hear a question asked by someone in the front? Repeating the question allows the entire audience to hear it clearly and also gives you a moment to gather your thoughts before answering.

Fourth, be honest. If you're unable to answer a question, it is best to respond transparently: "I'm not sure about that, but I'll look into it and follow up with you." Alternatively, if an expert or collaborator is present, you may invite them to respond on your behalf.

Fifth, address your answer to the entire audience, not just the person who asked the question. You may have seen presenters who focus solely on the questioner, inadvertently ignoring the rest of the audience. This is particularly problematic when the questioner appears to be intentionally confrontational, as it can create an isolating dynamic.

Sixth, apply the 25%–75% rule. Maintain eye contact with the questioner for about 25% of your response, while directing the remaining 75% toward the rest of the audience. This strategy is especially useful when managing challenging or aggressive questions, as it helps you retain control and maintain engagement with the broader audience. It is important not to ignore the questioner, but also not to overlook the rest of the audience.

Seventh, stay focused on the point. While your answer should be complete and informative, avoid rambling. Long-winded answers may cause the audience to lose interest, so aim to be concise but thorough.

20 Evaluating Research Reports

It is practically impossible to read all of the numerous scholarly articles that are published in large volumes. Therefore, the first step in reading the literature efficiently is to identify and select journals that are most likely to provide reliable and relevant information in a given field of interest. When seeking information on a specific topic, it is often helpful to visit a library to consult recent textbooks or review articles. Such sources are valuable in that they offer foundational and comprehensive background information necessary to understand a subject. However, it is important to remember that the information presented in reviews reflects the interpretation of the review authors and is thus secondary or indirect. As a result, there is a risk that the original research may be misinterpreted or oversimplified. To minimize such issues, readers are encouraged to consult the original research articles whenever possible.

20.1 Evaluating Scientific Papers

The first factor to consider when evaluating a research paper is the reputation of the journal in which it is published. Articles submitted to scholarly journals typically undergo peer review by experts in the field. The editor-in-chief, associate editors, and reviewers assess manuscripts according to established criteria before selecting those that meet the journal's standards. These criteria may include the importance and originality of the research, the appropriateness of the study design, the rigor of the experimental procedures, the validity of the results and their interpretation, the soundness of the discussion, and the clarity of writing. The more prestigious the journal, the more rigorous and selective the review process tends to be. In highly ranked journals, it is not uncommon for the time from submission to publication to exceed two years.

Title and Abstract

The title of a research article should use concise language that effectively conveys the core focus of the study. It must reflect the essential information of the paper without being vague or overly general. The abstract should provide a scientifically accurate summary of the study's objective, methodology, results, and main conclusion. It should not be written in vague terms, but must be expressed in scientific terms. From the reader's perspective, the abstract should not be accepted at face value. Instead, readers should always consult the full text of the article to evaluate the validity and reliability of the study's findings.

K.-H. Yi, *Statistical Research Methods for Dermatologists and Plastic Surgeons*,
https://doi.org/10.1007/978-981-95-5668-7_20

Introduction

When reading the Introduction, the reader should be able to clearly understand the research questions the study aims to address. The following are key questions that can be used to evaluate the quality of an introduction:

1. Does the study address a research problem of significant importance?
2. Is the problem stated clearly and precisely?
3. Has the author used literature effectively to build a clear and logical theoretical framework?
4. Is there a well-defined theoretical rationale for conducting the study?
5. Are the cited references appropriate, relevant to the topic, and sufficiently comprehensive?
6. Is the type of research (e.g., experimental, correlational, descriptive) clearly indicated?
7. Are the specific objectives of the study explicitly stated?
8. Is the research hypothesis clearly articulated?

At the beginning of the introduction, the author should inform the reader what the central research issue is, so that the reader can understand why the study is necessary. The most critical element is to clearly state the specific aims of the research. While authors may not always include a detailed hypothesis in the introduction, the writing should be sufficient for the reader to infer the expected hypothesis.

If the answers to the questions listed above are mostly affirmative, the reader is likely to view the study as well-directed and meaningful. However, if even one of these questions receives a negative answer, it may raise concerns about the author's critical thinking skills and the validity of the subsequent stages of the research process.

Methods

The Methods section provides the fundamental information that enables readers to evaluate the validity of the research.

Subjects

To assess the validity of the study's conclusions and determine its clinical applicability, readers must be fully informed about the characteristics of the study participants. The following questions are essential in evaluating the subject-related information:

1. Who were the subjects included in the study?
2. What were the specific inclusion and exclusion criteria for selecting subjects?
3. How were the participants recruited, and from which population were they drawn?
4. What was the total number of participants?

These questions help identify the potential presence of sampling bias and reveal possible confounding variables. Participant characteristics, such as age, sex, diagnosis, and functional level, can influence both the internal and external validity of the study. To clearly define the source population, authors must explicitly list the selection and exclusion criteria. If a reader intends to apply the study results to their own clinical population, the characteristics of the study subjects must match those of the target patients.

In many student-led studies, participants are often healthy individuals, which limits the direct applicability of findings to patient populations. Therefore, researchers must provide sufficient detail about their subjects to allow readers to judge the scope of clinical generalizability. It is also important to specify the sampling method used in the study. Knowing the sample size is crucial for interpreting the results of statistical analyses. In particular, sample size affects the risk of Type II error, which refers to the likelihood of failing to detect a real effect when one exists.

Research Design

The reader must evaluate whether the researcher has selected a research design that is appropriate and effective for addressing the stated research problem.

1. Is the type of research design (e.g., experimental, quasi-experimental, or nonexperimental) clearly described?
2. Is the selected design appropriate to the research question?
3. How many groups were included in the study?
4. Was randomization used in the allocation of participants?
5. Was there a control group?
6. How many independent variables were there, and how many levels did each have?
7. How frequently were treatments and measurements administered?

In experimental studies, the method of group assignment and the presence or absence of a control group greatly influence the internal validity of the research. There are three main reasons why readers should pay close attention to research design when reviewing a study.

First, it allows the reader to assess how well the researchers managed the inherent tension between internal validity and generalizability. When a tightly controlled experimental design is used, the reader must consider how well the findings translate to real-world settings. In laboratory-like conditions, where confounding variables and internal threats are strictly controlled, the effect of the independent variable may appear stronger. However, actual clinical environments are rarely so controlled or artificial. If a quasi-experimental design was used, the reader should consider the potential influence of extraneous variables on the interpretation of results.

Second, the number of groups, the number and levels of independent variables, and the number and timing of dependent variable measurements can all influence the choice of statistical procedures used for data analysis.

Third, if a single-subject (single-case) design was employed, the study must be evaluated based on the unique principles and standards applicable to that design type.

Instrumentation

This section describes the experimental instruments and tools used in the study.

1. Are the instruments described in sufficient detail?
2. Has the author addressed the reliability and validity of the instruments?

Readers need to know whether the researcher used any specialized equipment or instruments. If the instruments are standardized and commercially available, the model number, product name, and manufacturer contact information should be provided. If standardized questionnaires or survey tools were used, the source must be cited.

The reliability of an instrument relates to the consistency and reproducibility of measurements. Three aspects of reliability should be considered.

1. Instrument reliability itself must be clearly documented. Readers should look for evidence that supports the instrument's reliability.
2. Intra-rater and inter-rater reliability should be reported, particularly if human raters were involved in measurements.
3. The reliability of the instrument should be verified in the specific population under study. For example, a corneometer may demonstrate high reliability in measuring skin hydration in healthy volunteers, but it cannot be assumed that the same level of reliability will apply to patients with severe xerosis or barrier-damaged skin following chemical peels. Similarly, a cutometer may reliably measure skin elasticity on the forearm, but it is uncertain whether it would yield equally reliable results when used to assess periorbital elasticity, where skin thickness and biomechanical properties differ significantly.

From the reader's perspective, it may be difficult to directly verify the validity of the instruments used. However, the reader should be able to assess whether the instruments were used in a manner that was accurate, appropriate, and methodologically sound for collecting the intended data.

Procedures

This section provides a detailed account of the experimental procedures, from the beginning to the end of the study.

1. Are the procedures described in enough detail that another researcher could replicate the data collection process?
2. Are the operational definitions of the independent and dependent variables clearly stated?
3. Were potential threats to internal validity adequately controlled?

The methods used to collect data should clearly specify who performed the measurements, what was expected of the participants, what actions were taken by the data collectors, as well as when and how frequently the measurements were conducted. In experimental studies, the control group may be asked to follow specific protocols, such as refraining from food intake or resting for a certain period prior to testing. The experimental group, by contrast, is exposed to the independent variable as defined operationally. All procedures must be described in enough detail that other researchers could replicate the study using similar participants and similar conditions.

Most authors do not explicitly refer to internal validity when describing procedures. However, researchers should consider potential extraneous variables that may influence the results, such as history, maturation, instrumentation, testing effects, and selection bias.

Data Analysis

The data analysis section must clearly specify the statistical methods used in the study.

1. Was the data analysis process appropriate for the type of data collected?
2. Did the author provide justification for the chosen statistical techniques?
3. Were the statistical methods clearly linked to the specific research questions they were intended to address?
4. Was the level of significance reported?

The author must report the alpha level explicitly. Statistical procedures should not simply be listed by name; rather, the analysis should include a detailed description of how each method was applied to the respective data. This information is critical for the reader to evaluate the appropriateness of the statistical techniques selected. The appropriateness of statistical methods depends on several factors, including the level of measurement, the reliability of the instruments, the linearity of the data, and the research design (e.g., number of groups, variables, or measurement occasions). The reader should be able to determine, for example, whether a parametric test was inappropriately applied when a nonparametric test would have been more suitable, or whether a t-test was used when analysis of variance (ANOVA) was warranted.

Results

In the Results section, the author should not interpret or explain the findings; rather, only the outcomes of the data analysis should be presented.

1. Are the results clearly reported?
2. Are the figures and tables accurate and appropriate?
3. Are the results for all stated hypotheses fully addressed?
4. Are the findings statistically significant?

Through the Results section, the reader should be able to identify the outcomes related to each research question or hypothesis. Each result should provide a clear and direct answer to the corresponding research question and be reported using statements, graphs, or tables, with appropriate statistical values (e.g., t-values, F-values, degrees of freedom, p-values). Results are often presented using tables or figures, and readers should examine these carefully. Visual elements must be clear and not overly complicated. A single table or figure should not be overloaded with too much information, as this can make it difficult to interpret. It is also essential for readers to determine whether all participants were included in the final statistical analysis. If some subjects were excluded, the author must provide a clear explanation for their exclusion.

Discussion and Conclusion

Before reading the Discussion and Conclusion, the reader should carefully review the Methods and Results sections once again to evaluate the validity of the study and gather the necessary information to answer the following questions.

1. How does the author interpret the results?
2. Did the author clearly state whether each hypothesis was accepted or rejected?
3. Did the author consider plausible explanations for the findings?
4. Is the discussion supported by relevant literature?
5. Did the author acknowledge the limitations of the study?
6. If the findings were not statistically significant, did the author discuss the possibility of a Type II error?
7. Regardless of statistical significance, do the results have clinical relevance?
8. Did the author discuss how the findings could be applied in clinical practice?
9. Did the author suggest directions for future research?
10. Is the conclusion logically derived from the findings of the study?

The reader should be able to identify the author's main conclusions, based on the stated research hypotheses and the interpretation of results. Did the author compare the findings with those of previous studies? Do the results support current clinical theory, or does the author propose alternative explanations or approaches? Has the author acknowledged factors that may have complicated the interpretation of the results? Were the limitations of the study adequately addressed, and were future research directions clearly articulated? Finally, is the evidence presented in the study compelling enough to suggest changes to current clinical practices? To answer these questions, the reader must carefully evaluate the Discussion and Conclusion sections to determine whether the author's claims are supported by the data (Table 20.1).

Table 20.1 Evaluation criteria for research reports

1. *Title* 1. Is the title easy to understand? 2. Is it concise? 3. Does it provide sufficient information about the study? 4. Is the English title grammatically correct?
2. *Abstract* 1. Is the research problem clearly and concisely stated? 2. Is the methodology described? 3. Are the key results summarized? 4. Is the conclusion presented? 5. Is the word count within the journal's specified limit? 6. Are the keywords appropriate? 7. Is the English abstract grammatically accurate and focused on essential content?
3. *Introduction* 1. Is the research problem clearly defined? 2. Is the problem statement concise? 3. Is the research problem of significance? 4. Is the hypothesis clearly articulated and appropriately framed for testing? 5. Is the importance of the problem discussed, and is the research design appropriate to address it? 6. Are the variables clearly defined? 7. Are the variables categorized by type? (e.g., dependent, independent, predicted, predictor). 8. Are operational definitions provided for key terms?
4. *Literature review* 1. Are appropriate references cited in relation to the stated research problem? 2. Are the cited works relevant to the study? 3. Are the references drawn from credible academic sources? 4. Is the literature review logically structured? 5. Are related studies concisely summarized?

(continued)

Table 20.1 (continued)

5. *Methods*
   A. Participants
      1. Is the target population described?
      2. Is the sampling method explained?
      3. Is the sampling method appropriate (especially for hard-to-reach populations)?
      4. Is participant protection described (e.g., informed consent)?
   B. Instruments
      1. Are the instruments appropriate for the research setting and objectives?
         (a) Is construct validity established?
         (b) Is content validity addressed?
         (c) Is criterion-related validity described?
      2. Are the instruments reliable for the intended use?
         (a) Internal consistency coefficients
         (b) Equivalence coefficients
         (c) Stability coefficients
         (d) Interrater reliability
         (e) Intrarater reliability
      3. Is the instrument development process through pilot testing described?
   C. Research design
      1. Is the research design relevant to the theory and hypothesis?
      2. Does the design support internal validity?
      3. Are proper controls included?
      4. Are confounding variables minimized or acknowledged with justification?
      5. Is the design described in sufficient detail for replication?

6. *Results*
   1. Are the results presented clearly and accurately?
   2. Do the findings adequately address the research questions?
   3. Are the reported statistics appropriate for the research design?
   4. Are the statistics relevant to the research hypotheses?
   5. Are all tables and figures clear and complete?
   6. Are the titles of tables and figures concise?
   7. Are measurement units indicated?
   8. Are tables and figures arranged in a logical, comprehensible order?

7. *Discussion*
   1. Are the results discussed in relation to the original research questions?
   2. If hypotheses were stated, are they addressed in the discussion?
   3. Are the conclusions supported by the results?
   4. Is the relevance of the findings discussed?
   5. Are limitations acknowledged and suggestions for future research provided?

(continued)

Table 20.1 (continued)

8. *Conclusion*
   1. Are the key findings highlighted?
   2. Are the conclusions appropriately drawn without overgeneralization?

9. *References*
   1. Are references formatted according to submission guidelines?
   2. Are all in-text citations included in the reference list?
   3. Are there any references listed that were not cited in the text?

10. *Writing style*
    1. Are spacing and spelling correct?
    2. Are the sentences concise and well-structured?
    3. Are author names and year citations accurate?
    4. Are there any redundant or repetitive sentences?

21 How to Write a Research Proposal

At the initial stage of the research process, the investigator formulates the research question and outlines the method of data collection. The success of a research project depends largely on how well these elements are developed and defined, how effectively the necessary resources are assembled, and whether the study begins with methodological rigor in terms of reliability and validity. A research proposal serves to organize and communicate these foundational elements. It describes the purpose of the study, the significance of the research question, and the overall protocol of the project. Research proposals fulfill several important functions.

First, a well-prepared proposal demonstrates the researcher's critical thinking and scientific reasoning. By thoroughly reviewing the literature, the researcher establishes that the study addresses a question worth investigating. The proposal should present a theoretically justified and methodologically sound approach for testing the research assumptions.

Second, research proposals serve as essential documents when applying for funding from grant agencies or sponsoring organizations.

Third, proposals are reviewed by an Institutional Review Board (IRB)—particularly in the United States—when the research involves human or animal subjects. The IRB evaluates the proposal to ensure that the research poses no undue harm to participants and adheres to ethical standards. Researchers must submit their proposals for ethical approval through their institution's IRB before beginning data collection. Upon completion of the study, investigators are typically required to submit a final report as well.

Fourth, the research proposal promotes communication and collaboration among colleagues, particularly those with shared research interests or those seeking guidance and feedback.

Finally, a proposal provides a clear framework for conducting the study, including a detailed description of data collection methods and the overall structure of the research process. In this way, the research proposal is a crucial planning tool in the early stages of study development.

When a proposal is submitted to a research institute or funding agency as part of a formal request for financial support, the investigator must adhere to the specific guidelines provided by that organization. Although the core components of a research proposal are generally consistent across settings, proposals must often be reformatted to meet the submission criteria of a given institution or grant program.

21.1 Essential Elements of a Research Proposal

Before writing a research proposal, the investigator should engage in thorough reflection and planning, collect relevant background information, and seek advice from experts who are well-

K.-H. Yi, *Statistical Research Methods for Dermatologists and Plastic Surgeons*,
https://doi.org/10.1007/978-981-95-5668-7_21

versed in the subject matter and research methodology. If the proposal is being prepared for grant application purposes, it may be helpful to review previously approved proposals from the same funding agency. Although proposal guidelines vary by institution, the following outlines the most commonly used components found in research proposals.

Title

The title of the proposal serves as the reader's first impression. It may be determined in the early planning stage or after the research design has been finalized. The title should clearly reflect the content and focus of the study, providing sufficient information in a concise format.

For example, a title such as "Skin Pigmentation" may be simple, but it leaves the reader unclear about the specific focus of the study. A slightly more informative title like "Skin Pigmentation and Laser Treatment" provides some context, but still does not fully convey the core of the research. A more appropriate title would be: "The Effects of Laser Treatment on Skin Pigmentation in Adults with Melasma." This version clearly presents the independent variable, the dependent variable, and the population being studied (adults with melasma), making it a suitable and informative title.

Abstract

A one-page summary of the research proposal should be prepared and included when submitting the proposal to funding agencies, Institutional Review Boards (IRBs), or as part of a graduate thesis proposal. Review committees typically begin their evaluation by reading this abstract, and often only a select group of reviewers will proceed to examine the full proposal in detail.

The abstract should emphasize the purpose of the study and the importance of conducting the research. It should also include a brief description of the study population, procedures, methods of data analysis, anticipated duration, and estimated costs. Because reviewers will read the abstract before reading the full proposal, it is essential to write this section in a way that makes a strong and positive impression. In particular, the abstract should clearly convey why the research is important and what contribution it is expected to make.

Body of the Proposal

The body of the research proposal provides a detailed explanation of the purpose and significance of the study, as well as the planned procedures.

Statement of the Problem

The research proposal should begin by situating the topic within the relevant field of inquiry. The introduction must emphasize why the issue is worth studying, and whether it is likely to produce clinically meaningful outcomes. The discussion should start with general background information and progressively narrow in focus to guide the reader toward the specific topic of interest in a logical and structured manner.

For example, in a study comparing the effects of two different skincare approaches following a cosmetic laser procedure, the researcher should begin by defining the nature of laser-induced skin sensitivity and describing the increasing frequency with which post-laser care is required in clinical dermatology settings.

The importance of this issue is related to factors such as the cost of follow-up care and how long it takes for patients to resume normal daily activities or return to work. Post-laser skin management can include a wide range of approaches—from simply advising rest and barrier protection, to recommending hydrating treatments or active formulations that aim to accelerate skin recovery. In such cases, the researcher would need to evaluate and define the effectiveness of these different strategies.

When presenting the problem, the proposal should include a theoretical rationale related to the topic.

In this example, the rationale might compare the outcomes of in-clinic skin recovery protocols to those of at-home regimens, possibly addressing differences in effectiveness, cost, or accessibility.

Therefore, the proposal should clearly describe how the study is clinically relevant and why a specific approach may be warranted in the given context.

Purpose, Hypotheses, and Specific Aims

This section should provide a concise description of the research plan. The purpose of the study must be clearly stated and scientifically justified. In the case of experimental or correlational research, the purpose may be framed as a research hypothesis. The hypothesis should be written in a positive and directional form, expressing the expected relationship or outcome. A null hypothesis should also be included to fulfill the requirements of statistical testing. In studies examining relationships between variables, the purpose is to determine the correlation among those variables. In descriptive research, on the other hand, the goal is to identify and report specific characteristics or behaviors observed in the target population.

In many cases, researchers are expected to specify their particular aims. For instance, the stated purpose may involve determining which of two known treatments is more effective, or identifying relationships between a particular variable and the reliability of a tool or the structure of a treatment plan. Clearly stating the hypothesis also helps to clarify the purpose of the research. By articulating the purpose in this way, the researcher will be better prepared to describe the methodology and develop a meaningful discussion of the findings upon completion of the study.

Theoretical Background

The theoretical background section of a research proposal should include the rationale for the study, relevant and verifiable facts, objective findings, and the key questions or uncertainties identified by the researcher. Such information is typically derived from a thorough review of prior research and relevant literature. Funding agencies often evaluate the theoretical foundation of a study when reviewing submitted proposals.

Although conducting a literature review may seem straightforward, summarizing it effectively can be challenging, especially when previous studies have explored the topic from multiple perspectives. Researchers will often consult more literature than they ultimately cite in the proposal. If the review attempts to include too much information, it may lose focus. Therefore, it is advisable to present only what is essential to understand and address the research problem, including relevant theories, the independent and dependent variables, and how they might influence the study's results.

When reviewing the literature, researchers should continually ask themselves questions such as "Is this reference directly related to my research question?" and "Is the theoretical rationale valid and appropriate for the proposed study?" If a source does not meet these criteria, it should be excluded from the proposal without hesitation. In the background section, the researcher should aim to concisely summarize the key findings, unresolved issues, contrasting viewpoints, and their own relevant experiences related to the topic.

Methods

The Methods section is one of the most important parts of a research proposal and should be written clearly and concisely. The researcher should aim to provide sufficient detail to demonstrate the soundness and feasibility of the study. This section is often used by Institutional Review Board (IRB) members to evaluate the ethical and practical viability of the proposed research. At the beginning of the section, the type of research design should be clearly stated. The methodology is typically organized into four components such as subjects, materials, procedures, and data analysis.

In studies involving human participants, many factors must be described in detail. The researcher must specify the inclusion and exclusion criteria, explain how subjects were selected, and describe how many were enrolled and how they were assigned to each group. Relevant information such as age, sex, height, weight, diagnosis, severity of condition, or length of hospital stay should be included when applicable. Among these variables, the researcher should clearly indicate which factors are expected to influence the study outcomes.

The materials section refers to the equipment and measurement tools used in the study. Important characteristics such as the manufacturer, model number, and details about the reliability and validity of each tool should be reported. If a newly developed, unfamiliar, or previously unused instrument is employed, it should be described in full, and photographs or diagrams may be included if needed to ensure clarity.

The procedures section should describe, in chronological order, what was done from the beginning to the end of the study. In addition to outlining what occurred, it should explain when, how, and by whom the data were collected. Operational definitions of the independent and dependent variables must be clearly stated. If the study was conducted over a long period or involved complex steps, references to other sources or an appendix may be used to provide additional detail while keeping the main text concise.

The data analysis section explains how the data were collected, coded, and prepared for statistical analysis. It should identify the variables used in the analysis, specify the types of statistical procedures planned, and justify the appropriateness of those procedures for the study design and level of measurement. When reviewing a proposal, evaluators must determine whether the descriptive and inferential statistical methods are appropriate for the research design and measurement levels used in the study.

Documentation of Informed Consent

A copy of the informed consent form must be attached to the research proposal at the time of submission. This is a standard requirement for Institutional Review Boards (IRBs) and research funding agencies (see appendix for an example).

Budget

Every research proposal must include a detailed budget estimate to demonstrate the feasibility of the study. Typically, the budget should present both a summary of the total cost and a breakdown by category. Standard budget categories include personnel, equipment, facilities, supplies, and travel expenses.

The personnel section should specify who is involved in the project, the percentage of effort or time commitment, whether they are full-time or part-time, and the corresponding salary or stipend allocated to each role.

In the equipment section, only approved purchases should be listed. Each item should include the manufacturer, model name, and any specialized accessories required for the study. Sometimes, facility modification costs may be requested as part of the budget to support the research environment.

The supplies category typically includes consumable items such as paper, data collection forms, stationery, and experimental materials. These may also be listed under a general category such as "miscellaneous."

Travel expenses refer to costs incurred for data collection trips or attending research-related meetings or conferences. The items listed above are considered direct costs. In contrast, indirect costs refer to institutional overhead expenses necessary to support the research project, such as facility maintenance and administrative support.

Resources and Environment

This section refers to the laboratories, clinical research facilities, equipment, computer systems, and office space available to carry out the proposed study.

Personnel

Describing the qualifications of the researcher is not only a critical component of the proposal but also a required element when applying for external funding. Funding agencies will evaluate the researcher's academic background, relevant experience, scholarly achievements, and publication record, along with the proposal itself.

Presentation of the Proposal

Writing Style

A research proposal is a forward-looking document, so the research problem should be described using the present tense, the background in the past tense, and the methods in the future tense. Because the formatting and submission requirements vary by institution or funding agency, it is essential to follow the specific style guidelines provided by each. Only references that are cited in the text should appear in the reference list, and a consistent citation format must be used throughout. Tables, figures, and appendices must be clearly labeled and titled.

The overall tone of the proposal should be positive, persuasive, and scholarly, convincing reviewers of the significance of the study and the research team's capability to carry it out successfully. Avoid vague or tentative expressions such as "The results may possibly contribute..." or "We hope to observe such outcomes...," as well as overly exaggerated claims. The proposal should be sensible, fact-based, and realistic in scope and tone.

Printing and Formatting

The final version of the proposal should be clearly and legibly printed, with formatting that enhances readability and comprehension. All sections should be thoroughly proofread to eliminate typographical errors, which may suggest a lack of attention to detail. Some reviewers may significantly penalize proposals with errors, interpreting them as a sign of poor preparation or insufficient care.

Appendix 1: List of Abbreviations for Journals in Cosmetic Dermatology and Plastic Surgery

Subject area	Name of journal	Abbreviation
Aesthetic surgery	Aesthetic Surgery Journal	Aesthet Surg J
	Aesthetic Plastic Surgery	Aesthetic Plast Surg
	Journal of Plastic, Reconstructive and Aesthetic Surgery: JPRAS	J Plast Reconstr Aesthet Surg

K.-H. Yi, *Statistical Research Methods for Dermatologists and Plastic Surgeons*,
https://doi.org/10.1007/978-981-95-5668-7

Subject area	Name of journal	Abbreviation
Clinical dermatology	American Journal of Clinical Dermatology	Am J Clin Dermatol
	Anais Brasileiros de Dermatologia	An Bras Dermatol
	Annales de Dermatologie et de Venereologie	Ann Dermatol Venereol
	Archives of Dermatological Research	Arch Dermatol Res
	Australasian Journal of Dermatology	Australas J Dermatol
	BMC Dermatology	BMC Dermatol
	British Journal of Dermatology	Br J Dermatol
	Clinics in Dermatology	Clin Dermatol
	Clinical and Experimental Dermatology	Clin Exp Dermatol
	Current Problems in Dermatology	Curr Probl Dermatol
	Dermatologic Clinics	Dermatol Clin
	Dermatology Online Journal	Dermatol Online J
	Dermatologic Surgery	Dermatol Surg
	Dermatologic Therapy	Dermatol Ther
	Dermatology (Basel, Switzerland)	Dermatology
	European Journal Of Dermatology: EJD	Eur J Dermatol
	Experimental Dermatology	Exp Dermatol
	Giornale Italiano di Dermatologia e Venereologia	G Ital Dermatol Venereol
	Hautarzt; Zeitschrift fur Dermatologie, Venerologie, und verwandte Gebiete	Hautarzt
	Indian Journal of Dermatology, Venereology and Leprology	Indian J Dermatol Venereol Leprol
	International Journal of Dermatology	Int J Dermatol
	Journal of the American Academy of Dermatology	J Am Acad Dermatol
	Journal of Dermatology	J Dermatol
	Journal of Dermatological Science	J Dermatol Sci
	Journal of Dermatological Treatment	J Dermatolog Treat
	Journal of Drugs in Dermatology: JDD	J Drugs Dermatol
	Journal der Deutschen Dermatologischen Gesellschaft = Journal of the German Society of Dermatology: JDDG	J Dtsch Dermatol Ges
	Journal of the European Academy of Dermatology and Venereology: JEADV	J Eur Acad Dermatol Venereol
	Journal of Investigative Dermatology	J Invest Dermatol
	journal of Investigative Dermatology. Symposium Proceedings	J Investig Dermatol Symp Proc
	JAMA Dermatology	JAMA Dermatol
	Pediatric Dermatology	Pediatr Dermatol
	Photodermatology, Photoimmunology and Photomedicine	Photodermatol Photoimmunol Photomed
	Veterinary Dermatology	Vet Dermatol
	International Journal of Cosmetic Science	Int J Cosmet Sci
	Journal of Cosmetic Dermatology	J Cosmet Dermatol
	Journal of Cosmetic and Laser Therapy	J Cosmet Laser Ther
	Journal of Cosmetic Science	J Cosmet Sci

Subject area	Name of journal	Abbreviation
Plastic & reconstructive surgery	Acta Chirurgiae Plasticae	Acta Chir Plast
	Annals of Plastic Surgery	Ann Plast Surg
	Clinics in Plastic Surgery	Clin Plast Surg
	Facial Plastic Surgery Clinics of North America	Facial Plast Surg Clin North Am
	Female Pelvic Medicine and Reconstructive Surgery	Female Pelvic Med Reconstr Surg
	Journal of Plastic Surgery and Hand Surgery	J Plast Surg Hand Surg
	Journal of Reconstructive Microsurgery	J Reconstr Microsurg
	JAMA Facial Plastic Surgery	JAMA Facial Plast Surg
	Neural Plasticity	Neural Plast
	Ophthalmic Plastic and Reconstructive Surgery	Ophthal Plast Reconstr Surg
	Plastic and Reconstructive Surgery	Plast Reconstr Surg
	Scandinavian Journal of Plastic and Reconstructive Surgery and Hand Surgery. Supplementum	Scand J Plast Reconstr Surg Hand Surg Suppl
	Zhongguo xiu fu chong jian wai ke za zhi = Zhongguo xiufu chongjian waike zazhi = Chinese Journal of Reparative and Reconstructive Surgery	Zhongguo Xiu Fu Chong Jian Wai Ke Za Zhi
Skin biology	Skin Pharmacology and Physiology	Skin Pharmacol Physiol
	Skin Research and Technology	Skin Res Technol
	Skin Therapy Letter	Skin Therapy Lett
	Skinmed	Skinmed

[a]Only journal abbreviations registered in Index Medicus are listed.

Appendix 2: Questionnaire on Occupational Risk Factors Among Aesthetic and Cosmetic Practice Professionals

Dear Participant,

Hello. I am a doctoral student currently enrolled in the Graduate School of Public Health at **OO University**. This questionnaire has been designed to investigate occupational risk factors that may affect musculoskeletal health and skin exposure among professionals working in the fields of aesthetic dermatology and cosmetic surgery in Korea. We sincerely thank you for taking the time out of your busy schedule to participate in this research.

The information you provide will serve as valuable data in identifying the working conditions of aesthetic and cosmetic professionals in Korea and the extent to which those conditions may contribute to physical strain or skin-related symptoms. All responses will be entered into a computer and processed collectively, so no individual record will be disclosed to outside parties. Furthermore, the data will be used exclusively for research purposes. Your honest and sincere responses will greatly contribute to the reliability and validity of this study.

Once again, thank you for your cooperation despite your busy schedule. If you are interested in receiving information related to occupational health or prevention strategies in your field, please feel free to contact me. I would be happy to share relevant materials collected during the course of this research.

Sincerely,

2025. 05.

Graduate Program in Public Health

OO University

(Your name)

*(Phone number)
*(Postal code)

I. The following questions pertain to your general characteristics.

Please read each item carefully and either answer the question or check the appropriate box.

1. Sex: ☐ Male ☐ Female
2. Age: ______ years
3. Highest level of education: ☐ High school ☐ Associate ☐ Bachelor's ☐ Graduate or above
4. Type of workplace: ☐ Dermatology clinic/hospital ☐ Plastic surgery clinic ☐ Aesthetic clinic ☐ Other (_______)

K.-H. Yi, *Statistical Research Methods for Dermatologists and Plastic Surgeons*,
https://doi.org/10.1007/978-981-95-5668-7

5. Job role: ☐ Esthetician ☐ Assistant nurse ☐ Laser technician ☐ Other (______)
6. Years of experience in the current field: _____ years _____ months
7. Average working hours per week: _____ hours
8. Average number of clients treated per day: _____ persons
9. Approximate hours per day spent with head tilted downward during procedures: _____ hours
10. Approximate hours per day involving repetitive wrist or hand movements: _____ hours
11. Approximate hours spent standing per day: _____ hours
12. Have you experienced skin irritation or allergy symptoms from gloves, cosmetics, or chemicals used in practice? ☐ Yes ☐ No
13. If yes, which areas were affected? ☐ Hands ☐ Arms ☐ Face ☐ Other (______)
14. What types of protective gear do you typically use during work? (Check all that apply)
☐ Cotton gloves ☐ Face mask ☐ Protective gown ☐ None

II. The following questions ask how often you practice proper body mechanics during work or daily activities. Please think carefully about your posture and movements during treatments or tasks, and check the number that best represents your behavior.

Question	Never	Rarely	Sometimes	Often	Very Often
1. *When working in a standing position*:					
1.1 Do you keep your back straight while working?	**0**	**1**	**2**	**3**	**4**
1.2 Do you keep your knees slightly bent?	**0**	**1**	**2**	**3**	**4**
1.3 Do you place one foot slightly forward?	**0**	**1**	**2**	**3**	**4**
1.4 Do you use a footrest or place one foot on a raised object?	**0**	**1**	**2**	**3**	**4**
2. *When working in a sitting position*:					
2.1 Do you rest your arms on an armrest or desk while working?	**0**	**1**	**2**	**3**	**4**
2.2 Do you lean back against the chair support?	**0**	**1**	**2**	**3**	**4**
2.3 Do you position your knees slightly higher than your hips while sitting?	**0**	**1**	**2**	**3**	**4**
3. *When lifting equipment or supplies from the floor*:					
3.1 Do you lift items while keeping them close to your body?	**0**	**1**	**2**	**3**	**4**
3.2 Do you bend your knees while lifting?	**0**	**1**	**2**	**3**	**4**
3.3 Do you keep your back straight while lifting?	**0**	**1**	**2**	**3**	**4**

III. The following questions are designed to assess your experiences related to skin exposure and chemical-related risks in your occupational environment. Please read each item carefully and select the number that best corresponds to your experience.

No.	Question item	Never	Rarely	Sometimes	Often	Always
1	I experience skin dryness or irritation after performing procedures.	(0)	(1)	(2)	(3)	(4)
2	I am exposed to chemical substances (e.g., peels, disinfectants, topical anesthetics) without protective equipment.	(0)	(1)	(2)	(3)	(4)
3	I experience redness or itching after contact with gloves or cosmetic products.	(0)	(1)	(2)	(3)	(4)
4	I skip the use of protective gloves or masks during short procedures.	(0)	(1)	(2)	(3)	(4)
5	I continue wearing gloves or masks even when they cause discomfort or sweating.	(0)	(1)	(2)	(3)	(4)
6	I regularly wash or sanitize my hands during work hours (10+ times/day).	(0)	(1)	(2)	(3)	(4)
7	I use hand sanitizers or cleansing products that worsen my skin condition.	(0)	(1)	(2)	(3)	(4)
8	I experience dermatitis or eczema symptoms during work.	(0)	(1)	(2)	(3)	(4)
9	I feel that the skin on my hands has deteriorated since working in this profession.	(0)	(1)	(2)	(3)	(4)
10	I feel that protective equipment interferes with treatment accuracy or speed.	(0)	(1)	(2)	(3)	(4)

Appendix 3: Sample Institutional Review Board (IRB) Form

University and Medical Center Institutional Review Board
Human BioMedical Internal Processing Form
SUBMISSION FOR UMCIRB review
Full and Expedited research

DEMOGRAPHIC INFORMATION

Type of application: x New Modification Date: UMCIRB #:

Title of proposed research (this title must match protocol, funding application and consent form):
Effects of Seat Surface on the Biomechanics of Sit-to-Stand Movement in Healthy Adults

Principal Investigator, credentials, department, section and school:
Chung Hwi Yi, PhD, PT, Department of Physical Therapy, CAHS
Check the institutions for which the principal investigator is associated: x ECU PCMH Other

Subinvestigators, credentials, department, section and schools:
D*** B******* EdD, PT, Department of Physical Therapy, CAHS

*** Investigators not associated with ECU or PCMH require submission of an Unaffiliated Investigator Agreement.

List all items related to this research study submitted for UMCIRB review and approval:
Human Biomedical Internal Processing Form
Informed Consent Form
Conflict of Interest Disclosure Form

SOURCE OF FUNDING

Government Agency, Name:
Private Agency, Name:
Institution or Department Sponsor, Name:
x No funding
Grant: include 3 copies of the final grant application for full committee reviews or 1 copy for expedited reviews
NOTE: The UMCIRB Conflict of Interest Disclosure Form needs to be submitted for expedited and full review.

CHECK ALL INSTITUTIONS OR SITES WHERE THIS RESEARCH STUDY WILL BE CONDUCTED
:
x East Carolina University
Pitt County Memorial Hospital, Inc
Heritage Hospital
Other
Beaufort County Hospital
Carteret General Hospital
Boice-Willis Clinic

K.-H. Yi, *Statistical Research Methods for Dermatologists and Plastic Surgeons*, https://doi.org/10.1007/978-981-95-5668-7

CHECK THE FOLLOWING INVOLVED IN THIS STUDY:

Population Specifically Targeted	Methods/Procedures
Normal volunteers	Surveys / Questionnaires
x Adults (› 18 yrs old)	Interviews
Minors (‹ 18 yrs old)	Standardized Written / Oral / Visual Tests
Institutionalized Participants	Videotaping / Voice Recording / Photography
Students	Deception
Inpatient participants	Randomization
Prisoners	Drugs
Pregnant Participants	Placebo (s)
Participants of child bearing potential	Medical Devices
Embryos or fetuses	Sterile Surgical / Invasive Procedures
Neonates	Non-sterile Invasive Procedures
Wards of the State	Surgical or otherwise discarded Tissue/Samples
Minorities	Autopsy or cadaver tissue
Non-English speaking	Therapeutic Radiation
Desperately / Terminally Ill Participants	Diagnostic Radiation
Traumatized/Comatose Participants	Banking of biological materials
Communicable Disease	Genetic testing
Outpatient participants	HIV Testing
International research	Registry / Database
Cognitively or emotionally impaired	Recombinant DNA / Gene Transfer Technology

INVESTIGATIONAL TEST ITEMS

Does your proposal involve investigational drugs?	x No	Yes
Does your proposal involve approved drugs for non-approved uses?	x No	Yes
Does this proposal have an IND	x No	Yes

Name:
Manufacturer:
IND No:
IND Filing date:
Drug study phase:

Does your proposal involve investigational devices, instruments, machines?	x No	Yes
Is this device exempt from the requirements of 21CFR812?	x No	Yes
Does your proposal involve approved devices for non-approved uses?	x No	Yes
Is this a significant risk (SR) device?	x No	Yes
Does this proposal have an IDE?	x No	Yes

Name:
Manufacturer:
IDE No., device study type:
Device study phase:
Provide the FDA letter of SR/NSR designation or the sponsor letter of risk designation.
Attach a copy of the FDA approval letter of the IDE.

Research Risk and Level of Review Required

Research participants will be placed at as defined below:

x No more than minimal risk

More than minimal risk

Minimal risk means that the probability and magnitude of harm or discomfort anticipated in the research are not greater in and of themselves than those ordinarily encountered in daily life or during the performance of routine physical or psychological examinations or tests. 45 CFR 46.102(i) The definition for prisoners differs and is located at 45 CFR 46

What level of review does your proposal require?

x Expedited

Full

Those research studies utilizing Pitt County Memorial Hospital resources, Brody School of Medicine resources or involving ionizing radiation should complete the Institutional Approval for Research Form.

Research Questions

1. Subject Selection

Describe how participants will be selected or recruited for the research, including enrollment procedure.

Participants will be healthy volunteers. The subjects recruited for this study are students of the Physical Therapy Department at the ECU. The investigators will request the participation of the subjects and a writ ten consent form will be completed by the subjects.

Identify the projected number of participants to be enrolled. 20 Outline the inclusion and exclusion criteria for this research study. None of the included subjects reports any recent history of any neuromuscular or orthopedic disorder. All participants are able to clearly hear and understand the instructions given. Observational sit-to-stand motion analysis of the participants will be performed to ensure the absence of movement disorder.

Provide a justification for the sample size selected.

The sample size is based on the calculated statistical power to find differences between groups in the biomechanical variables of interest.

Describe the safeguards in place to protect the rights and welfare of any vulnerable participants enrolled in this research study.

All subjects' data will be assigned a code and stored in a locked cabinet. All subjects will be closely guarded by a physical therapist or physical therapy student during data collection to prevent falls. Subjects may rest at any time to avoid fatigue. Subjects may withdraw from the study at any time by informing the investigators they wish to withdraw.

Are there any advertisements (public display in written, radio, or TV form) for participant recruitment?

Yes x No If yes, attach the advertisements to the processing form.

Does the research include any monetary inducements, compensation or reimbursement for participation in this research study?

Yes x No If yes, attach the payment schedule to the processing form or provide specific. Protocol reference.

Will the sponsor reimburse for any items or procedures or supply any items at no cost involved in this research study?

Yes x No If yes, attach written documentation of the items that will be reimbursed or supplied by the sponsor unless this information is specifically noted in the research protocol.

Are there any associated costs that participants will incur as a result of participating in this research study?

Yes x No If yes, describe these costs.

2. Researcher Qualifications

Name and list the duties of the research team members and describe the qualifications of each member to perform their duties. Dr. Yi and Brunt will oversee the data collection.

Both have considerable experience in a biomechanics setting.

Include the completion date of the human protections modules located on the UMCIRB web site.

B*****—09/08/2006

Yi—03/17/2008

3. Risk Determination

Describe the research setting, listing any safeguards in place for participant safety.

The Gait and Balance Laboratory in the Department of Physical Therapy is used by the PI for collection of motion analysis data. It occupies a space of approximately 1,000 sq. ft. with a 30-ft walkway the length of the room. In the center of the walkway are situated two AMTI OR6-7 2000 force plates. The dimensions of each plate are 464 x 508 mm. Thc laboratory also contains an 8-camera motion analysis system, which can monitor the motion of a moving body in three-dimensional space. The lab has a 12 channel surface EMG system. There is ample seating for participants and family members, if necessary. Participants will be guarded by a physical therapist or physical therapy student to reduce the likelihood of a fall. Participants may rest at any time to avoid fatigue.

4. Risk Determination

Describe all foreseeable physical, psychological, economic, social, legal and dignitary risks to the participants, with steps outlined to minimize those risks. Risks should be described in terms of probability or likelihood, magnitude and duration when possible. Possible risks include fatigue and a fall. Both are minimal risks. Participants will be allowed to rest between trials or when requested. Participants will be guarded by a physical therapist or physical therapy student to reduce the possibility of a fall.

Outline the mechanism for reporting adverse events or unanticipated risks to participants or others for this study. Adverse or unforeseen events occurring in the lab will be reported to the UMCIRB on the appropriate form.

Specifically address any risk associated with the use of placebo, if applicable. N/A

5. Data/Safety Monitoring : Data monitoring includes activities such as interim analysis or other opportunities for both individual and aggregate study data to be reviewed to ensure the safety and efficacy of a research test item. A plan for this type of data monitoring is required to meet the criteria for IRB approval in order to ensure the protection of participants involved in the research, to review the risk-benefit analysis, and to ensure there are no new findings for which current or future participants should be apprised. Describe any additional data monitoring challenges when the principal investigator or another research team member is not directly involved in data collection or monitoring because they are not available on the research site. Describe the data monitoring plan according to Good Clinical Practices (and Data Safety Monitoring Board/Committee, if applicable) to ensure safety of subjects. Data is monitored in real time to ensure accurate data collection. In addition, a participant's data will be analyzed immediately. This data monitoring will allow us to determine if specific elements of the data collection can be eliminated or modified and/or whether variables need to be added to the protocol.
6. Anticipated Benefits

Describe the benefits of the research study to participants or others. The sit-to-stand (STS) movement is one function people frequently use as they change from a sitting position to standing position. And the STS ability is an important skill in elderly people and people with disabling diseases in their activities of daily living. Assessment of the STS movement has been done using quantitative techniques. The ability to do an STS movement, according to the research reviewed, is strongly influenced by the height of the chair seat, use of armrests, and foot position. However, more study of the interaction among the different determinants is needed. Although wheelchair has been used for the disabled and the elderly for a long time, STS study about rising from wheelchair using kinematic and kinetic analysis could not be found from the literature review. Failing to consider the characteristics of seat surface may lead to erroneous measurements of changes in STS performance. Therefore, the purposes of this study are to determine whether the characteristics of seat surface affect the STS movement and to describe their influence on the performance of the STS movement while the subjects are rising from a wheelchair. With information obtained from this study we will be able to:

Provide the clinician with precise information on the STS characteristics analyzed by using kinematic and kinetic techniques. This information will be useful to select proper technique and seat surface to train STS from a wheelchair and assess the performance of the STS movement in clinical settings.

7. Data Confidentiality and Subject Privacy

Describe how confidentiality will be maintained by providing details about the storage facility, duration of storage, data destruction method, and persons with access to the data. All data will be stored on password-protected computers and stored in locked file cabinets with coded files. The investigators and graduate assistants will have access to data. By the nature of the data, there are no potentially harmful uses.

How will subject privacy be maintained during recruitment, data collection and data analysis?

All data sheets and files will be coded to protect subject confidentiality.

If the participants' data or samples will be used for future research, describe how their privacy will be protected. N/A

Describe any additional safeguards in place to manage illegal, significantly intimate or potentially embarrassing information gathered in this research study. N/A

Include steps to handle information that requires mandatory reporting to officials, for example physical abuse, emotional abuse or health problems. N/A

If the research study involves HIV testing, describe the plans for pre/post-test counseling and other related considerations. N/A

8. Obtaining Consent or Parental Permission

Describe the consent process, including members of the research team that will be obtaining informed consent from study participants.

Dr. Yi and Dr. B****** will request the students' participation in the study. One of the investigators will ask. the subjects to read and sign an informed consent document.

Describe the setting in which the consent will be obtained.

Gait and Balance Lab, ECU Department of Physical Therapy, Health Sciences Building.

Describe the process to minimize undue influence and coercion during the consent process.

Participants will be given ample time by themselves to read the consent form, and will be asked if they. have any questions before signing. Their role as volunteers in this project will be stressed, as well as their right to withdrawal at any time.

Outline procedures for obtaining informed consent from participants with limited or low literacy. N/A

Describe the process for determining cognitive impairment or other conditions that may make a participant more vulnerable. It is expected that all participants in this study will be of average or above cognitive abilities.

Describe the process for identifying the legally authorized representative and the process to debrief and. subsequently obtain consent from the study participant, when feasible. N/A

9. Minor Assent Related Issues

Describe the assent processes given the range of ages intended for this research study. N/A

If a separate assent is not being used, how will assent be documented? N/A

How will custody changes during participation in the study be determined? N/A

Describe the processes as required for enrolling wards of the state if they are a target population for this. study. Note: If a child becomes a ward of the state, the IRB must be notified immediately to seek advice on further protections that may be required. N/A

Background

Describe the current state of knowledge surrounding the research questions to be addressed in this study. The literature indicates that the chair has an influence on the performance of the STS movement. Most research has been focused on the height of the seat, and few studies tried to clarify the influence of the armrest position, use of armrests, or the type of chair on the STS movement (Janssen 2002; Etnyre et al. 2007). The evaluation of STS performance involves a variety of measurements to include joint angles and moments, speed of time to rise, functional reach and sway, and perception of patient stability (or perceived safety) in rising from a chair (Edlich et al. 2003). These studies reported that chair seat height, use of armrest, and foot position had a major influence on the ability to do a STS movement. The use of higher chair seats resulted in lower moments at the knee and hip level. Investigators reported that lowering the chair height increased the need for momentum generation or repositioning of the feet to lower the needed moments. They found that the use of an armrest reduced the moments needed at the hip without altering the range of motion of the joints. Displacement between the person and the wheelchair seating surface is one measure of the shear forces (Cooper et al. 2000). The goal of the present study is to determine the thus far unstudied effects of seat surfaces on the kinematics and kinetics of sit-to-stand (STS) motion in healthy adults, in a wheelchair.

Describe the uncertainty to be addressed by this research study (research question). The questions to be asked in this pilot study are:

Will the seat surface of a wheelchair affect the kinematics of sit-to-stand motion in healthy adults?

What the seat surface of a wheelchair affect the kinetics of sit-to-stand motion in healthy adults?

Describe the rationale for the type of research design chosen for this study. Because there are two advantages of the within-subjects design: a) power and b) reduction in error variance associated with individual differences, we chose within-subjects design. Although within-subjects design has a fundamental disadvantage of "carry-over effects (practice and fatigue)", we will avoid the problem using random order technique and application of enough rest time between trials.

Protocol Description

Provide a brief, one page description of the research study. All more than minimal risk research studies or research requiring full UMCIRB review must have a separate protocol.

Twenty participants will be tested. Prior to the experiment, all subjects will sign informed consent forms. Testing will require about two hours in the Gait and Balance at East Carolina University. Retroreflective markers (at least three per segment) will be placed bilaterally on the segments of the rearfoot, shank, thigh, pelvis, shoulders and head. Kinematic data will be collected using an 8-camera, motion analysis system. A standing calibration trial will be collected. A force plate mounted in the gait walkway will record ground reaction forces as the subject performs sit-to-stand task. Kinematic data will be sampled at 120 Hz, and force data will be collected at 960 Hz. Kinematic and kinetic data will be time-synchronized. Surface electrodes will be placed on selected lower extremity muscles to collect electromyographic (EMG) data. These electrodes will be taped onto the skin with hypoallergenic tape.

The three-dimensional coordinates of each marker are reconstructed using a direct linear transformation method. The reconstruction errors in a volume of approximately 1m X 1m X 2m are typically on the order of 1.5 mm. The 3-dimensional coordinates will be filtered using a 2nd order recursive Butterworth filter with an 8 Hz cutoff frequency. These data will then be used to calculate relative three-dimensional joint angles in an anatomical reference frame. This is achieved via transformation matrices between the local and global coordinate systems. The combination of the kinematic data and the force data will allow the calculations of joint forces, moments and powers through inverse dynamics. EMG data will be collected on line and pre-amplified on site. Specialized software will allow the calculation of both timing and amplitude events of muscle activity.

Subjects will be asked to complete 10 trials in each of the following tasks during each visit to the Gait and Balance lab:

1. Sit-to-stand from a standard chair
2. Sit-to-stand from a standard wheelchair without cushion
3. Sit-to-stand from a standard wheelchair with Roho cushion
4. Sit-to-stand from a standard wheelchair with Jay cushion

The biomechanical variables can be subdivided into three categories: tri-dimensional joint kinematics (position and velocity), joint kinetics (moments and powers), and ground reaction forces. Peak and excursion (total range of motion) values for the above kinematic and kinetic variables will be calculated unilaterally for the ankle, knee, hip, and trunk. Onset of EMG, relative to movement initiation, seat off (sit-to-stand), and amplitude of EMG will be analyzed. Comparisons between mean values will be performed with one-way repeated ANOVA techniques. Independent variable is seat surface. Significant level will be set at alpha=0.05.

Required Research Approvals

Is it reasonably foreseeable that studies will be done on participants of attending physicians other than investigators listed on the proposal?

Yes x No

If yes, obtain their signatures below or describe the method for obtaining their approval prior to the involvement of their patients.

The following physicians acknowledge their willingness to participate in the above named research study, have read the enclosed documents describing the study, and agree to allow their patients to participate.

Signature Print Date

Signature Print Date

Signature Print Date

CHIEF OF SERVICE OR DEPARTMENT CHAIR APPROVALS STATEMENT

I have reviewed this project. I believe that the research is sound, the goals are scientifically achievable, and does not involve any significant human rights issues. There are appropriate departmental resources (financial and otherwise) available to conduct the research. The investigator is qualified to conduct all aspects of this research project based on education, training or experience, and has the necessary authorizations or privileges to conduct all outlined procedures. I endorse the investigator and outlined research project as indicated by my signature below.

I have reviewed the UMCIRB Conflict of Interest Disclosure Form and evaluated the principal investigator of this project for risk related to conflict of interest according to the UMCIRB Standard Operating Procedure Manual. I endorse the investigator and the attached plan (if required) for managing conflict of interest related to this research study as indicated by my signature below.

NOTE: (1) A department chair may not sign this statement if listed as an investigator, and should seek the signature of the division chair/dean. (2) If you don't have a department chair (such as a private practice investigator) then attach a current CV.

Signatureof Chief of Service/Department Chair Print Date

Contact Information

Mailing address for all correspondence: Department of Physical Therapy, HSB
Telephone Number: 744-6244 Fax Number: 744-6240
e-mail: yi***@ecu.edu
Study coordinator: Dr. Yi Telephone number: 744-6244

RESPONSIBLE FACULTY MEMBER: For any Principal Investigator that has an undergraduate, graduate, post-graduate student status including residents and fellows, or visiting status to serve as a responsible individual in the oversight of the research study.

Responsible Faculty: Dr. Yi
Mailing address: Department of Physical Therapy, HSB
Telephone Number: 744-***** Fax Number: 744-****** e-mail: yi***@ecu.edu

I have reviewed the study proposal and all documents and materials to be used in the study.

Signature responsible faculty as above. Print Date

Investigator Responsibilities

The principal and subinvestigators agree to:

1. To obtain UMCIRB approval prior to undertaking any aspect of this research study.
2. To obtain UMCIRB approval prior to instituting any change in the research study, unless it is necessary to protect the safety and welfare of human participants. An action instituted to protect the safety and well-being requires immediate reporting to the UMCIRB.
3. To engage in a continuing exchange of information or advice with the UMCIRB ensuring a continuing review process for the protection of human participants, including submission of a closure form upon completion of the study.
4. To engage in a continuing exchange of information with the appropriate departments within the institutional study site, the institutional officials, the department chairs when appropriate, and the research study sponsor.
5. To ensure the research study is conducted only within the periods of UMCIRB approval.
6. To inform the UMCIRB, research site institution, sponsor or appropriate federal regula-

tory agency, in writing of any serious adverse events and unanticipated problems involving risks to study participants or others as soon as possible.

7. To maintain all study records for 3 years after completion of the study at all sites or longer if required by a professional organization, sponsor, regulatory body or others. To regard participant informed consent as an ongoing process.
8. To enroll participants only after obtaining ethically and legally effective informed consent, using only the most currently approved UMCIRB consent document, when required.
9. To obtain minor assent from children prior to enrollment as outlined.
10. To notify the UMCIRB if any relationships develop that may be considered a conflict of interest.
11. To abide by the UMCIRB Standard Operating Procedures, all applicable federal regulations, Good Clinical Practice, state laws, respective institutional policies to conduct this research study. Ethical standards include the Belmont Report and other professional standards for an individual research area.
12. To comply with regulatory reviews, data audits, and 3rd party observation for the consenting process by appropriate institutional regulatory officials.
13. To notify the UMCIRB prior to relocating employment to provide for the orderly study closure or to transfer the study to another investigator.

Signature Principal Investigator	Print	Date
Signature Subinvestigator.	Print	Date
Signature Subinvestigator.	Print	Date
Signature Subinvestigator.	Print	Date
Signature Subinvestigator.	Print	Date

Appendix 4: Sample Informed Consent Form

INFORMED CONSENT FORM

Principal Investigator: [Your Name]
Department: Department of Public Health
Institution: [OO University]
Address: Graduate School of Public Health, [OO University], [Address Line]
Telephone: [Your Phone Number]

Occupational Risk Factors Related to Musculoskeletal Strain and Skin Exposure Among Professionals in Cosmetic Dermatology and Plastic Surgery Clinics

INTRODUCTION

You are invited to participate in a research study conducted by [Your Name] at the Graduate School of Public Health, [OO University]. The purpose of this study is to investigate occupational risk factors-specifically musculoskeletal strain and skin exposure-among professionals working in the fields of cosmetic dermatology and plastic surgery in Korea.

You have been selected as a participant because of your professional role in a dermatology or cosmetic surgery clinical setting. Your insights will be valuable in understanding how work conditions affect skin and musculoskeletal health in this professional group.

PLANS AND PROCEDURE

If you agree to participate, you will be asked to complete a structured questionnaire that consists of approximately 40–50 questions regarding:

- Your general demographic and occupational background
- Your daily posture, body mechanics, and physical workload
- Your exposure to skin irritants and protective behaviors
- Your level of perceived work-related stress

The survey will take approximately 15–20 minutes to complete.

RISKS AND DISCOMFORTS

There are no known risks or physical discomforts associated with this questionnaire. Some questions may involve reflecting on your physical health or working conditions, which could cause minor psychological discomfort. You are free to skip any question or discontinue participation at any time without penalty.

POTENTIAL BENEFITS

While there may be no direct benefit to you from participating, your input will help us better understand occupational health risks in cosmetic medical practice. The findings may help develop guidelines or interventions to improve working conditions in clinical settings.

Subject's Initials______

K.-H. Yi, *Statistical Research Methods for Dermatologists and Plastic Surgeons*,
https://doi.org/10.1007/978-981-95-5668-7

COST AND COMPENSATION
I understand that there is no cost to me for participating in this research. I understand that I will not be compensated for my participation. I understand that the level of exercise required by this study is minimal. I understand that in the event of physical injury resulting from the research, OO University will assume neither financial compensation nor free medical treatment beyond immediate emergency care.
CONFIDENTIALITY
I am giving permission for my data to be used in future publications but I understand that a code number will be assigned to my data so that total anonymity will be maintained in reporting all of the results. All data will be stored in the OO Department at OO University. Dr. Yi and Dr. ****** and his research associates will have access to the data. After the study is complete, the data will be permanently stored at the same facility.

VOLUNTARY PARTICIPATION
My participation in this project is totally voluntary; there has been no coercion (overt or implied) to force my participation in this project. I understand that I can withdraw from the project at any time by simply informing the Principal Investigator of my desire to terminate participation: no explanation will be required. In addition, I can decline to answer any questions that may arise. I have read and understand the above explanation of the procedure to be used.

PERSONS TO CONTACT WITH QUESTIONS

I may contact the Principle Investigator, Dr. Yi at (252) 744-***** (weekdays). If I have questions related to physical injury resulting from the research you may contact the ECU Risk management Office at 252-328-*****. If questions arise about my rights as a human subject, I may contact the Chairman of the University and Medical Center Institutional Review Board at (252) 744-******.

Subject's Initials ________

TITLE OF PROPOSED RESEARCH

Occupational Risk Factors Related to Musculoskeletal Strain and Skin Exposure Among Professionals in Cosmetic Dermatology and Plastic Surgery Clinics

CONSENT TO PARTICIPATE

I certify that I have read all of the above, asked questions and received answers concerning areas I did not understand, and have received satisfactory answers to these questions. I willingly give my consent for participation in this research study. (A copy of this consent form will be given to the person signing as the subject or subject's authorized representative).

NAME (please print)

SIGNATURE

DATE

AUDITOR WITNESS: I confirm that the contents of this consent form were orally presented.

AUDITOR'S NAME (please print)

AUDITOR'S SIGNATURE

PRINCIPAL INVESTIGATOR'S NAME (please print)

PRINCIPAL INVESTIGATOR'S SIGNATURE

MIX
Papier aus verantwortungsvollen Quellen
Paper from responsible sources
FSC® C105338

If you have any concerns about our products,
you can contact us on
ProductSafety@springernature.com

In case Publisher is established outside the EU,
the EU authorized representative is:
Springer Nature Customer Service Center GmbH
Europaplatz 3, 69115 Heidelberg, Germany

Printed by Libri Plureos GmbH
in Hamburg, Germany